Free Yourself from Pain

by Dr. David E. Bresler
Director of the UCLA Pain Control Unit
with Richard Trubo

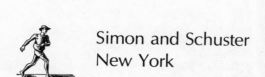

Simon and Schuster
New York

The names of the patients described in this book have been changed to protect their privacy.

1 2 3 4 5 6 7 8 9 10

Library of Congress Cataloging in Publication Data

Bresler, David E
   Free yourself from pain.

   Bibliography: p.
   Includes index.
   1. Pain. 2. Pain—Prevention. 3. Pain—
Psychological aspects.   I. Trubo, Richard, joint author
II. Title.
RB127.B72   616'.047   79-36

ISBN 0-671-24071-4

Acknowledgments

Dozens of people have made invaluable contributions to the development of this book. Ronald L. Katz, M.D., introduced me to the subject of pain, and has supported me constantly over the years. Alice Mayhew has generously provided editorial wisdom and perspective in the book's preparation. Michael Hamilburg's expert guidance was indispensable. Johnne Campbell, my personal secretary, nobly endured many long days and nights of typing and editing, usually under the pressure of deadlines. A special thanks is also in order for Eloise Fang.

Many people have been very generous in sharing their knowledge about their specialties. These include pain experts Verne Brechner, M.D.; Martin C. Brotman, M.D.; Richard Kroening, M.D.; Norman Levin, M.D.; Armin Sadoff, M.D.; and C. Norman Shealy, M.D. I have also often called upon acupuncture authorities Sheldon Altman, D.V.M.; Alice DeGroot, D.V.M.; Richard Glassberg, D.V.M.; Marshall Ho'o; Master Ju Gim Shek; William Prensky; Louis Prince; Steven Rosenblatt; and Master So Tin Yau. Information on biofeedback has been provided by Kenneth Pelletier, Ph.D.; Eric Peper, Ph.D.; and Melvyn Werbach, M.D. For my introduction to imagery, I am indebted to William Kroger, M.D.; Stephanie Matthews-Simonton; Irving Oyle, D.O.; Martin Rossman, M.D.; and O. Carl Simonton, M.D. Information on the family has come from James Gordon, M.D.; Dennis Jaffe, Ph.D.; and Nancy Solomon, M.D.; and nutritional contributions have been offered by Mark Bricklin, Robert Rodale, and Michael Volen, M.D.

Those responsible for much of my knowledge of alternative healing practices include Paul Brenner, M.D.; Rick J. Carlson, J.D.; Jack Drach; Arthur Gladman, M.D.; Raymond Gottlieb, O.D.; Brugh Joy, M.D.; Stanley Krippner, Ph.D.; Gay Luce, Ph.D.; Gladys McGarey, M.D.; William McGarey, M.D.; Richard Miles; Thelma Moss, Ph.D.; Jim Polidora, Ph.D.; Harold Stone, Ph.D.; Robert Swearingen, M.D.; and John Thie, D.C.

I am particularly grateful to my devoted staff at the UCLA Pain Control Unit. Although some are already cited above, others deserve special recognition, including Jack Booker; Hyla Cass, M.D.; Diane Chais; Caroll Dolan, M.D.; Howard Emory, M.D.; Rosalyn Englander; James Gagne, M.D.; Sharon Garrell; Herman Kattan; Larry Kattan; Attila Kemeny; Trinh Le; Barbara Moser; Ellen Murisaki; Terrence Oleson, Ph.D.; Barbara Pearce; How Chung Poon, C.A.; Jack Sandweiss; Anil Shah, M.D.; Susanne Shaw; Judith Stone; Oanh Tran; Yam Ying Tsai, C.A.; Diane Vega; Jacqueline Weinreb; Iris Weinstein; Caryle Wilson; and Kwong Wong, C.A.

I am also deeply grateful to James Fadiman, Ph.D.; Marvin Gelfand; Norman Levin, M.D.; and Eleanor Wasson, for critically reading the manuscript and making helpful recommendations.

Finally, I would like to thank the many patients who have shared their lives with me. Each has made a uniquely important contribution to the creation of this book.

D.E.B.

To our parents, wives and children—for enriching our lives

Contents

Foreword

Pain is one of the most misunderstood and neglected phenomena in modern medicine. It is a drain on the physical and emotional well-being of millions of people, making it difficult, if not impossible, for them to lead happy and fulfilling lives.

As an anesthesiologist, I've long had an interest in the terrible problem of pain. While medicine has made significant strides in preventing and treating many of the most serious diseases of man, pain still remains a mystery not only to the public, but to the medical profession as well. It has been said that pain is a humbling experience, both for the patient and the physician.

Until recently, the problem of chronic pain has been largely ignored. Typically, pain is treated with drugs and surgery which often neglect the complex psychological components of the pain experience. Too often, neither provide the long-term relief that is sought. The patient is left with agonizing pain and growing desperation.

The situation, however, is far from hopeless. I have closely observed the pioneering program of Dr. David Bresler at the UCLA Pain Control Unit in our Department of Anesthesiology. And I've been impressed. Dr. Bresler's patients, who often view his unit as "the last resort," are frequently helped by techniques generally unfamiliar to the Western world. The large, ongoing acupuncture treatment program at UCLA, for example, has clearly substantiated the value of this ancient technique. Other approaches—from biofeedback to guided imagery—are successfully exploring the important role of the mind in pain relief.

Significantly, many of the methods employed at the Pain Control Unit emphasize patient participation. They are intended to maximize to the fullest extent each individual's inner resources for pain control. As patients learn to manage their own discomfort, the devastating feelings of helplessness and hopelessness that once characterized their lives quickly fade into the past.

This book is founded on this self-help concept. The following pages not only describe and document the encouraging success of the UCLA Pain Control Unit, but also invite the reader who suffers from chronic discomfort to participate actively in the same, safe, carefully designed program.

Dr. Bresler encourages you to explore for yourself some of these exciting new approaches to pain control. You will discover the role that stress may play in your illness. By learning a Conditioned Relaxation exercise, you may be able dramatically to ease your discomfort for the first time. You'll be guided toward a nutritional program for maximum health benefits. And you'll see why the cultivation of pleasurable activities in your life is essential for managing the pain experience. In the process, you'll also learn why pain occurs in the body and how it is sensed and felt.

Because of therapeutic programs like Dr. Bresler's, this is an exciting time for pain patients and physicians interested in their problems. Self-control techniques are becoming increasingly reliable in reducing or even eliminating discomfort. And as researchers learn more about bodily substances called endorphins, which may naturally turn off pain, the path to healing may become even easier to find in the future.

I think you'll find this book extremely useful and significant. It will dispel some destructive myths about the problem of chronic pain. It will help you develop a new perspective on your discomfort, your body, and your entire life. And if you're willing to commit yourself to practicing diligently the techniques presented here, I believe you may be pleasantly surprised by the positive results you can obtain. With the help of *Free Yourself from Pain,* you may be closer than you think to achieving the productive, positive, and pain-free life you seek.

Ronald L. Katz, M.D.,
Professor and Chairman,
Department of Anesthesiology,
UCLA School of Medicine

Los Angeles, California
October, 1978

Introduction

By Richard Trubo

Pain.

It cripples tens of millions of Americans, crushing their spirits and destroying their lives. Although it has persisted since the beginning of time, it is still difficult to describe and even harder to relieve.

Everyone knows something about pain. We have all experienced it. Agonizing visits to the dentist's office. Excruciating headaches after a difficult day at work. A throbbing ankle, sprained while lunging awkwardly for a tennis ball.

But the worst kind of pain—chronic pain—can persevere literally for years. When it does, it becomes more than just an annoyance. It becomes a destructive way of life.

Like so many other people, I have seen chronic pain touch the lives of those I love. Such prolonged discomfort can influence literally all aspects of a person's life. And in the process, his pain can affect the lives of everyone around him.

Knowing of my personal and journalistic interest in such medical phenomena, Michael Hamilburg (my literary agent) suggested that I venture into the basement of Franz Hall at UCLA, where a Pain Control Unit had been established, helping patients who were once considered hopelessly ill. As part of the prestigious UCLA Medical Center, the Pain Control Unit occupies a section of the bottom floor of a large university building. Its operations are far from glamorous—an overworked staff, cramped offices, and aging furniture. But despite such obstacles, its pain-alleviation program has been quietly prospering with relatively little public notice.

During my first conversation with Dr. David Bresler, the unit's director, he explained the basic approach of his program. Drugs and surgery are deemphasized, he said. Patients are taught to draw upon their own inner resources to overcome their discomfort, with the assistance of unconventional therapies rarely used for people in pain. Each individual is asked to evaluate and deal with his discomfort in the context of his entire life.

Although open-minded, I was still somewhat skeptical after that initial visit. After all, I reasoned, could it be true that each patient was more capable of terminating his chronic pain than a physician, a drug, or a surgical procedure? Didn't this run contrary to everything that Western medicine has taught us?

In the ensuing days and weeks, I talked with Dr. Bresler many more times, interviewed other doctors at the Pain Control Unit, researched some of the medical literature, and most importantly, was granted permission to talk to the patients at UCLA.

I met people, young and old, who had spent many months and years hobbling from one doctor to another, frustrated in their desperate search for pain relief. They had tried all the wonder drugs and miracle surgeries, with little more to show for it than the complications often associated with these chemical and surgical assaults on the body. Time after time, they described their lives as agonizing, devoid of the friends and positive activities they had once enjoyed. Some had been simply close to giving up. A few even talked about suicide. They were, in short, miserable.

Interestingly, many of these patients were initially as skeptical of the Pain Control Unit's program as I was. They were referred there by personal physicians who were often convinced they were beyond help. These patients had been told that probably nothing could ever help ease the terrible, chronic pains in their head, neck, arms, or back. So how, they asked, after futilely trying the most sophisticated pain-alleviation techniques that Western medicine can offer, could these new approaches be any help at all?

Weeks later, after being treated by the doctors and psychologists at the Pain Control Unit, and attending classes in pain alleviation, their skepticism was gone. More importantly, so was their pain! That's right— no pain! Many claimed they were totally pain-free for the first time in years. Others reported, "I know it's still there, but now it doesn't bother me!" They had worked diligently with the staff at UCLA, and they no longer hurt. What more could they possibly hope for?

As one middle-aged man told me, "I threw my pain pills down the garbage disposal a month ago. The first few days after that were pretty rocky, but since then, every week I've felt better and better."

Dr. Bresler, a tall, dynamic man, possesses a medical wisdom far beyond his years (he is in his mid-thirties). But his youth and his unique experiences with unconventional therapies have provided him with an openness to new approaches that is so desperately needed in the field of pain control.

Even to Dr. Bresler and his colleagues, pain is still a complex and baffling phenomenon. They admit they don't have all the answers. But they are making very encouraging progress. Hundreds of patients can corroborate that.

In the upcoming years, I believe that medicine will have to rethink the ways it has approached pain for decades. Doctors from across the country, generally unfamiliar with the innovative techniques at the Pain Control Unit, have visited its facilities in recent years, and have left with new ideas, therapies, and beliefs. In their minds, there is now genuine hope for pain patients who once seemed to have very little cause for optimism.

This book, a self-help guide to both conventional and radically new approaches to pain alleviation, is an outgrowth of the success of the UCLA program. This success, however gratifying, has not been UCLA's victory. Nor has it been Dr. Bresler's victory. It's the victory of hardworking patients who refused to give up. They refused to accept themselves as they had been for so long—crippled by terrible discomfort that had drained them of the joys and pleasures that make life meaningful. They were determined to divest themselves of pain, and they did. It is their victory. If you hurt, perhaps it will soon be your victory, too.

I

The Pain Experience

1   The Control of Pain

"My pain is a screech against an open, black, ripped, upside down sky. And the sky is my head, jagged and tearing, tearing, tearing. Sometimes I think it's on backwards because my teeth are in the wrong place. How can your own teeth gnash your own temple otherwise? The same way your temple is a fist all doubled up to really smash you with those steel knuckles, first icy cold, then fire hot; then flashes out in tough, ragged mandarin nails to scrape that same spot over and over. And there's a bruise—blue and purple and blood red—in back of your eye. Your ear is being ripped off and the blood isn't blood but fire, stabbing in centimeter by centimeter down the back of your neck.

And your neck fights back. It wants to be the sky so it sends the lightning back boxerlike in stiff jabs and explosion punches. Your teeth erupt and pelt you in the face; your ear bursts open and pastes itself against your eye; your eye recoils and shoots out through your temple and the blades and the whistles and the symbols and the blackboard chalk and the bombs and the jets all go off at the same time in a piercing scream. Then the rocket attached to the electric drill attached to the razors zooms down exactly on target to the temple. And a minute has passed."

This is how Linda, a forty-two-year-old advertising executive, described the vicious headaches that have shattered her life for a decade. She had been seen by dozens of internists, neurologists, dentists, otolaryngologists, allergists, psychiatrists, and psychologists to no avail. When one of her doctors first referred her to me at the UCLA Pain Control Unit, she was heavily addicted to pain pills, tranquilizers, and sleeping pills, and so thoroughly helpless and depressed that she questioned whether life itself was worth living.

The Pain Epidemic

Linda is not alone, for chronic pain has become America's most common, expensive, and debilitating disorder. For instance, an estimated 8 to 10 percent of the population in most Western countries suffer from some form of migraine headache. Arthritis alone afflicts over fifty million Americans, twenty million of whom require medical care. Each year, arthritis claims six hundred thousand new victims, and its cost to the national economy is estimated to be nearly $13 billion. Low back pain—another of the most common pain complaints—has disabled seven million Americans and, according to the National Center for Health Statistics, generates nearly nineteen million visits to doctors annually. Add to these the many other pain-related disorders—facial and dental pain, neuralgia and neuritis, cancer, aching necks and shoulders, tennis elbow, muscle spasms, and other problems—and it's understandable how chronic pain can cost the nation's economy an estimated $50 billion annually. Its cost in terms of human suffering is incalculable.

These statistics shock me. If a mysterious new flu virus were expected to infect tens of millions of Americans and cost our country billions of dollars in lost wages, a national campaign would immediately be launched to mobilize our scientific resources for battle. Chronic pain runs rampant in our land, inflicting severe physical, emotional, intellectual, and economic damage upon its victims, their families, and society as a whole. But America has yet to respond.

Suicide: the Ultimate Painkiller

Although statistics may be helpful in identifying the magnitude of the pain problem, they cannot describe the anguish of lives shattered by pain. People with chronic pain often live in a self-destructive sea of negativity, which in time begins to infect their friends and their families as well.

Consider the plight of John. He is young, attractive, and intelligent, but his life hurts. Since he severely injured his back three years ago, he has lost his job, his wife and children, his friends, and his self-confidence. He eats and sleeps poorly and can no longer engage in the many activities he once enjoyed. No more tennis, no more surfing, no more sex. He has been subjected to countless diagnostic tests and injections, three surgical procedures, and over $80,000 in medical bills. He is addicted to pain pills and consumes enormous quantities of tranquilizers and sedatives. John is alone, broke, hurting, and suicidal. He will either get better or kill himself. Soon.

I rarely meet a person with chronic pain who is not also a victim of depression. In a sense, depression can be thought of as psychological pain, or the emotional component of the chronic pain experience. Depression is known to manifest itself following the loss of an important person in one's life, and John has lost himself. The medications he so desperately consumes have affected his alertness, emotional stability, and body image. He feels totally helpless and out of control, drowning to death in feelings that are matched only by the terrifying fear of future pain attacks. It's not hard to see why he wonders whether it is worth it to keep living.

Linda and John and countless others have asked me why doctors can't do more to help their chronic pain patients. Why has there been so little research conducted? Why isn't there a government-sponsored National Pain Institute? Why aren't medical students given specific training in the management of chronic pain? Why aren't there more pain control centers that specialize in helping its victims? Where are the major fund-raising efforts to support clinical and basic research studies? Why has the control of chronic pain been so cruelly ignored?

I wish I knew what to tell them. True, medical researchers have been busily seeking to identify the *causes* of pain-related illnesses—the *cause* of cancer, the *cause* of arthritis, the *cause* of headaches—but surprisingly little attention has been paid to the pain problem itself.

Laughingly, I used to tell the medical students who rotated through the UCLA Pain Control Unit about an imaginary Disease of the Year Pageant. This pageant was attended by various funding agencies, media representatives, medical research centers, patient groups, and power brokers, each of whom promoted his or her own particular nominee. Following fierce elimination trials that resembled a combination of an Ali-Norton fight and an episode of *Let's Make a Deal*, one disease emerged victorious to rule America until next year's pageant. Heart disease has been the big winner for several years, but cancer and diabetes are now looking stronger. Pain was never even nominated.

Pain and Modern Medicine

We live in an age of medical miracles. With the development of immunizations, antibiotics, and improved health conditions, we have witnessed the virtual elimination of infectious diseases that once decimated entire civilizations. Infant mortality has dropped dramatically, and almost daily we read of astounding medical advances that would have been unthinkable only a few years ago.

We have harnessed the atom and sent a man to the moon, but we have

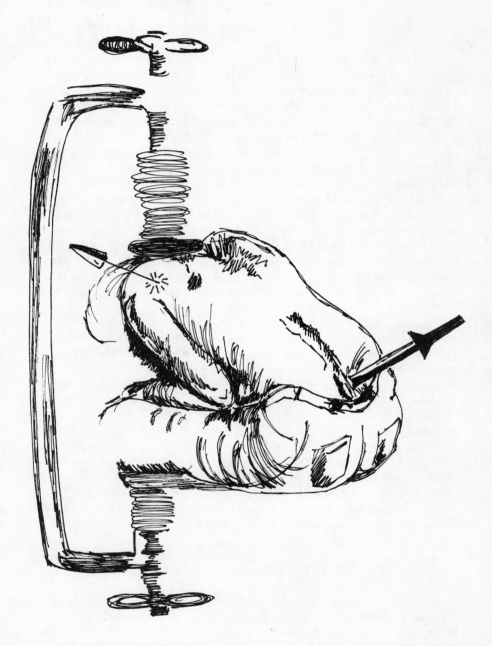

Fig. 1 *This self-portrait was drawn by a patient with low back and shoulder pain.*

yet to discover one single form of therapy that is completely safe and effective for alleviating pain. Many of the techniques that our doctors most frequently use were developed by ancient civilizations, not modern man, and they have remained fundamentally unchanged over thousands of years.

Morphine, modern medicine's most effective painkiller, is derived from opium, which was widely used as an analgesic forty centuries ago by the Egyptians. The ancient Romans relied on a combination of opium and wine. Primitive tribes of India and South Africa employed willow leaves, which are rich in salicylic acid (an ingredient of aspirin), to ease joint discomfort as well as the pain of childbirth.

The Incas chewed on the leaves of the coca plant centuries before cocaine was isolated by a German scientist in 1860. Transcutaneous electrical stimulation—a technique for controlling pain by applying small amounts of electricity—was utilized by Scribonius Largus, a surgeon with Nero's armies, who applied a torpedo fish as a source of electricity. Even before that, Plato and Aristotle had written about the numbing effects of the electric fish to treat gout and headaches.

Acupuncture, herbs, and various physical therapies (heat, cold, and massage) have been an integral part of Chinese medicine for at least five thousand years. Acupuncture needles carved from stone have been found in China, and have been dated back to the Stone Age.

By refining and expanding the insights of ancient civilizations, modern technology has created an almost endless variety of pharmaceutical products, many of which are available over the counter. For management of short-term or *acute* pain, these agents are often highly effective. If, for example, you were to sprain your ankle or have a tooth pulled, there are several types of medications which can make you more comfortable while your injury heals. Since acute pain is by definition self-limiting, temporary relief is all that's required. Perhaps our most dramatic achievement is the development of modern anesthetic procedures that can usually spare the surgical patient even the slightest degree of discomfort.

Yet the sophisticated pharmacologic approaches which have proven so successful in the management of acute pain are often ineffective for controlling *chronic* or long-term pain. Although acute pain will usually get better by itself as the body heals, chronic pain often becomes worse with time. As a rough rule of thumb, chronic pain refers to any pain problem that lasts longer than six months. Its victims are referred endlessly from doctor to doctor, for even if temporary relief can be obtained, the pain frequently returns with time.

When medications and/or surgery fail, patients like John and Linda are often told "nothing more can be done. You'll have to learn to live with it." But in my opinion, there is always hope for someone in pain. Until *every* conceivable therapeutic approach has been attempted, no one should proclaim that "nothing more can be done."

In my experience, drugs and surgery are often found to be the *least* effective techniques for the control of chronic pain. Far more promising are the innovative new approaches described later in this book, for they acknowledge the amazingly complex nature of the chronic pain experience.

I find it helpful to distinguish between a painful *sensation* (mental awareness of a noxious stimulus) and the pain *experience* (the total subjective experience of suffering due to pain). Furthermore, it is important to recognize that there is not necessarily any direct relationship between the sensation and experience of pain. For example, although soldiers seriously wounded in battle are certainly aware of their injuries, they usually do not get caught up in the experience of pain, for they are elated to be going home alive, leaving the war behind them. Conversely, there are many patients who continue to suffer, even after the entire injured area has been totally anesthetized.

The chronic pain experience is known to be affected by childhood experiences, ethnic and cultural variables, socioeconomic factors, genetic predisposition, birth order, gender, and a host of other physical, perceptual, cognitive, and emotional influences. Thus, it's easy to see why no simple pill or shot can cure chronic pain. Only by developing a comprehensive understanding of the physical, mental, and spiritual aspects of each patient's life situation can an appropriate therapeutic program be created. Some doctors consider only the physical aspects of chronic pain, for they assume that the objective of therapy is to treat the *pain*. For me, however, the objective of therapy is to treat the *patient in pain*.

Although the pain problems of various patients may seem similar, every individual is different. For one person, drugs may be the best form of therapy. For another, acupuncture. For yet another, family counseling. Or nutritional therapy, hypnosis, biofeedback, or guided imagery. The list grows longer as new alternatives are developed and evaluated. Fortunately, there is still hope for *anyone* in pain. Including you.

The UCLA Pain Control Unit

The UCLA Pain Control Unit (PCU) was established on the premise that every pain patient who truly wants to get better can be helped to at least some degree, regardless of the prognoses of conventional medicine. This basic supposition has yet to be refuted.

The key to our success lies in the creation of a treatment program individualized for each patient. Such a program may include ancient techniques like acupuncture or yoga, as well as more modern forms of therapy such as biofeedback and ultrasonic stimulation. Although we prefer to use the most noninvasive and natural approaches whenever possible, we do utilize drugs or nerve blocks when we feel they are more appropriate. And how do we determine what's most appropriate? By getting to know as much as we can about each patient's unique life situation, and by enlisting the active cooperation of patients in the development of their own therapeutic programs.

Several thousand patients have now been treated at the PCU, and although only time can tell how effective we have been on a long-term basis, some of our initial results have been astounding to say the least. Our patients have come from all walks of life and have suffered from a wide variety of pain-related ailments. Typically, they have been living with pain for more than ten years and have already experienced everything that conventional medicine can offer, without success. It's therefore not surprising that they feel depressed, trapped, abandoned, and helpless. As a last resort, they have come to us looking for a miracle.

Although no miracles have occurred at the PCU, something just as exciting has become almost commonplace. Using an individualized combination of conventional and unconventional approaches, we have helped the majority of our patients significantly reduce their discomfort and often eliminate it altogether. While many patients come to the PCU dependent on their pain medications, most who complete our program end up using none. Many of our patients who were disabled because of pain have now returned to work without resorting to costly surgery, hospitalization, or long-term psychotherapy. This is often an incredible accomplishment, given their initial prognoses.

One Perspective on Chronic Pain

As a result of my experiences at the PCU, I now view the treatment of chronic pain in a very different light. My personal conclusions about the nature of the chronic pain experience can be summarized as follows:

All Pain Is Real

The pain experience involves a complex interaction of physical, mental, and spiritual factors. From this perspective, it is nonsensical to wonder if a patient has "real" versus "unreal" (imaginary) pain, "physiological" (organic) versus "psychological" pain, or "legitimate" versus "illegitimate" pain. Pain is an intense personal experience, and even if a doctor can find no physical reason for your pain, it is still *real*.

There are many mysteries that Western medicine has yet to solve.

Although we know a great deal about the nature of painful *sensations*, the physical basis of the pain *experience* remains an enigma. When a patient tells me he hurts—then he hurts. I demand no more proof than that simple pronouncement.

However, there is one exception to this rule. It involves the "malingerer"—the individual who pretends to have pain so as to avoid work or other responsibilities. Everyone is different, and since no one else can judge what is "real" for another person, it is almost impossible to determine if someone is "faking" pain. Knowledgeable therapists do everything possible to establish a strong sense of trust, rapport, and confidence, and if this is successful, most patients will candidly share their inner experiences. True, a convincing malingerer may be able to fool even the most experienced therapist, but I prefer to give my patients the benefit of the doubt. I would rather "waste" my resources on someone who doesn't need them than deny help to someone who might benefit from my care.

Pain Is a Positive Message

Since the dawn of creation, pain has provided important information concerning man's relationship to his inner and outer environments. Your pain is conveying the message that "something is wrong," and it is encouraging your body to take action to prevent further injury. From an evolutionary point of view, it is one of the most powerful ways to ensure the survival of an organism in a dangerous world.

While most authorities acknowledge the positive aspects of acute pain, many believe that chronic pain is a "biological mistake" serving no useful purpose. In order to compensate for this "mistake," they recommend strong drugs or surgical procedures to obliterate the sensation of pain. To me, artificially suppressing or "masking" pain before its message is heard may not be in the best long-term interest of the patient. To do so is like coping with a fire by cutting the wires of a ringing alarm, rather than leaving the burning building.

Chronic pain is usually not a disease or mistake; rather, it is a symptom generated through the wisdom of the body. In my opinion, symptoms are the way that the body tries to heal itself or prevent further injury. Once their message is heard and appropriate action taken, symptoms will usually disappear, for they are no longer needed.

What is your pain trying to tell you? What is "wrong" in your life? What sort of action do you need to take? The techniques presented later in this book are designed to help you find answers to these questions.

Effective Therapy Is Most Seriously Blocked by
Unrealistic Beliefs and Expectations

If a doctor has ever told you, "I'm sorry, but there's nothing more that can be done for you," you probably found it devastating. The prospect of a life of endless pain, pills, and inactivity is understandably depressing. Like millions of people, you may have resigned yourself to such a bleak existence—on doctor's orders.

But your doctor may have been overly pessimistic. Even though he may genuinely believe that your condition is hopeless, he should not proclaim that "nothing more can help you." To be totally accurate, he should have said, "There is nothing more that *I* can do for you, but possibly other doctors or treatments may be more successful."

By declaring your case as hopeless, he has given you the negative and unrealistic expectation that you must live with pain for the rest of your life. If you really believe that, it will very likely come true.

It is essential for you to be realistic about the possibilities still available to you—and there *are* still possibilities. I'm not trying to tell you that one acupuncture treatment or one magic pill is going to cure all your ills. That's unrealistic, too, and underestimates the complexity of the pain experience.

I simply want your expectations to be accurate. There's an old saying in medicine, "The conviction of illness leads to illness; the conviction of cure leads to cure." How you see your reality affects how you experience it. If you see yourself as your doctor does—a helpless, hopeless victim of an incurable illness—this may become a self-fulfilling prophecy.

I am reminded of a dramatic illustration many years ago involving a cancer patient, whose condition varied with each change in the way he perceived his treatment. The case was related by Dr. Arthur K. Shapiro thusly:

> The patient was febrile, gasping for air, required oxygen by mask, and every other day required a thoracentesis which produced 1 to 2 liters of milky fluid. Masses, the size of oranges, were present in the neck, axilla and groin, chest, and abdomen. The spleen and liver were greatly enlarged. The patient was resistant to all treatment, was completely bedridden, and his life expectancy was thought to be a matter of days or weeks. Despite this, the patient was not without hope because he had heard of the favorable publicity with which the newspapers had reported a new anticancer drug called Krebiozen. The patient learned that the drug was to be tried at the hospital at which he was confined. His entreaties for the drug were finally granted, although with reluctance and pessimism.
>
> The patient's response was astonishing. After one day of treatment, the tumor masses melted to half their original size. Within ten days all signs of

his disease vanished. He breathed normally, and he was discharged. After two months of almost perfect health, conflicting and pessimistic reports about Krebiozen began to appear in the newspapers. The patient lost hope and relapsed to his original state. The physician, however, rekindled the patient's hope by telling him not to believe what he read, that the drug deteriorated with standing, and that a new super-refined, double-strength drug was to arrive on the following day. The patient was then given water injections and his optimistic expectations were restored. Recovery was even more dramatic than before. He became ambulatory and was discharged, and continued symptom-free for over two months. The remission continued until a few days after the press published an American Medical Association announcement that nationwide tests showed Krebiozen to be a worthless drug in the treatment of cancer. Within a few days the patient was readmitted to the hospital and succumbed in less than 48 hours.

All of us have heard about people who experience "spontaneous remissions" from "incurable" illnesses. Even the medical literature occasionally reports such occurrences. For example, two surgeons, T. C. Everson and W. H. Cole, compiled a book, *Spontaneous Regression of Cancer* (1966), documenting numerous cases of cancer patients whose condition reversed without *any* therapy. When asked to explain such phenomena, most doctors typically shrug their shoulders in bewilderment.

Is "spontaneous remission" an accurate description of these surprising recoveries? Hardly. I'm convinced there must be some reason, some lawfulness, to this phenomenon, even if we don't yet fully understand it. As Saint Thomas Aquinas said more than seven centuries ago, "Nothing is contrary to the laws of nature, only to what we *know* about the laws of nature."

Dr. O. Carl Simonton, a radiation oncologist in Fort Worth, Texas, has developed a unique and successful program utilizing various psychological techniques to help inhibit the growth of cancer. Working together with his wife, Stephanie Matthews-Simonton, he reports that in most cases of so-called "spontaneous occurrence," the patients had visualized themselves being well. This image ultimately became a reality.

I agree with the Simontons. I've heard patients say, "I *can't* die; I have too much to do." It's more than not *wanting* to die or being *afraid* of dying—they can't!

The Mind Is the Safest and Most Powerful Pain Reliever

Anyone who has studied psychology is aware of the untapped potential of the mind. There are yogis who can walk on burning coals. There are people who, when hypnotized, can undergo surgery without anesthetic drugs, yet they feel no discomfort. There are still other techniques, such as biofeedback and guided imagery, which clearly demonstrate the power of the mind.

With hard work, many people with pain problems once thought "incurable" have learned to maximize their abilities to heal from within. In a later chapter, I'll describe some of the new techniques that they have used.

Self-Control Is the Key to Achieving Long-Lasting Relief

One of the most intriguing developments of modern medical science occurred in 1973, when two researchers discovered that the nervous system creates its own powerful pain-relieving substances. These complex substances are similar in many ways to morphine and they have therefore been called "endorphins" (inner morphines).

Does this surprise you? It shouldn't, for if you accept the hypothesis that the body is uniquely designed to promote its own survival, then its inner ability to control pain is not really so astonishing. In many situations, it is essential for the body to turn off pain so that the organism can respond to the demands of the environment.

Millions of people with pain continue to swallow pills that have the potential to kill them, unaware of the natural substances within that could control their discomfort more safely and more effectively. Like you, these pain-plagued patients must learn to encourage their nervous systems to secrete more of these endorphins—to maximize their body's abilities to turn off the pain from inside.

Can a doctor help you in this search for self-control? Perhaps. Medical researchers specializing in pain control are now discovering that some of their most effective techniques may involve the secretion of endorphins. There is preliminary evidence, for instance, that acupuncture releases endorphins.

But rather than relying solely on doctors, there are things *you* alone can do to maximize your body's ability to relieve pain. With diligent practice, you can learn to relax yourself on command, even in the face of overwhelming stress. By eating more nutritious foods, you can provide your body with the essential materials needed to activate its inner pain control system and to maximize its self-healing potential. As you rediscover the pleasures of the world, your entire life can change in a positive, long-lasting way. Certain self-control techniques, such as relaxation and guided imagery, may involve the endorphin system or some other physiological mechanism yet to be discovered. What is important is that *you* may be able to do more than anyone else can to overcome your discomfort.

Once you've begun to achieve self-control over your discomfort, you will no longer feel at the mercy of your pain problem. And you will certainly be able to deal more effectively with the feelings of hopelessness and helplessness that often accompany chronic pain. One of my patients recently wrote to me: "I used to be totally immobilized by my headaches. But now I recognize that it's not necessary for that to happen. Now when I wake up in the morning with a headache, I do the relaxation exercise, and then jump into the swimming pool for a leisurely swim. Within 20 minutes, the headaches are under control. An hour after that, they're gone. They don't frighten me anymore. I still get headaches occasionally, but they don't control me anymore. *I* control *them*."

When you think about it, all healing is self-healing. Even the most skillful surgeon can't create scar tissue or cause nerves to regenerate. All he can do is facilitate the process. More than any external factor, your own body has the ultimate power to regenerate and heal itself.

No Pain Problem Is Hopeless

No one is beyond help. Pain has been a problem since long before the birth of modern medicine. Earlier civilizations utilized a multitude of approaches, many of which were highly effective. Though once considered eccentric or esoteric, these techniques are being rediscovered and reevaluated, and many are becoming an integral part of the most modern approaches to pain control. Therapeutic systems like acupuncture, hypnosis, and yoga might help you. If they don't, something else might. We are just beginning to appreciate the wide range of possibilities that can mobilize our inner resources for controlling pain.

For instance, did you know that a simple food substance—an amino acid called tryptophan—may help ease your pain if it's consumed in larger-than-normal amounts? And did you ever think that your own vivid imagination could recruit your body's intrinsic healing forces and even help you understand on a subtle level the message your pain is trying to communicate?

In talking to thousands of people with pain in recent years, I've concluded that their "hopeless" state of mind has often been aggravated because they've attempted to smother pain's symptoms instead of trying to understand and effectively deal with them. Only when you fully understand pain's message—from a physical, mental, emotional, and spiritual viewpoint—can long-lasting improvement in your condition occur. And it will.

Your situation is *not* hopeless. But I wonder how many lives have been wasted because patients have been convinced that "nothing more can be done."

A Plan of Action

If you are afflicted with chronic pain, the information in the following chapters could conceivably change your life. This book is a self-help guide that will provide you with information about your pain, including many things your doctor never told you. It will describe why you hurt, and how to extricate yourself from the tragic circumstances in which you find yourself. Both conventional and unconventional approaches to pain relief will be explained.

This book will teach you to maximize the power of your mind. You'll learn how to speak the language of the nervous system and comprehend the message your pain is trying to communicate. The essence of this therapeutic program is to help you develop a consciousness incompatible with the chronic pain experience.

The book is richly illustrated with case histories so you can see how other people afflicted with problems just as distressing as yours confronted and overcame them. My father used to say, "Smart people learn from their mistakes; wise people learn from the mistakes of others." You'll learn how other people stumbled and fell but ultimately rose to conquer their chronic pain problem.

In every chapter, you will be encouraged to participate in exercises designed to make the new facts you're learning relevant to your own life. Some of these exercises may help you control your pain better than you ever thought possible.

Keep in mind that I'm not offering any magic formulas. No promises. No guarantees. As in any self-help program, your success will be determined primarily by *you*—by the extent to which *you* master the techniques presented here. To obtain the fullest benefit from this book, you must be willing to take some responsibility beyond simply reading it. More than anything else, your progress will depend upon the effort and energy you're willing to invest in the program. No matter how agonizing your present situation is, if you have a strong desire to get better and are willing to dedicate yourself to that goal, your chances are good. In fact, very good.

I encourage all my patients to be scientific. I'm not asking you to accept blindly any of these new approaches; instead, I'm asking you to *try* them in order to determine whether they might benefit you. They are useful only if you validate them through your own personal experience. Knowledge alone doesn't change anything. You must combine that knowledge with personal experience in order to achieve a new understanding of your life situation and to make that grueling pain a growthful part of your past.

Become a participant in this book. As you read, have a pencil and paper by your side, jotting down notes and underlining passages you can refer back to. I also encourage you to buy a cassette tape recorder, which will be invaluable when practicing many of the relaxation and guided imagery exercises presented in the later chapters. Commit yourself now to spending thirty minutes each day practicing the techniques you'll learn.

Let me back up for just a moment, because some readers are probably thinking, "This program may be OK for people who only *think* they have pain. Those people are crazy and they might be helped by some of these unconventional ideas. But I'm different. My pain is *real*. I have a positive myelogram. None of this is going to help me."

I cringe when I hear such comments. Let me repeat—*all* pain is real. And if you're thinking, "This won't help me," it may turn out to be true. Keep an open mind. Give it a chance.

Actually, you may be surprised to learn that you've already been successful in turning off your chronic pain at one time or another. Everyone has. Can't you recall moments in the past months when your pain seemed to disappear while you were totally engrossed in a TV show or enjoying making love? If you've ever experienced even just one second of pain relief since your discomfort first began, there's no longer any question as to whether or not your pain can be turned off. You *know* it can. All that remains is to learn how to extend that painless moment into hours, days, weeks, months, and years. Others have done it. So can you.

A few precautionary notes: As I will repeat many times throughout these pages, pain is a message that something is wrong. If you have pain, consult a physician to obtain as full an understanding of your specific malady as possible. I feel that it is unwise to utilize the techniques described in this book until as clear a diagnosis as possible has been made of your particular pain problem.

Also, be aware that my patients are introduced to the material in this book over a six-week period. Thus, I urge you to take your time in proceeding through this book, as if you were participating in a program that lasts several weeks. If you read the entire book in one sitting, don't expect instant results. It takes time and a lot of hard work over many weeks or even months for this approach to be fully successful. Be willing to reread parts of the book over and over, and share and discuss some of what you have learned with your family. (Family members are as affected by your pain as you are.) Be patient, diligently practice what you learn, and you might be amazed to see what happens.

One doctor recently cautioned me that perhaps this book is a bit premature. After all, he reasoned, the pain-alleviation program described here has only been implemented at UCLA for a few years. Where are all the long-term, double-blind, placebo-controlled, counterbalanced research studies that *prove* the program is effective?

I am very sensitive to his concerns. In fact, I share many of them. I deliberated for quite some time before eventually deciding to write this book. If I had decided to write it five or ten years from now instead, perhaps some things in it would be different. The volume you hold contains my own current thoughts, based on my recent experiences with these new approaches.

This book has been published now because there are millions of people suffering from grueling chronic pain at this very moment. For these people, programs like this one might give renewed meaning to lives now filled only with agony.

The techniques presented in this book are noninvasive and safe. Unlike drugs, no one has died from an overdose of them. Nor are there any of the risks that accompany major surgery or many of the more conventional methods now used to treat patients with pain.

So what have you got to lose? Nothing. Except perhaps your pain.

Exercise One: Starting a Personal Journal

As you proceed through this book, you may undergo many changes in your way of thinking and feeling. My patients have found it very useful to chronicle their experiences in order to help them understand these transformations and what they may mean. A journal is one effective way of keeping these notations organized.

I encourage you to buy a notebook that will serve this function. Commit yourself to keeping your journal active for at least ninety days. There should be two aspects to your journal:

Part One: *Daily Comfort Log*

The first part will be a daily comfort log. Each day, I want you to keep track of your pain and pleasure. What time of day did you have pain and for what duration? What made you feel good? At what time and how long did this last? In each case, what activity were you engaged in, or what were you thinking about when you experienced pleasure or pain?

After several days or weeks, try to spot some patterns in these experiences. For instance, perhaps your pain occurs only at certain times of the day, or only during particular activities. If your migraine headaches begin regularly at 8:15 every morning, just as you are getting ready for work, there may be a message there. If you're feeling bored, frustrated, or anxious just before the onset of your back pain, this may be an indication of what is triggering your discomfort. Likewise, there may be some cyclic pattern or special activity associated with the times when you feel extraordinarily good.

SAMPLE

EXERCISE ONE: PART ONE:
Daily Comfort Log

DATE: ___feb. 3___

Time	Activity	Feeling	Duration	Rating	Comments
8:30 a.m.	shower	weak	10 min.	−1	still trying to wake up; feeling very 'average'.
8:50 a.m.	eat breakfast	relaxed	15 min.	0	
9 a.m.	watch TV	amused	1 hour	+1	takes my mind off my problems
10:15 a.m.	read the mail	angry	10 min.	−5	doctor bill arrived, his fee is more than expected
10:40 a.m.	balance checkbook	anxious	20 min.	−3	we're spending too much money
11:30 a.m.	housework	depressed	45 min.	−2	can't do the things I used to
12:30 a.m.	phone call from my daughter	elated	15 min.	+5	during the entire call I was barely aware of discomfort
1 p.m.	planning for summer vacation	hopeful	40 min.	+2	maybe there still is room for pleasure in my life
3 p.m.	call from women's club	frustrated	5 min.	−1	had to turn down request to help at charity lunch
5:40 p.m.	cooking dinner	bored	35 min.	−3	it's so monotonous
6:25 p.m.	Bill comes home from work	relieved	5 min.	−1	he showed me a lot of affection; made me feel better
6:30 p.m.	eat dinner	stimulated	20 min.	+1	good conversation about taking our vacation soon
8 p.m.	watch TV	lethargic	2 hours	−2	my mind wanders; thinking about future
11 p.m.	get ready for bed	fatigued	10 min.	−4	very weary, really need to sleep

NOTES:

EXERCISE ONE: PART ONE: **DATE:** _____
Daily Comfort Log

Time	Activity	Feeling	Duration	Rating	Comments

NOTES:

I also want you to rate the intensity of your pain or pleasure on a −10 to +10 scale. When you have very minimal discomfort, rate it as a −1. When it's the worst it's ever been, give it a −10. Anything in between should be so rated. Use a +1 to +10 scale for pleasure. When you feel just slightly good, rate it +1. Although the times you feel magnificent may be rare, rate them +10. Your other pleasurable experiences can be rated somewhere between these extremes. Don't feel as though you must be restricted to the limits of −10 to +10. If you need to use lower or higher numbers to express what you are experiencing, do so.

When you look back at these ratings several weeks from now, you may be able to spot other patterns that you didn't know existed. For instance, what were you doing every time you experienced a pain intensity of −9 or −10? Is there an activity or a feeling that seems to trigger your worst pain? What seems to produce consistently a +5 rating? A +8? A +10?

Part Two: *Life Chart*

The second part of your journal should focus on more general notations about your life experiences. It should include notes about what you have been experiencing, significant conversations you've had with others, and your interpretation of messages from within. Once again, by keeping such a running record, you will probably detect patterns developing. You'll also see very clearly whether the energy you're investing in this program is paying off.

While it is valuable to record the events that occur, it is more important to document the *significance* of the events, and your awareness of their meaning in your life.

Several journal categories are listed below as a guide. However, feel free to use other categories or to create personalized ones of your own as well.

Under the Emotional Status category listed below, you can insert notes about your emotional experiences (both painful and pleasurable) and how other people are influencing your state of being. Under the Recent Dreams category, describe what your subconscious is trying to tell you during dream periods that reveal insights from within.

The section on Intuitions may include the instinctive feelings you have about how your life is changing. Check them out later to see which hunches are fulfilled. Document the changes in your life when you describe your Plans, list the things you want to try tomorrow or next week—such as relating more honestly to your family about your discomfort, or starting to paint or swim again. Enter anything else you wish to document under Notes.

Don't censor your journal entries because you're ashamed of certain actions or feelings, or because you don't understand them. This journal is for *your* use; it is for no one else's eyes. Only if you are honest and thorough in your entries will you be able to see how your life progresses over an extended period of time.

Make the notations in your journal as soon after an experience occurs as possible. Our memories are not always as keen as we'd like, and the description of an event usually becomes less accurate and vivid with the passing of time. Entries should be made into the journal at least once a day without fail.

Remember to keep your journal as concise as possible. Usually a few words is all that you'll need to make a record of a particular experience. If your notes become lengthy, you may soon find yourself running out of enthusiasm for the project. The journal should be something you look forward to keeping. By doing so, you'll have a permanent record of significant changes in your life.

Set aside a large section of your journal for recording the self-learning exercises that are presented throughout this book. You may wish to refer back to them periodically, so keep them permanently on file.

Exercise Two: Your Goals

One of the first entries I'd like you to make in your journal is a list of the goals you hope to achieve as a result of the program in this book. What exactly would you like to accomplish in, say, the next ninety days? What do you want to do, have, or become? Also, how will you know when you've accomplished each goal? By referring back to this list frequently, you will gain an important perspective of how well you're doing. Your most important goal should be listed first, your second most important goal next, and so forth.

Of course, if you're a victim of chronic pain, I know that you want to stop hurting. That's taken for granted, so it needn't be included here. Instead, these goals should reflect the ways you wish to improve the quality of your life, and what you would specifically like to accomplish once your pain has been alleviated.

For instance, one of your goals might be to return to work. Or perhaps you'd like to have an active social life again, or be able to climb stairs. Or maybe you hope to drive a car, or remove yourself from the terrible economic pressures that your pain problem has caused.

Through this exercise, you'll gain a better understanding of the ways in which your pain has affected your life. Refer back to your list of goals

SAMPLE

EXERCISE ONE: PART TWO: Life Chart   **DATE:** feb. 5

                                               TIME: 9:30 p.m.

Experiences of importance

I walked five blocks to the market, and five blocks back, for the first time in over a year. I didn't know I could do that.

Conversations of importance

Melanie called. She says she loves talking to me, and that I seem a lot more hopeful than I used to. She's right.

Messages from within

There might be a lot of unrealistic thinking inside of me. I want to get better overnight.

Emotional status

I wish Bill would stop pushing me into trying to drive again. He says I'm "chicken". Doesn't he know I'm just scared?

Recent dreams

Last night, I dreamed about Mary's graduation from high school. I was so happy and proud and excited.

Intuitions

I really think that that everything is going to get better. I'm thinking a lot more about trying to do things again.

Changes

I'm trying to be more outgoing. I invited the neighbors over for coffee tomorrow.

Plans

I really want to go back to work. I'm going to start putting together a job résumé.

Notes

Today was one of the best days I've had in a long time. I hope I keep on feeling this way.

EXERCISE ONE: PART TWO: Life Chart   **DATE:** _____

                                           TIME: _____

Experiences of importance

Conversations of importance

Messages from within

Emotional status

Recent dreams

Intuitions

Changes

Plans

Notes

SAMPLE

EXERCISE TWO: Your Goals

DATE: _feb. 7_

TIME: _12 noon_

	I want to	I've reached my goal when
1	return to work	I'm well enough to begin working at least 3 days a week
2	make love with Bill like we used to	I'm able to enjoy sex without pain
3	sleep more soundly	I sleep eight consecutive hours without awakening
4	stop taking pain pills	I can throw <u>all</u> my medications away
5	drive a car	I can drive by myself to Don's school
6	go to a movie	I can sit in a crowded theater comfortably for 2 straight hours
7	go to a nightclub and dance	I can stand the loud noises and dance without pain
8	not have to depend on doctors	I can stop seeing Dr. Carlton
9	travel to see my sister	I can visit Martha in Oregon at Christmas
10	climb stairs more quickly	I can climb 20 stairs, one right after the other

EXERCISE TWO: Your Goals

DATE: _____

TIME: _____

	I want to	I've reached my goal when
1		
2		
3		
4		
5		
6		
7		
8		
9		
10		

SAMPLE

EXERCISE THREE: Corresponding with Your Discomfort

DATE: _feb. 11_

TIME: _6 p.m._

From: _Peggy_

To: PAIN

Dear Pain:

Why are you causing me so much misery? You've been interfering with my life for three years now, and I don't understand why. Sometimes I feel like I'm reaching the breaking point, like if you stay with me one more day, I'm just going to crack. I hope you'll be a lot more considerate of what I'm going through.

You've really messed things up. My husband and I don't get along very well anymore, mostly because I just can't do the things I used to do. I had to quit my job because of you and I resent you for that. When will you go away? Why won't you leave me alone? I can't afford to have you around anymore, either physically, psychologically or emotionally.

You've warped me into a different person. I feel sorry for myself. I'm depressed. My few remaining friends tell me I look terrible. I'm lonely. You're my most constant companion. And you're not making my life easy.

If you have something to tell me I'd like to hear it. If there's something I'm doing wrong for you to hurt me like this, let me know. You exhaust me and use up all my energy, but I'll find some energy to do whatever I have to do to get you out of my life. Please contact me soon, but gently.

Sincerely,

Peggy

**EXERCISE THREE: Corresponding with
Your Discomfort**

DATE: _____

TIME: _____

From: _____

To: PAIN

Dear Pain:

Sincerely,

SAMPLE

EXERCISE THREE: Corresponding with Your Discomfort

DATE: feb. 11

TIME: 6:30 p.m.

From: PAIN

To: Peggy

Dear Peggy :

    I'm sorry for what you're going through. Life is not always easy, and I realize that it is very unpleasant for you now. But there's a reason for it. I hope we can open up a dialog with one another, because I think I have a lot to tell you.

    First of all, I hope you will trust me. Although I may be making your life difficult, there is a reason for it. And when this experience is all over (which I hope it will be soon), I hope you'll truly understand it.

    In some ways, I think you've become a better person because of me. I think you've become a more sensitive person, and I know you've come to appreciate the people who stand by you when once you took them for granted.

    But there are other reasons why I have become part of your life. It wasn't just a quirk of fate that brought us together. I have many more things to tell you as we get to know each other better. You have within you the ability to make your life what you want it to be, and I hope I can show you some of the ways to do that.

    I'm so glad you contacted me. Please write again.

Sincerely,

PAIN

**EXERCISE THREE: Corresponding with
Your Discomfort**

DATE: _____

TIME: _____

From: PAIN

To: _____

Dear _____ :

Sincerely,

PAIN

often, for they will serve as an important source of motivation and encouragement for the remainder of the program.

When you have at least tried to complete Exercise Two, you may refer to the sample page that follows it. Then go back and try the exercise again.

Exercise Three: Corresponding with Your Discomfort

As one of your journal exercises, I'd like you to write a letter to your discomfort. If you could tell your pain anything you wanted to, what would you say? Be totally honest. Tell your pain how you feel about it, and what you'd like it to do.

Second, whenever you feel so moved, have your pain write you a letter back. Write this letter on behalf of your pain, addressed to you. What do you think your pain would tell you about yourself and why it is causing you so much misery? What does *it* want? Begin a dialogue with your discomfort and initiate communication about what is happening within you.

Although this exercise may seem unnecessary or even silly, it may give you important insights into your pain experience. I encourage you to complete it, for you'll never discover what it might reveal until you do so.

Oasis

This is a good place to stop and rest for a while. I strongly recommend that you begin your journal by completing the first three exercises during the next twenty-four to thirty-six hours. Then continue with chapter 2.

2 *What Is Pain?*

Pain is not evil, unless it conquers us.

—Charles Kingsley

Throughout the history of mankind, pain has been a perplexing phenomenon. In early times it was blamed on demons or hostile spirits that could be exorcised only by witch doctors or priests. In the Book of Genesis, Eve was condemned to bear children in pain because of her sin of disobedience. In other cultures, pain resulted from a block in the natural flow of "life energy." Although we have accumulated considerably more information about pain over the past several thousand years, our understanding of pain is really not much more sophisticated than these early conceptualizations.

The Language of Pain

Charlie Brown, in the "Peanuts" comic strip, once proclaimed, "Pain is when it hurts." But beyond a general statement like that, there is little agreement over precisely what pain is. The sharp discomfort of a pinched nerve in the neck can be very different from the stinging pain of a severely burned hand. They both can be quite unlike the wrenching pain of an arthritic knee or the crushing ache of a back injury. To add to the confusion, one person's headache (or sprained ankle or slipped disk) can feel very different from the same disorder in another individual.

Although friends or family can observe a person in pain and feel empathy for him, only the sufferer himself knows exactly how his agony really feels. Although they can try to identify with what his pain might be like by recalling experiences of their own that may have been similar, no one can better describe pain than the person who is feeling it.

The language of pain has been thoroughly studied by Ronald Melzack and W. S. Torgerson, pain researchers at McGill University and the Johns Hopkins Hospital, who compiled a comprehensive list of over one hundred words used to describe various aspects of the pain experience. Yet my patients continue to add new terms to this list as they desperately grope for the words to describe their own unique discomfort. If you are in pain, only you and you alone know exactly how you feel.

Exercise Four: Describing Your Discomfort

Below is a list of words that people use to describe their pain experiences. Check the words that apply when you experience your discomfort at its *worst* (− 10 rating in your Daily Comfort Log), and those that describe it at its *best* (− 1 rating). When you have completed this part of the exercise, write a few sentences or a short paragraph that encompasses the essence of your discomfort at its worst and at its best. Feel free to choose words from the list or to create descriptions of your own. This exercise will provide important information for evaluating your progress later on.

The Pain Experience

According to *Dorland's Medical Dictionary*, pain is "a more or less localized sensation of discomfort, distress or agony, resulting from the stimulation of specialized nerve endings." Adds Dorland, "It serves as a protective mechanism insofar as it induces the sufferer to remove or withdraw from the source."

Although any attempt to define a subjective experience like pain is noteworthy, this definition—like all others I've seen—is incomplete. Almost everyone knows what pain is, but I have not yet found a definitive description of pain. No two people, it seems, view the phenomenon quite the same way.

Many individuals, for instance, think of pain as a *thing*, much like a splinter is a thing—that is, an object or substance from the outside that infiltrates the body. Thus, if you accidentally strike your thumb with a hammer, you might say you have "pain *in* the thumb."

Such a notion is inaccurate, for there is no pain *in* your thumb. When you injure it, you stimulate neural receptors that send a barrage of electrical and chemical messages up through the nerves in your hand and arm to your central nervous system (your spinal cord and brain). *Whether or not a given sensation becomes painful depends upon the way it is interpreted by your nervous system.* If your nervous system decides that the messages from your thumb are urgent, it may create an experience of pain that is *identified* with your thumb. However, the main pain receptor is between your ears, for that is really where pain resides.

If pain were solely "a . . . localized sensation . . . resulting from the stimulation of specialized nerve endings," as Dorland's suggests, every time you injured yourself, you would feel it. And it would hurt with about the same intensity as it did the last time you sustained a similar injury. But have you ever accidentally cut your finger while so deeply engrossed in an activity or thought that you weren't even aware of it right away? Doesn't this experience run counter to Dorland's definition?

What about the football player who breaks his arm during a game, but continues to play with unrestrained vigor, feeling no pain at all? Only in the locker room does he experience the initial sharp pangs of discomfort. Although he sustained the injury much earlier, his nervous system did not interpret the condition as painful until the game was over.

Joe Namath, former quarterback for the New York Jets and the Los Angeles Rams, played with injuries most of his football career. Although he would frequently limp on and off the field, his pain was buried somewhere in his nervous system while the game was actually in progress. *Life* magazine (November 3, 1972) even ran an article on Namath's dilemma with the headline: "Namath—the Juicy Rewards of a Painful Life."

Jerry West, one of the purest shooters in professional basketball history, was also an injury-prone athlete, playing at various times with pulled muscles, jammed thumbs, and a broken nose. But the pain that tormented him off the court was somehow forgotten during each forty-eight-minute game, when his mind was distracted from his discomfort.

Sometimes soldiers exhibit an uncanny tolerance to injury-related pain. During World War II, Dr. H. K. Beecher noted that only one of every three severely wounded soldiers experienced enough pain to need morphine. Most of the others denied the existence of pain or experienced so little of it that they did not want any analgesics. When the war had ended, and Beecher returned to his clinical practice, he found that 80 percent of his patients with surgical wounds similar to those of the soldiers requested morphine for their discomfort.

According to Beecher, the soldiers were not in shock, nor were they **incapable** of experiencing pain, for they complained violently of an

SAMPLE

**EXERCISE FOUR: Describing
Your Discomfort**

DATE: ___feb. 14___

TIME: ___4:30 p.m.___

At Worst	At Best	
−10	−1	
✓		abominable
		aching
✓		acute
		aggravating
✓		aggrieving
		agitating
✓		agonizing
		anguishing
	✓	annoying
✓		appalling
✓		awful
		beating
		binding
✓		biting
✓		boring
		bruising
		burning
		caustic
		chafing
		cold
		constant
		consuming
		contemptible
		convulsing
		cool
		corroding
		cramping
		cringing
		cruel
✓		crushing
		cutting
		debilitating
		desolating
✓		despicable
✓		disastrous
		disquieting
	✓	distressing
	✓	disturbing
		drawing
✓		dreadful

At Worst	At Best	
−10	−1	
✓		drilling
		droning
	✓	dull
		exasperating
✓		excruciating
✓		exhausting
✓		fearful
		flashing
		flickering
		flinching
		forbidding
		foul
		fragile
		freezing
✓		frightful
	✓	gnawing
		grating
		grave
		grievous
		grinding
		grim
✓		gripping
✓		grueling
		harassing
		hard
		harrowing
✓		harsh
		heavy
		heartbreaking
✓		horrible
✓		horrid
✓		horrifying
✓		hot
✓	✓	hurting
		infesting
		insufferable
✓		intense
✓		intolerable
	✓	irritating
		itching

EXERCISE FOUR: Describing Your Discomfort

DATE: _____

TIME: _____

At Worst	At Best	
−10	−1	
		abominable
		aching
		acute
		aggravating
		aggrieving
		agitating
		agonizing
		anguishing
		annoying
		appalling
		awful
		beating
		binding
		biting
		boring
		bruising
		burning
		caustic
		chafing
		cold
		constant
		consuming
		contemptible
		convulsing
		cool
		corroding
		cramping
		cringing
		cruel
		crushing
		cutting
		debilitating
		desolating
		despicable
		disastrous
		disquieting
		distressing
		disturbing
		drawing
		dreadful

At Worst	At Best	
−10	−1	
		drilling
		droning
		dull
		exasperating
		excruciating
		exhausting
		fearful
		flashing
		flickering
		flinching
		forbidding
		foul
		fragile
		freezing
		frightful
		gnawing
		grating
		grave
		grievous
		grinding
		grim
		gripping
		grueling
		harassing
		hard
		harrowing
		harsh
		heavy
		heartbreaking
		horrible
		horrid
		horrifying
		hot
		hurting
		infesting
		insufferable
		intense
		intolerable
		irritating
		itching

SAMPLE

EXERCISE FOUR—*Continued*

At Worst −10	At Best −1	
		jumping
✓		killing
		lacerating
		lancinating
✓		miserable
		molesting
		mortifying
	✓	nagging
✓		nasty
		nauseating
		noxious
		numb
		obnoxious
		odious
		onerous
✓		oppressive
		penetrating
	✓	pestering
✓		piercing
		pinching
		piquing
✓		plaguing
✓		pounding
		pressing
		pricking
	✓	pulling
		pulsing
		puncturing
✓		punishing
		quivering
✓		racking
		radiating
		rasping
		repugnant
		repulsive
		revolting
		scalding
✓		screaming
✓		searing
✓		sharp
		shocking

At Worst −10	At Best −1	
		shooting
✓		sickening
		smarting
	✓	sore
		spasming
✓		splitting
		spreading
		squeezing
✓		stabbing
		stinging
✓		suffering
✓		suffocating
		taut
		tearing
	✓	tender
✓		terrible
✓		terrifying
✓		throbbing
		tight
	✓	tingling
	✓	tiring
✓		tormenting
✓		torturing
		troublesome
	✓	tugging
		twinging
		twisting
✓		unacceptable
✓		unbearable
		unending
		unendurable
	✓	unpleasant
		vexing
✓		vicious
		weighty
		wincing
		worrisome
✓		wrenching
		wretched
✓		writhing

EXERCISE FOUR—*Continued*

At Worst −10	At Best −1	
		jumping
		killing
		lacerating
		lancinating
		miserable
		molesting
		mortifying
		nagging
		nasty
		nauseating
		noxious
		numb
		obnoxious
		odious
		onerous
		oppressive
		penetrating
		pestering
		piercing
		pinching
		piquing
		plaguing
		pounding
		pressing
		pricking
		pulling
		pulsing
		puncturing
		punishing
		quivering
		racking
		radiating
		rasping
		repugnant
		repulsive
		revolting
		scalding
		screaming
		searing
		sharp
		shocking

At Worst −10	At Best −1	
		shooting
		sickening
		smarting
		sore
		spasming
		splitting
		spreading
		squeezing
		stabbing
		stinging
		suffering
		suffocating
		taut
		tearing
		tender
		terrible
		terrifying
		throbbing
		tight
		tingling
		tiring
		tormenting
		torturing
		troublesome
		tugging
		twinging
		twisting
		unacceptable
		unbearable
		unending
		unendurable
		unpleasant
		vexing
		vicious
		weighty
		wincing
		worrisome
		wrenching
		wretched
		writhing

SAMPLE

EXERCISE FOUR—*Continued*

DATE: feb. 16

TIME: 9 p.m.

At its worst, my discomfort is

absolutely horrifying. It's impossible for me to think about anything but the vicious, grinding pain in my head.

It feels like it's going to envelop my face and suffocate me. It's the worst torture imaginable.

At its best, my discomfort is

unpleasant, but still somehow tolerable.

The discomfort in my head is a nuisance, pestering me with its tingling, itching sensations.

My head is sore, as if someone had been tugging and pulling on my brain.

EXERCISE FOUR—*Continued*   **DATE:** _____

                                        TIME: _____

At its worst, my discomfort is

At its best, my discomfort is

improper puncture of a vein. So how can this situation be explained? In *The Measurement of Subjective Response*, Beecher reasoned:

> The data state in numerical terms what is known to all thoughtful observers: there is no simple direct relationship between the wound *per se* and the pain experienced. The pain is in very large part determined by other factors, and of great importance here is the significance of the wound . . . In the wounded soldier, [his response to his injuries] was relief, thankfulness at his escape alive from the battlefield, even euphoria; to the civilian, his major surgery was a depressing, calamitous event.

Just as astonishing are the fakirs who walk on burning coals or lie on beds of nails. One of them, an American cheesemaker named Vernon Craig (aka Komar), has been tested by pain authorities like C. Norman Shealy, a neurosurgeon who directs the Pain Rehabilitation Center in La Crosse, Wisconsin. Craig has showed amazing ability to distract the most punishing types of pain from his mind. He has walked on a twenty-five-foot bed of coals burning at 1830 degrees Fahrenheit, and has lain on a bed of six-inch nails for more than twenty-five hours. To most of us, such experiences would be intolerable. But individuals like Craig have become very sophisticated at self-regulating their awareness of painful stimuli.

An anthropologist in Africa has described a tribesman who approached him with severe injuries and no signs of pain, calmly stating, "A lion has just ripped my arm off; can you stop the bleeding?" The episode was the result of an initiation ritual in which the tribesman confronted the pride of lions without showing fear. Such pain would be torturous in our culture, but it was quite a different phenomenon for the tribesman.

In some cultures, childbirth is considered painless. Girls are raised to envisage the birth experience as a natural and pleasurable event. Expectant mothers often work in the fields until the moment of birth, and then return to their crops almost immediately after their baby is born.

By comparison, the delivery of a child in Western society is a very different phenomenon. Many women fear the entire process, regard it as the most painful and stressful event of their lives, and demand an anesthetic to help them tolerate the pain associated with the birth experience. No wonder they feel as they do: they have been taught that childbirth may be a life-threatening process, requiring hospitalization. It is interesting to note that the Bible mentions that the suffering of childbirth is the will of God ("In sorrow thou shalt bring forth children").

Our understanding of pain becomes even more tangled when we recognize that a sensation painful in some circumstances can be quite pleasurable in others. Sexual stimulation, for instance, is usually very pleasurable, but in certain situations, the same sensations could be agonizing.

Or how about when you play with a child? If you playfully slap him on the behind as you run through the park, it will probably provoke laughter from him. But the exact same slap administered in the context of punishment will usually cause tears and pain.

The fallacy of thinking of pain as a "thing" or sensation becomes even more apparent when we consider the experience of pleasure. When you taste something enjoyable, do you say "Ummmmm, I've got a mouthful of pleasure," as if the pleasure were *in* your mouth? Of course not. There is no pleasure in your mouth. The gratification you're feeling is simply your interpretation of taste-bud stimulation, which generates a complex combination of salty, sour, bitter, and sweet sensations.

Pain is more than a sensation or "thing." To some extent, part of it may be a perception, like vision and audition. The way we perceive pain is known to be affected by a myriad of influences—including early learning experiences; ethnic, cultural, and economic factors; birth experience, gender, sibling order, and age; right- or left-handedness; and frame of mind and environment.

As a result, the same stimulus can be perceived in many different ways. If while playing touch football you bruised your shoulder and developed a strong ache because of it, you would interpret it in a very different way than had you obtained the same sensation when attacked and robbed by a mugger. The way you perceive a stimulus greatly affects how you experience it. But unlike other perceptions, pain has an affective, emotional quality that signals its urgency and importance to the organism. This is the "flavor" of pain that distinguishes it from all other perceptions.

More than twenty-three hundred years ago, Aristotle suggested that pain was also an *emotion*, as pervasive as anger, joy, and terror. In defining pain, many of the early philosophers simply labeled it as "the opposite of pleasure." Pain is clearly an emotional experience, for it is usually accompanied by anxiety, anger, resentment, depression, and other types of emotional feelings.

Often the emotional aspect of pain is its most significant component. For some people, the *fear* of future pain (an emotion) is much worse than the pain sensation itself. Morphine is an effective pain reliever because it usually suppresses those emotions, leaving the patient with the attitude, "It hurts, but I'm not worried about it. I'm not worried about *anything*."

But that's not all. Pain is also a *cognition*, communicating the message that "something is wrong." Until this message is recognized and heeded, the pain experience may continue unabated.

Pain is also a *motivation*, for it moves you to take action that will reduce or prevent further damage. Pain provides the incentive that makes you remedy a dangerous situation.

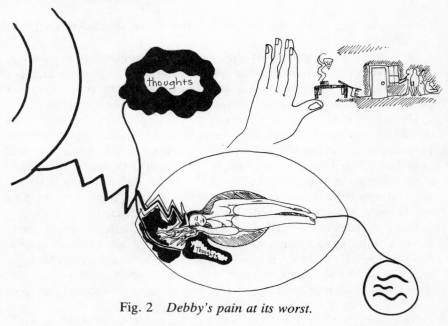

Fig. 2   *Debby's pain at its worst.*

Finally, in some cultures, pain is thought of as an excessive accumulation of *energy*. This is what the ancient Chinese Taoists believed, and accordingly, their treatment was directed at the energetic rather than the material aspects of pain. Acupuncture needles and herbs were used to correct the blockage of energy flow in the body, thus relieving pain. Modern physicists, such as Einstein, by demonstrating that energy and matter are two forms of the same thing, may have lent some credence to the Taoistic point of view.

I believe that chronic pain includes *all* of these components to some extent. It is a sensation, a perception, an emotion, a cognition, a motivation, and an energy. I find it difficult, if not impossible, to isolate the individual components of pain, since it is such a highly integrated, multifaceted phenomenon. How can you distinguish the pain sensation from the pain emotion, the pain perception from the pain cognition, and so forth? Hurting encompasses them all, and I prefer to use the term "pain experience" to indicate this holistic perspective of the problem.

The pain experience can often be described more graphically in pictures than in words. Figure 2 was drawn by one of my patients, an attractive woman named Debby who suffered from blinding migraine headaches. This picture was a representation of Debby's pain experience at its worst. Note its rich symbolism. Clearly, words are inadequate to describe what Debby feels when her headaches flare up.

At other times, though, Debby is able to enjoy her life. The picture in Figure 3 is her representation of her pain at its best. Note the symmetry and balance of this picture. In time, Debby learned how to help her

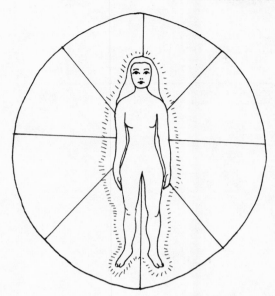

Fig. 3   *Debby's pain at its best.*

nervous system convert her pain from its worst to its best. With hard work and persistence, you may soon be able to convert your discomfort, too.

Exercise Five: Drawing Your Discomfort

A picture is worth a thousand words. In Exercise Four, you were asked to use words to describe your discomfort at its worst and at its best. Review your descriptions and try to sense their shortcomings due to the limitations of words.

In Exercise Five, I would like you to draw two pictures: one that represents your pain experience at its worst and another that represents it at its best. Try to encompass not only the pain sensation, but all other aspects of the experience as well—the perceptual, emotional, motivational, cognitive, and energetic components. Let your imagination run free. Use different-colored pens or pencils if that will help, but try to express the entire experience as you sense it, see it, feel it, and live it.

The Mind Versus the Body Revisited

When you first saw a doctor for treatment of your pain problem, one of your questions might have been, "Is something really wrong with my body, or am I just making all this up?" In other words, is there really a disorder in your body or is it all in your mind?

EXERCISE FIVE: Drawing Your Discomfort   **DATE:** _____

                                                TIME: _____

My discomfort at its worst

EXERCISE FIVE: Drawing Your Discomfort

DATE: _____

TIME: _____

My discomfort at its best

Quite possibly, one of your doctors has said that your pain is "psychosomatic." Such a conclusion might have shocked you. After all, wasn't that just a polite way for him to tell you that you're crazy?

Not at all. Although many people think that "psychosomatic" means "imaginary" or "nonexistent," that's not really the case. The term psychosomatic means that both the mind *and* the body are involved. From this perspective, I believe that *all* pain is psychosomatic—that is, it always embraces both mind and body.

Some people disagree with me. For example, I've talked to many doctors who think that pain is always a physiological function of the body. To them, the mind is nothing more than an epiphenomenon of the brain, a bodily organ. Everything that occurs in the mind, they say, can be reduced to physical processes such as nerve discharges and chemical secretions.

Other researchers argue that pain exists *solely* in the mind. My friend, Dr. Irving Oyle, director of the Bolinas (California) Headlands Healing Service, assumes this ultimate stance, even hypothesizing that there is no body! He suggests that your mind may be creating the fantasy that you have a body! According to Dr. Oyle: "The mind projects out a three-dimensional hologram in quadraphonic sound. Everything we see around us is a mind-created illusion. In reality, it's all painted on the back of our eyeballs. There's nothing else out there." Can you prove him wrong?

The mind-body problem has been pondered by philosophers down through the ages. In some ways, its inherent ambiguity is similar to questions debated by scientists in other fields as well. In physics, for example, there's a perpetual controversy over whether an electron is a wave or a particle. In some kinds of experiments, an electron acts like a particle, for when it bombards other particles, it causes them to split apart. But in another type of experiment, an electron was fired at a thin, metal screen containing two minute holes. The results suggested that it passed through both holes at precisely the same instant, which only a wave can do. What, then, is an electron? A wave or a particle? Is it energy or matter?

Physicists have developed very sophisticated theories in their attempts to deal with these types of questions. From the point of view of relativity theory, energy and matter are considered to be two different aspects of the same thing ($E = mc^2$). Thus, an electron can be thought of as both a particle *and* a wave.

The theory of quantum mechanics provides additional insight to this problem. According to the Principle of Complementarity, the same event can be viewed through two entirely different frames of reference. Although these two frames mutually exclude each other, they also complement each other. Only when taken together do they provide a complete view of the phenomenon.

In other words, what you see depends upon how you look at it. In some situations, an electron acts like a particle (matter); in others, it appears to be a wave (energy). It is the act of observing that influences what is seen.

A classic illustration of this notion involves a small tank of water at an unknown temperature. How can you determine the *exact* temperature of the water?

Use a thermometer, you might be thinking. But the instant the thermometer touches the water, the temperature of the water is changed, even if the thermometer's temperature differs from that of the water by only a millionth of a degree! Clearly the act of observing always influences what is seen. As Werner Heisenberg, one of modern physics' greatest theorists, has stated, "The universe is not completely knowable or predictable."

Thousands of years before the dawn of modern physics, Chinese Taoist philosophers postulated remarkably similar insights concerning the nature of reality. According to Taoist principles, man is a miniature reflection of the universe, a microcosm in the macrocosm. Both man and the universe are composed of energy, matter, and movement ($E = mc^2$), and both are subject to the same universal and divine law—the law of the Tao. To live according to the Tao is to adapt to the "order of nature," and to live in accordance with "the Way."

Everything in the universe (including man) lies upon a constantly changing continuum between two polarities, yin and yang. Yang is the more masculine, positive, active, and hard polarity, whereas yin is more feminine, negative, receptive, and soft. Please note that although Taoist philosophy describes yin as "negative" and "feminine," and yang as "positive" and "masculine," you should not consider this to be sexist. The terms "negative" and "positive" are used in the same way that physicists describe an electron as "negative" and a proton as "positive." A proton is not in any way superior to an electron! Yin and yang describe the extreme polarities, forces, or tendencies that are contained in "everything under the sun."

Yang	*Yin*
Positive	Negative
Masculine	Feminine
Active	Receptive
Sky	Earth
Sun	Moon
Splendorous	Plain
Hard	Soft
Odd	Even
Light	Dark
Warm	Cold
Fullness	Emptiness

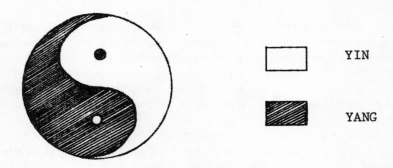

Fig. 4 *The relationship of yin and yang.*

The Taoist version of the Principle of Complementarity is described in terms of yin and yang as follows: "Nothing is purely yin, and nothing is purely yang. Within each yang, there exists yin, and within each yin must be yang." Thus, for example, no one is completely male or female; rather, masculinity and femininity are both present to varying degrees in each individual. Likewise, nothing is pure day or pure night. Nothing is pure matter or pure energy. And nothing is purely in the mind or purely in the body.

As a scientist, I have spent a great deal of my life trying to determine what is real. It now seems clear to me that reality itself is vague and ambiguous, for how you view reality determines how you experience it.

Let me give a simple illustration of this idea. Imagine that two of your friends have just had a serious argument. After talking with the first friend, you feel outraged by the other friend's behavior. Yet, after talking with the second friend, you now see his position as well. Who is right? Both and neither. The reality of the situation is ambiguous, and the question of "who is right" depends upon your frame of reference.

Returning to the mind/body question, then, is your pain all in your mind or all in your body? According to the Principle of Complementarity, the pain experience is in both. It's how you see it that determines how you experience it.

Perhaps you're thinking, OK, I agree that my pain is *now* both in my mind and in my body, but it *started* in my body only. Let me suggest that from the point of view of an egg, a chicken is just the way one egg makes another egg. Does it matter which came first?

If you hurt, the pain experience involves *all* of you. In my opinion, it is impossible to separate fully the psychological aspects of pain from the somatic (bodily) ones. All pain is "psychosomatic," and therapy should therefore be directed toward both the mind and the body. By following the program presented in this book, you'll get a better sense of how powerful such an approach can be.

Pain and Pleasure

> Our sincerest laughter with some pain is fraught.
> —Shelley

For the past several years, the emphasis of my research has been on the relationship between pain and pleasure. I believe that there are at least two fundamentally different ways that humans (and perhaps other mammals) experience both these phenomena. For the sake of clarity, I'll discuss the experience of pleasure first.

One type of pleasure is characterized by feelings of power, confidence, control, and excitement. It's what you experience when you feel on top of your world and totally in control of yourself and your outer environment. This type of pleasure is regulated by an *excitatory* system in the brain that enhances sensations from the world around you. Interestingly, this system is also activated by drugs such as amphetamine.

Although it is no less intense, the second type of pleasure is quite different, characterized by feelings of serenity, security, tranquillity, and safety. This relaxed sense of well-being is regulated by an *inhibitory* system in the brain that minimizes sensations from your outer world. At a high level of inhibitory activation, it produces sleep. This system is mobilized by drugs such as morphine.

In a similar fashion, there are also two fundamentally different types of pain. When the excitatory pleasure system shuts down, you experience the opposite of power, confidence, control, and excitement; namely, helplessness, worthlessness, futility, and lethargy. If these feelings, which reflect a lack of excitatory pleasure, persist for too long, the person who experiences them soon lapses into a state of hopelessness and despair, convinced that he will have to live in pain forever.

Conversely, a very different kind of pain develops when the inhibitory pleasure system is inactivated. This type of pain is characterized by feelings of tension, agitation, anxiety, and hypersensitivity. In essence, you lack the ability to inhibit or shut out excessive stimulation, so that environmental input becomes excessive, and bodily aches become ex-cruciatingly painful.

Perhaps you've experienced this type of hypersensitivity, where you were so nervous and agitated that ordinary lights seemed blinding, everyday noises seemed deafening, common substances smelled "funny," and normal sensations like the taste of food were terribly exaggerated. In such a state, your natural response was probably to run away, to hide somewhere, and to isolate yourself from the world.

This model of pleasure and pain is diagrammed in Figure 5. Depending on the relative degree of excitatory and inhibitory activation, pain may be experienced as a sense of helplessness and futility, or as anxiety and tension. Some chronic pain patients alternate from one extreme to the other in an endless cycle of suffering. Others, who are even less fortunate, experience both types of pain simultaneously.

But there is hope. Did you notice the close similarities between excitatory pleasure and the type of pain related to a lack of inhibition? For instance, when you are very excited and enthusiastically looking forward to something, isn't that very close to the experience you feel when anxious, tense, and agitated? Your body responds the same way in both situations, even though you interpret them differently. Likewise, when you're feeling secure, serene, and mellow, isn't that very close to a feeling of submission and lethargy? The crossed arrows in Figure 5 note these relationships.

Seneca, the Roman philosopher and statesman, once proclaimed, "there is a certain pleasure akin to pain." He was sensitive to the close relationship of these two apparent opposites. Earlier, I cited some examples of moderate forms of pain that we often interpret as pleasure. You can probably think of others—like a lover's playful biting, or the exhilarating ache and exhaustion that accompany running a mile. Or how about moving quickly from a hot sauna to a cold shower? What about tickling—is it painful or pleasurable? How about the experience of being terribly hungry, and knowing you're about to eat—is that painful or pleasurable? And what about when you furiously scratch an itch? Does it hurt or feel good?

Even in the animal kingdom, there are many examples of this fine line between pleasure and pain. Male cats and lions, for instance, bite the neck of their mate prior to mating. Without this very physical, aggressive, almost sadistic/masochistic ritual, they won't mate.

The point is that pleasure and pain run hand in hand. To paraphrase the Taoist philosophers, "Nothing is pure pain, nothing is pure pleasure; there is always some pleasure in pain, and some pain in pleasure."

From this perspective, pleasure and pain are not opposites, but complements, for they represent two different aspects of the same

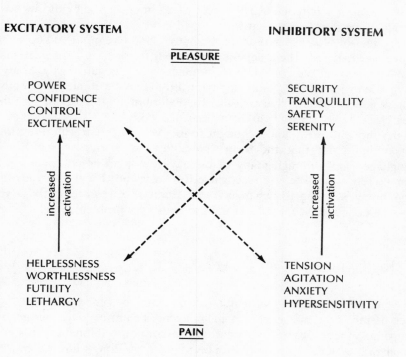

EXCITATORY SYSTEM

INHIBITORY SYSTEM

<u>**PLEASURE**</u>

POWER
CONFIDENCE
CONTROL
EXCITEMENT

SECURITY
TRANQUILLITY
SAFETY
SERENITY

increased activation

increased activation

HELPLESSNESS
WORTHLESSNESS
FUTILITY
LETHARGY

TENSION
AGITATION
ANXIETY
HYPERSENSITIVITY

<u>**PAIN**</u>

Fig. 5 *A model of pleasure and pain.*

process. Pleasure and pain keep you intimately in touch with your inner and outer worlds. The opposite of both is total insensitivity.

To experience both pleasure and pain is natural, normal, and healthy. I used to believe that "health" was the absence of illness and the full actualization of well-being. Ivan Illich, the philosopher-author, has helped to clarify my thinking on this subject, for he points out that "health is the ability to deal effectively with both pleasure and pain." In other words, both experiences are a natural consequence of life.

In a sense, pain lets you see pleasure. One of the most unhappy people I know is a man who seems to have everything. He is extraordinarily wealthy, successful, influential—and bored to death. The simple pleasures in life have long since lost their meaning, and even an impulsive flight to the French Riviera aboard his private jet no longer "turns him on." I have seen far more excitement in the eyes of an impoverished child who was thrilled by a twenty-five-cent toy.

Feelings of pleasure and pain are relative, and like mind and body, the way you experience them depends upon your frame of reference. Perhaps you've seen your pain problem in an unnecessarily negative way. Many of my patients have said, "I *hate* my pain. I'd like to cut it out of my body!" These patients would give anything to "exterminate" their pain, and they search endlessly for a "painkiller" that will work.

In other cultures, pain is thought of in a very different way. Ivan Illich has pointed out that the term "painkiller" is unique to the English language, and although many of us may view pain as an enemy to be conquered, other societies recognize it as a friend that warns you when something is wrong. By changing your frame of reference, perhaps you, too, can begin to see a positive side to your pain problem.

The Purpose of Pain

Some people see the world as a hostile, dangerous enemy that is "out to get them." Others see it as a magnificent, beautiful place designed to maximize their sense of personal enjoyment and fulfillment. At a given moment, either frame of reference may be accurate, for the world is constantly changing in a waxing-and-waning movement of ebb and flow, danger and safety.

Pain and pleasure are essential for survival in an ever-changing world. At the deepest level of instinctual functioning, they keep us responsive to our inner and outer environments. Pain warns us that something is wrong, and it is nature's way of helping us to prevent further damage.

From an evolutionary perspective, only the fittest members of a given species will survive the various predators and other dangers around them. Man's greatest predator is disease, and pain usually alerts us the instant that trouble strikes. If we listen to its message and take appropriate action, we are often able to prevent the problem from becoming worse. In some cases, removing ourselves from a source of danger is all that is needed, for the body has a remarkably powerful ability to heal its own injuries. From this point of view, pain is clearly a positive, healthy, and *adaptive* phenomenon.

When I suggest to my patients that there may be a positive side to their pain, a few seem ready to walk out the door. But give it a moment's thought. Pain is not a disease: it is a *symptom*. James Fadiman, one of the founders of transpersonal psychology, defines symptoms as "the way the body tries to heal itself."

For example, a low-grade fever (under 103 degrees Fahrenheit) represents the body's attempt to raise its temperature in order to "burn out" an invading microbe. Practitioners of Oriental medicine consider fever to be a *healthy* response to danger, and they make no attempts to reduce it unless it rises to injurious levels (over 104 degrees Fahrenheit). But in the Western world, we quickly reach for aspirin.

Another good example is the "workaholic" who suffers from high blood pressure. The stress of his day-to-day life is intense, and each time he is checked by his physician, he appears more agitated and his blood pressure climbs to higher and higher levels. Does he get the message to slow down? Maybe. If not, his blood pressure may continue to rise, and he may begin to experience pain in his chest as well. Soon, he may be unable to climb stairs or walk long distances without shortness of breath and severe chest pain. If he continues to rush through life, his heart may attack him, for a major coronary finally makes the message quite clear: Slow down! Stop! Let yourself enjoy life a little!

Pain is a message that alerts you to danger. Through the primitive, survival-oriented wisdom of your nervous system, it also motivates you to correct the situation by changing something in your life. Pain shows that you are alive, and that some part of you is attempting to adapt to the shifting demands of your environment.

Think back to the times when you've said, "I'd give anything to never feel pain again." Although it may have sounded like an ideal situation, consider the consequences of such a pain-free existence. For example, picture yourself fracturing a bone after slipping in the rain, but being completely oblivious to it. Or severely burning yourself by lying in the sun too long, without any recognition of the damage it's done to your body.

Unfortunately, there are people congenitally insensitive to pain. They are normal in all other respects, but from birth they have no pain responses. Consequently, they sustain cuts, burns, and bruises without ever being aware of them. One man almost died from a burst appendix, because he didn't feel the typical abdominal pain conveying the message that something was terribly wrong. Another man continued walking on a cracked bone in his leg until it completely broke.

A Canadian girl bit off her own tongue while chewing her food, and was never aware of what she had done. She once seriously burned herself by leaning on a hot radiator while peering out a window. She suffered many bone fractures during her life because she was not conscious of the amount of pressure she was putting on her joints. A month before she died at age twenty-nine, she finally began experiencing normal pain sensations. Doctors said that the many years of excessive skin and bone trauma directly contributed to her death.

For these individuals, pain would be a blessing. So stop cursing your discomfort, and start accepting it as an ally. Your pain may be trying to help you to survive.

Many of my patients believe that their discomfort is related only to an injury or disease. Such patients may say, "If only my back (or legs, or head) didn't hurt, my life would be perfect." Although this may be true in some cases, I typically find that other problems of living also become projected onto the area of injury. Thus, it's not just their backs, legs, or heads that are involved; it's their *lives* that hurt. Frequently, these other unresolved life problems must also be dealt with before the full weight of the pain experience can be lifted.

Through pain, your nervous system warns you about *all* of the dangers you face, and if you continue to ignore them, the intensity of your pain will increase. Perhaps this is why many chronic pain patients receive only temporary relief after symptomatic treatment. Drugs, nerve blocks, and neurosurgical procedures can fool your nervous system for a while, but if some subtle danger still lurks unknown, instinct will remind you by causing your pain to break through. The pain will continue to return until you finally understand what's wrong, deal effectively with the problem, transform your life in an appropriate way, and adapt to the changing world around you.

It has always amazed me to witness how people with the same problem experience their illness so differently. For example, one patient with severe, crippling arthritis lives a life of constant agony. Another with the same type and degree of arthritis appears to experience little, if any, discomfort. Perhaps the first patient has other problems that haven't been properly dealt with, whereas the second has his inner life in order.

What's really wrong in your life? Are there unresolved personal problems that could be contributing to your pain experience? Perhaps deep inside, you can find the answer. Accept your pain as a friend, not an enemy, and begin to work *with* it, rather than against it. For as you come closer to discovering and resolving the unknown problems in your life, your nervous system well tell you so by reducing your discomfort or by turning it off altogether.

Try it. All you stand to lose is your pain and suffering. If you win, you may regain a meaningful, pleasurable life.

Exercise Six: Discovering Pain's Message

As I've emphasized in this chapter, pain may be a warning about other serious problems in your life. In this exercise, I would like you to try to find at least ten possible messages that your pain may be trying to convey. What has gone wrong in your life that may be contributing to your discomfort? Do you have certain insecurities and fears that may be involved? What are you doing wrong? And what do you need to stop doing? What attitudes and beliefs do you need to change? In short, what is your pain trying to tell you? Have you any hints or clues? (If not, I'll suggest several ways to help you find answers to these questions later in the book.)

SAMPLE

EXERCISE SIX: Discovering Pain's Message DATE: <u>feb. 21</u>

TIME: <u>8 p.m.</u>

My pain is trying to tell me that
1 I'm working too hard; I've got to balance my time better between work and play
2 I should stop being so self-critical, and see my good side too
3 I should stop being so frightened about the possibility of having a headache
4 I don't express my emotions enough; too much is being kept locked up inside me
5 I should stop being so perfectionistic, and should accept my weaknesses
6 I'm not taking enough time for my own needs
7 I'm not exercising or nourishing my body as I should
8 I'm not having enough fun in my life
9 I'm too suspicious of everyone and not as trusting as I need to be
10 I should stop being so angry about my doctors' inability to help me
Notes:

EXERCISE SIX: Discovering Pain's Message   **DATE:** _____

TIME: _____

My pain is trying to tell me that
1
2
3
4
5
6
7
8
9
10
Notes:

3 *Why Do You Hurt?*

When patients ask me, "Why do I hurt?" I suggest that they consider at least three possible explanations:

Theory #1 maintains that your pain is a punishment for your sins. According to this theory, God is responsible for your discomfort and it was Divine Fate that has placed you in the predicament you're in. You've lived an evil life, and you are being penalized for it. Or as comedienne Joan Rivers has said, "When things get bad, and your whole world looks like it's going to fall apart—never forget that you're basically a rotten person and you deserve it all!"

Theory #2 holds that it was an accident, and that your pain was caused by a force beyond your control. Who knows? Perhaps the Martians did it. You may have been walking down the street minding your own business when you accidentally stepped into a Martian pain ray and got zapped. If this is the case, there's not much your doctors can do about it, for they have not yet learned to communicate with extraterrestrial beings.

Theory #3 maintains that your own nervous system is responsible. Perhaps something is wrong in your life, and pain is the way your nervous system is trying to warn you about it.

The implications of the first two theories are terrifying to me, for they suggest that pain is beyond your control and therefore you may have to remain its helpless victim. I need not point out that modern medicine is totally in the dark when it comes to treating the effects of Martian pain rays or the dictates of God.

But if your pain was activated by your own nervous system, if it's a warning signal about the way you are living your life, if it has both meaning and purpose, if it's your friend, not your enemy—then perhaps you can discover what's wrong in your life and correct it. For if pain is no longer needed, your nervous system may have the power to turn it off naturally.

Why do you hurt? What is your nervous system trying to tell you? There are no simple answers. However, in my experience with pain patients, several major problem areas have emerged. Your pain may or may not be related to them, but let's at least consider the possibilities.

Are You Malnourished?

"You are what you eat."

It's more than just a catchy slogan, for the way you nourish yourself significantly influences how you feel.

Although food is essential for survival, other sources of energy are also required to sustain life in an ever-changing world. How long can you live without oxygen, water, heat, and sensory input?

In our modern world, there is great variability in the quality of the essential nutrients we consume. If you hurt, one part of your pain's message may be, "You are malnourished. Something that you're consuming is poisoning you." It could be emotional poison, food poison, air poison, or even electromagnetic poison. But your pain may be saying, "Something's wrong here. You're taking in something that's bad for you. Stop!"

Every disease is probably related in some way to environmental factors. Let's discuss some of the environmental poisons—the sources of destructive energy—that may need to be excluded from your life.

Food

Examine your own diet for a moment. It probably contains some instant foods that were nonexistent a generation ago. Many of these "convenience foods" are highly deficient in nutritional value, yet we consume them at the expense of food that is essential for good health.

For example, nutrients such as vitamin C are necessary for the body to develop strong connective tissue. But suppose that over many years, you haven't had sufficient amounts of these nutrients in your diet. If this is the case, your connective tissue may not have developed properly, causing weak tissues that can produce problems like a slipped disk. Although you might think that your slipped disk is the result of lifting a heavy object improperly, another individual with better nutrition and stronger tissues might make the same movement with no injury at all to the body. So what's really to blame for your pain in this case? Your diet.

And how about individuals with hypoglycemia? When they eat the wrong kinds of food, their body often tells them so with pain. A hypoglycemic who consumes foods too rich or too starchy will soon find his blood sugar level dropping dramatically. In the process, symptoms such as painful headaches are common.

There are literally thousands of food additives in the marketplace that your body has to battle against, day after day. These chemicals, designed to make food look better and last longer on supermarket shelves, may also be making you ill. No one really knows to what extent these additives may affect the onset and severity of pain, but when chemicals like preservatives and stabilizers accumulate in your body over a period of ten years, twenty years, or more, they could conceivably affect your nervous system in an adverse way.

There is evidence, for example, that certain food additives may cause hyperkinetic behavior in children. Dr. Ben F. Feingold, a prominent San Francisco allergist, believes that many children who have been classified as "hyperactive-learning disabled" or who have "minimal brain dysfunction" are actually genetically incapable of defending against the negative effects of synthetic colors and flavoring agents. Feingold, the author of *Why Your Child Is Hyperactive*, reports that when these children are placed on a diet free of all synthetic colors and flavors, their behavior often improves dramatically within one month.

Nitrates (chemicals found in hot dogs, bacon, etc.) have been directly connected to migraine headaches and may be cancer causing as well. And you've probably read the headlines in recent years linking a coloring agent called Red Dye #2 to cancer, and monosodium glutamate (MSG) to brain-cell impairment in children and burning chest pains in adults.

Allergic reactions to food additives may be far more common than we know. A Pennsylvania woman recently felt very weak and fatigued after eating a bowl of cornflakes. She knew she wasn't allergic to either milk or corn and was puzzled by the reaction. However, the mystery was solved when tests revealed she was allergic to beta-hydroxy acid, a chemical added to cornflakes to maintain freshness.

Artificial flavors have been reported to cause everything from headaches to asthma. One man fell into a severe anaphylactic shock when he ate ice cream artificially flavored with chocolatin and strawberrin.

Although food industry spokesmen insist that the minute quantities of chemicals added to foods cause little, if any, harm, the American Medical Association's Council on Pharmacy and Chemistry disagrees. No one knows the extent of damage that occurs when even small quantities of chemicals are consumed regularly over a long period of time. And no one knows what health hazards result when *combinations* of additives are taken together. According to the AMA, "the resultant injury may be cumulative or delayed, or simulate a chronic disease of other origin, thereby making identification and statistical comparison difficult or impossible."

At UCLA, we use techniques such as hair analysis (described in Chapter 4) to determine the impact that nutrition may have on a patient with pain. We also recommend nutritional supplements that will enhance our patients' health, not damage it. In Chapter 8, I'll discuss in detail specific foods and vitamin supplements that may help you to combat the pain in your life.

Water

Just as the food you consume can affect your well-being, so can the water you drink. Water is the most common substance on the planet, and for centuries has been thought to have a multitude of therapeutic benefits—from bathing in mineral and sitz baths, to drinking spring or mineral water.

However, there is recent evidence that the water coming through your faucet could be making you sick. The Environmental Protection Agency announced not long ago that it had found traces of organic chemical pollutants, including some suspected of causing cancer, in the water supplies of seventy-nine selected American cities. In Cincinnati and Philadelphia, thirty-six such compounds were found. In Miami, traces of thirty-five were detected, and New Orleans had sixty-six. High levels of cadmium and nitrate were discovered in some drinking water supplies. Cadmium has been linked to heart disease and high blood pressure, and nitrate to a rare blood disease.

Almost nothing is known about how drinking water affects chronic pain, but perhaps unrecognized contaminants in our water supplies may be involved. That's a frightening possibility, since Americans collectively drink about nineteen billion gallons of water a day, most of which come from public water systems.

If you are concerned about the water you drink, try switching to bottled spring water for a short time. If you notice no difference in your pain after a while, switch back. But if you seem to have less discomfort, you might benefit by staying with the change.

Air

A recent U.S. Public Health Service report proclaimed, "With every breath we take, an increased percentage of us comes a little closer to a diagnosable diseased condition."

Each day, tons of "aerial garbage" spew into the atmosphere of the United States. Because of factories, power plants, incinerators, homes, apartment buildings, and 100 million motor vehicles, our skies are contaminated with 180,000 tons of carbon monoxide, 100,000 tons of sulfur dioxide, 17,000 tons of nitrogen oxide, and 33 tons of hydrocarbons daily.

The air is something we have contact with continuously. We inhale and exhale hundreds of times every hour, and if the air is clogged with poisons, the long-term effect upon our bodies can be devastating. Add to that the negative psychological effect of looking at skies that are gray instead of blue, and it's not surprising that people who live in major metropolitan areas are often more depressed than those who live in rural communities.

Certainly, inhaling large quantities of carbon monoxide, lead particulates, ozone, and smoke is a phenomenon our forefathers never had to concern themselves with. "Progress" has given us diseases (such as emphysema) that were largely unheard of even a generation ago. More and more studies are indicating a definite link between bad air and bad health.

According to the National Tuberculosis Association, "Polluted air can make your eyes water and burn. It can blur your vision. But even worse, it can upset your breathing. You may have to make an effort to breathe. And you may not get all the oxygen your body needs to stay healthy.

"Air pollution has been known to kill, to sicken and to destroy. It is particularly hard on people with serious chest conditions—chronic lung or heart disease. Such people have to work harder to breathe the impure air."

In one frightening experiment in New York City, coronary patients briefly exposed to expressway traffic soon developed angina (severe chest pain caused by lack of oxygen in the heart). Some of these same people also experienced abnormal electrocardiograms in the smoggy environment.

The exact relationship between contaminants in the air and chronic pain remains unknown, but we hope that scientists will soon begin to conduct research in this area. In the meantime, there are many things you can do to help improve this situation. In the strongest possible terms, tell your legislators how you feel about air pollution. Avoid cigarette smoking and other obvious contaminants. In Chapter 7, I will describe a series of breathing exercises that have proved to be remarkably beneficial for people in pain. With practice, they may help you, too.

Sensory Impressions

Sensory stimulation is also an important source of nourishment, for if deprived of all stimuli, we quickly lose our ability to function as human beings. Many years ago, a team of psychologists tested the length of time an individual could survive with only a minimal amount of stimulation. Volunteers were placed in isolation, floating in a tank of salty water with their eyes and ears covered and their arms immobilized. Within forty-eight hours, all the volunteers found themselves in serious trouble. Their nervous systems had become so hungry for stimulation that they cannibalized their own inner sensations. As a result, these individuals began to hallucinate vividly, sensing their own blood corpuscles rushing through their veins and arteries, and hearing their thunderous heartbeat as it vibrated throughout their entire body.

Interestingly, sensory overload can be just as devastating. It so disorients people that neither their minds nor their bodies can function properly. Hyperstimulation is one of the essential components of brainwashing, as well as both mental and physical torture.

Your senses have a tremendous impact on your well-being, for everything you see, hear, smell, taste, and touch influences you in some way. These sensory impressions are constantly being absorbed by both the conscious and subconscious minds, and as a result they significantly affect the way you feel and the way you behave.

Consider something as ordinary as music. Throughout history, music has been incorporated into many healing rituals. In recent scientific studies, music has been shown to accelerate body metabolism, muscular activity, and respiration. It also influences pulse rate and blood pressure, and minimizes the effects of fatigue. Other studies suggest that music may even break down cholesterol in the bloodstream.

Although some types of music can be therapeutic, others can have the opposite effect. Harsh or jarring sounds may damage the body rather than help it. Two German psychiatrists recently concluded that 75 percent of the musicians in an orchestra playing modern music were frequently ill because of "noise levels and discord which make them nervous, irritable and aggressive, resulting in sleepless nights, headaches, stomach pains and bowel disorders."

Other types of noise may be even more destructive. People who live near airports report a variety of physical and mental problems that have been scientifically linked to excessive jet plane noise. Perhaps you, too, have felt aggravated by your inability to control the endless rumbling, droning sounds of jet planes flying overhead. When continued over a period of many months or years, this type of noise pollution can be devastating.

Many other common sources of stimulation are known to have subtle effects on your health. For example, there is evidence suggesting that television commercials may be related to certain types of illnesses. A study by Charles Atkins, a Michigan State communications professor, indicates that many children develop more colds and stomachaches after heavy doses of TV ads for nonprescription medicines. Why? Perhaps the commercials convey to them the message that such ailments are normal. Atkins, analyzing the reactions of 775 children in the ten-to-fourteen age range, divided the youngsters into two groups—heavy and light TV watchers. Interestingly, the heavy viewers reported 20 percent more stomachaches and colds than the light watchers. About 62 percent more of the heavy watchers worried about becoming ill.

All input has an effect upon us, whether or not we're consciously aware of it. For example, it is generally assumed that when patients are given general anesthesia they have no knowledge of the world around them, for they are in a certain type of sleep state. But in an astounding series of reports, David B. Cheek, M.D., a San Francisco obstetrician and an innovative researcher of unconscious perception, has demonstrated that this may not be the case. When he hypnotized surgical patients after their operations, they were able to recall minute details of their doctors' conversations during surgery. This information was absorbed subconsciously, and it may have significantly affected their rates of postoperative recovery.

According to Cheek, "Meaningful sounds, meaningful silence, meaningful conversations are registered and may have a profound influence upon behavior of the patient during surgery and for many years after."

Cheek's research uncovered the case of a nurse who "misunderstood the intended meaning of 'five-year survival' after mastectomy for breast cancer and died of a bowel obstruction on the fifth anniversary of her operation. Autopsy showed no evidence of recurrence of her cancer. Her sister was a nurse and had repeatedly tried to change the conviction of this patient, but conscious-level explanations could not alter the subconsciously fixed impression."

I believe that Cheek's findings are critically important. Imagine a surgeon, while operating on a cancer patient, saying, "There's nothing more we can do for him; the disease has spread too far; he's only got three months to live." The patient, having subconsciously absorbed this information while on the operating table, may subsequently die within several days of this three-month period, as if programmed by the doctor's prognosis. The evidence from Cheek's studies and other research indicates that stimuli perceived subconsciously may be capable of influencing the brain and the body to that significant a degree.

For people in pain, the quality of their sensory impressions is of particular importance. If, for example, everything you see, hear, and feel is negative, you may very well have "sensory malnutrition." When someone says, "You look awful," it often produces a kind of emotional indigestion that can accentuate your pain.

Remember, you are what you "eat," and if your environment is a cold and dreary ocean of negativity, it may be severely limiting your body's ability to overcome your discomfort. In Chapter 9, I'll discuss some of the things you can do to obtain the positive sensory nourishment that stimulates good health and self-healing.

Electromagnetic Influences

Although what we see, hear, and touch dramatically affects how we feel, the energy that stimulates these sensations represents only a tiny portion of the electromagnetic spectrum. Our bodies are constantly being bombarded by other electromagnetic radiations that we are unable to perceive. Although relatively little is known about the biological effects of these invisible and inaudible radiations, there is recent evidence suggesting that they may have profound effects upon our health.

For instance, if you work, live, or travel near ultrahigh-voltage power lines (now in use in Indiana, Kentucky, Michigan, Ohio, Virginia, and West Virginia), your body may be affected by these 765,000-volt lines. Scientists in the Soviet Union studied forty-five people who had worked in ultrahigh-voltage switchyards two to five hours a day for years. They found that, as a result of this exposure, more than 90 percent of these workers suffered from an "instability" of pulse and blood pressure, excessive perspiration, and arm and leg tumors. About 30 percent of the male subjects complained of reduced sexual vigor, and at least 10 percent showed signs of diminished electrical conduction in their heart. This is a frightening report, particularly since electric utility companies in the United States are now planning to erect many more of these ultrahigh-voltage lines.

Anxiety over such electromagnetic pollution is not new. It also existed in the late 1960s when the U.S. Navy announced plans for Project Sanguine, a sophisticated communications system to ensure continued contact between the continental United States and the Navy's submarine fleet in the event of a nuclear attack. If Project Sanguine had been implemented, high-intensity electromagnetic cables would have been buried under thousands of acres of land in western Wisconsin. Acting as a powerful antenna, they would have emitted extremely low frequency (ELF) waves—in the same range at which the human brain operates.

When plans for Sanguine were announced, environmentalists complained loudly that the ELF transmissions might disrupt the earth's geomagnetic field as well, with possibly horrendous results. Their objections were taken seriously, and Sanguine was squelched.

However, the concept was revived by the Navy in 1975, this time under the name Project Seafarer. Under the new plan, the antenna was to be erected aboveground. Despite strong protests, a Seafarer test project was implemented at the U.S. Navy Wisconsin Test Facility. Although the

Navy has publicly argued that Seafarer would produce few, if any, harmful effects, a 1973 paper by a Navy scientific panel indicated that some of the people who were exposed to ELF radiation experienced high levels of triglycerides in their blood—a condition often related to heart attacks and high blood pressure.

Evidence of Seafarer's impact was also revealed in a study by William E. Southern, a biological scientist at Northern Illinois University. He found that birds which entered the electromagnetic field created by the Seafarer test project were significantly disoriented by it. For decades, researchers have known that, during migration, birds use various geomagnetic cues to direct them to their destination. But because of Seafarer, they were noticeably diverted from their normal course. If birds are influenced by ELF waves, are people and other animals affected as well?

Dr. Robert O. Becker, an orthopedic surgeon at the Veterans Administration Hospital in Syracuse, New York, has hypothesized that the process of tissue repair may be regulated by a special electromagnetic control system in the body. This system may be subtly affected by electromagnetic forces in the external environment. In testing his theory, Becker has shown that when certain types of electromagnetic stimulation are applied to the body, the healing time of broken bones can be significantly reduced. Using frogs and other laboratory animals, Becker found that certain frequencies of electromagnetic stimulation could even cause limbs and organs to regenerate following amputation. In another series of studies, Becker has suggested that this electromagnetic injury control system may be partly responsible for the therapeutic effectiveness of acupuncture.

There are many theories of how electromagnetic energy may be associated with disease. One intriguing notion suggests that when excess electromagnetic forces accumulate within the body, they must be "grounded," or illness can result. This theory was postulated by George Starr White, M.D., author of *Cosmo-electric Culture*. White claimed that "the further humans departed from natural living, the less they lived grounded and the more prone they were to illness."

It is true that modern man is not as electrically grounded as his forefathers were. Thousands of years ago, man literally had "both feet on the ground." Today, we are separated from the earth by rubber-soled shoes, and houses made of wood and other nonconductive materials.

Many centuries ago, the Chinese theorized that pain resulted from an excess accumulation of energy within the body. If there is any validity to White's hypothesis, it may provide a modern explanation for this ancient belief.

In the contemporary world, there are an ever-increasing number of electromagnetic energy sources, including ultrahigh-voltage power lines, sophisticated communications devices, microwave ovens, and modern weapons systems. However progressive these new developments may seem, some of them may also be hazardous to your health.

No one knows for certain how prolonged exposure to electromagnetic energy may ultimately affect your body. While some sources of this energy may be highly destructive, others may have therapeutic value. Becker's research tends to support this hypothesis. So does the successful use of ultrasound. These very high frequency sound waves are helpful in treating problems like soft-tissue injury, for they facilitate tissue regeneration by stimulating protein synthesis. In the future, it is hoped we will learn how to maximize the therapeutic value of electromagnetic energy, while minimizing or neutralizing its harmful effects upon the body.

Cosmic Influences

Probably the most controversial of all the possible influences upon man and his well-being are the cosmic forces upon us. Sometimes I feel a little uncomfortable about even discussing this phenomenon. After all, is it really practical to suggest that the sun or the moon may be affecting your pain, either positively or negatively?

While scientific research on cosmic influences is still in its infancy, some of the initial studies in this area suggest that these distant forces play an important role in how we feel and behave.

The cyclic rhythms of the sun and moon are correlated with many changes in health, personality, and behavior. For example, during the earth's annual journey around the sun, the winter months produce a significantly greater incidence of earaches, sore throats, tonsillitis, and similar ailments. Not only does your body absorb less of the sun's vital nourishment during the shorter days of winter, but the cold weather can also reduce your body temperature, leaving you more vulnerable to certain types of viruses.

The season of your birth can also affect your physical and mental health. Several studies indicate that people born in the winter months have a greater incidence of schizophrenia, manic-depressive illness, and mental retardation than general population samples.

As the moon revolves around the earth, its lunar cycle (approximately twenty-nine and a half days) is correlated with several types of antisocial behavior. For instance, in studying criminal offenses committed in the year 1969 in Cincinnati, Jodi Tasso and Elizabeth Miller, psychologists at Edgecliff College in Cincinnati, Ohio, discovered that the frequency of crime in eight of nine categories (rape, robbery and assault, burglary, larceny and theft, auto theft, offenses against family and children, drunkenness, and disorderly conduct) increased significantly during the full phase of the moon. Only homicides did not rise in number.

Other reports suggest that accidents increase in number during the full moon, and as a result, the patient load at hospital emergency rooms also increases dramatically at that time. Some physicians have even suggested that elective surgery be avoided while the moon is full, because they believe that doctors are more prone to commit mistakes, and that patients on the operating table are more susceptible to complications.

But perhaps we are most affected by the nocturnal (nightly) and diurnal (daily) cycles of the earth's rotation, for they may influence the body's own circadian (approximately twenty-four-hour) rhythm. Nearly every physiological and psychological function in your body fluctuates according to this rhythm.

For example, research indicates that heart patients may be up to forty times more sensitive to digitalis, a drug used to treat congestive heart disease, at 4:00 A.M. than at certain other times of the day. Diabetics are most sensitive to insulin at that hour, and in many people, sensitivity to pain is at its lowest at 4:00 A.M., and increases to its maximum by 6:00 P.M.

Are there cycles to your own pain? Does it become more (or less) intense at certain times of the day? Perhaps you recognized such patterns many months ago, but never fully understood why they occurred.

If you're unaware of a rhythm to your discomfort, turn to your Daily Comfort Log (Exercise One), and analyze it for a few moments. Are there, in fact, certain times of each day when your pain intensity is stronger, or weaker, than at other times? Is your pain experience being influenced, at least to some degree, by your own circadian rhythm? The ultimate regulator of the circadian rhythm is unknown, but the diurnal and nocturnal cycles of the earth, interacting with the gravitational forces of the sun and moon, may well affect it.

What about the influence of other cosmic forces such as sunspot activity, solar and lunar tides, the gravitational pull of other planets in our solar system, and radiations that emanate from distant stars? What happens, for example, when an immense intergalactic body explodes in interstellar space, showering the earth with neutrinos, quarks, and other elementary particles? Can we reasonably assume that they have *no* effect on our planet or its inhabitants?

In short, could cosmic influences be affecting your pain? Frankly, we have barely begun to explore the possible impact of cosmic forces upon our well-being. But until more is known, I don't think we can ignore the role they may be playing. If man ever completely deciphers all the laws of the universe, then perhaps we will finally understand how cosmic influences affect illness and pain. Until then, I don't think that any possibility should be ruled out.

The Energy of Life

Thousands of years ago, the ancient Chinese described an invisible vital life-force called "Ch'i" that was thought to animate all living things. The

Hindus described a similar energy which they call "prana." Wilhelm Reich called it "orgone energy," and Soviet scientists speak of "bio-plasmic energy." Whatever name it's given, I find it a much easier phenomenon to experience than to explain. If you will allow yourself to be open to the possibility of its existence, the following exercise may make you briefly aware of this phenomenon:

Put this book down gently in your lap, and allow yourself to become as comfortable as possible. . . .

Now extend your arms straight out in front of you, with palms facing up. Wait a few moments. . . .

Soon you may begin to experience a light tickling or itching sensation in the palm or fingers of one or both of your hands. Some people even sense that their palms are becoming warm and heavy; others describe this feeling as a tingling sensation. Do you sense it? What is it that you're sensing?

Now turn your palms to face each other, about six inches apart, at eye level. Hold them there a few moments to see if you get a feeling of something moving from one hand to the other. . . .

Can you feel a sensation moving from your right hand to your left, or vice versa? The Chinese say that this energy moves from right to left in man, and from left to right in women. How does it move for you?

Next, point your fingertips toward each other, once again about six inches apart. Then slowly move your hands closer together, then farther apart, and repeat this several times. . . . Do you feel a tingling sensation in your fingertips? What's happening? Now slightly rotate your right wrist up and down. Can you see faint white lines traveling from the fingertips of one hand to the fingertips of the other? If so, what do you think is happening?

Finally, place your hands on opposite sides of your head, with palms about six inches from your ears. Do you feel any peculiar sensations? After a while, you may experience one hand becoming warmer than the other. Or perhaps one of your ears is becoming warm. What is happening?

Did you experience a tingling sensation during this exercise? If so, what was it? How can it be explained?

I recognize at least three possibilities. First, perhaps you made it all up. Maybe you were only imagining that something was there.

Or second, you might have actually been under hypnosis during the exercise, persuaded by the words themselves into believing that a sensation was there.

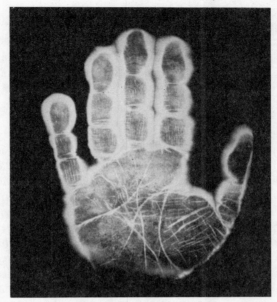

Fig. 6   *An electrophotograph of a hand using Kirlian techniques.*
(Courtesy of Stanley Krippner, Ph.D.)

Or finally, you may have been experiencing Ch'i, orgone energy, prana, or bioplasmic energy. For want of a better term, I'll call it "life energy." Some people dismiss this explanation since there is little scientific evidence to support it. But as all scientists know, the absence of data does not disprove a hypothesis. I find some of the initial research into this area encouraging enough at least to remain open to the possibility of its existence.

Using a specialized photographic technique developed by Semyon and Valentina Kirlian in the Soviet Union, some scientists claim that the effects of this invisible life energy can be documented on film. In *The Kirlian Aura*, edited by Stanley Krippner and Daniel Rubin, researchers from around the world postulate radically new ideas which, if true, may force us to take an entirely different look at the world in which we live.

For example, is life energy responsible for phenomena like telepathy? Perhaps it is this subtle energy that a mother senses when her child is in danger. Or perhaps it can explain some of the amazing experiences of psychics like Uri Geller.

Do healers who utilize "laying on of hands" transfer life energy to their patients? Do they somehow help them to generate their own?

The concept of life energy may also help define the attraction or warm feeling you have toward some people, even the first time you meet them. We call it "chemistry," or a "magnetic attraction." Study the people around you. There are probably some who energize you whenever you are with them. They make you feel good all over, for they seem to be bursting with a positive life-force. Such people provide the kind of stimulation that we all need in order to thrive.

By contrast, there are other individuals who always seem to exhaust you. At times, it appears that the only thing keeping them alive is the life energy they draw from those around them. They may be nice, friendly people, but often after just ten minutes, you feel totally drained of your own vitality.

The practice of medicine in ancient China was based largely on the concept of life energy, or Ch'i. Illnesses characterized by a deficiency of Ch'i included paralysis, weakness, and a variety of degenerative diseases, while those associated with excessive Ch'i produced pain. Might your pain be related in some way to an imbalance of Ch'i? In more modern terms, does excess tension or unexpressed anger make your discomfort worse? Are you suffering from an excess of negative life energy?

True, there is little, if any, scientific evidence that conclusively proves the existence of life energy. At present, we know little more about it than was known about gravity before Newton or about electricity before Franklin. But the curiosity of many outstanding scientists has been aroused. This is an exciting time in which to live, for hopefully, the basis of the life-force will soon be identified, and we will learn its critical relationship to the healing process.

Exercise Seven: Are You Properly Nourished?

The importance of proper nourishment cannot be overemphasized. One or more of the nutritional influences I've discussed may be related to your discomfort. If so, you may have to make some changes in the way you are now living your life.

In this exercise, carefully consider the *quality* of each source of energy you are consuming, how it may be positively or negatively affecting your discomfort, and what changes you need to make to overcome your "malnutrition."

Is Hurting a Bad Habit?

Although malnutrition is certainly important, other factors can also contribute to the pain experience. For instance, earlier in your life, you may have learned to feel discomfort whenever you were in a particular situation, and now hurting has become a bad habit. Even though your discomfort may no longer be appropriate or necessary, you may have programmed yourself to anticipate pain in certain circumstances. And when pain comes, you may have learned to accept it as inevitable.

I recall one of my patients who was the victim of a terrible accident in which his right arm had to be amputated. For six long years prior to this tragedy, he had experienced severe pain from arthritis in his right hand. Once he lost the limb, he still complained of pain in the hand that no longer existed! The pain, he said, was focused only in the area where his hand once was.

This particular patient had become so accustomed to feeling pain that, even after his hand was amputated, he could not adjust to the change. He had learned to see himself as a helpless victim of discomfort for so long that he was unable even to *try* to find the pain-free existence that might have been his for the taking.

Think for a moment about what happens when a hungry rat is placed in a Skinner box. To receive food, all he must learn to do is push a lever. But if by chance he runs to one corner, rears up, spins around, and then runs to another corner before pushing the lever for the first time, all these behaviors will become associated with the food he so desperately desires. When he wants more food, he may repeat each of the moves involved in this particular ritual, unaware that most of them are inappropriate and unnecessary.

In the same way, if you are victimized by, say, headaches, you probably have learned rituals of your own. Each time you awaken with pain, you play out these same rituals again and again.

For example, you may hold your forehead in your hands for a few minutes, then begin to gently massage the area that hurts. Next, you might go to the medicine cabinet, swallow a few pills, then lie down for a while. If there's no relief, you may try a cold (or warm) compress, stronger pills, screaming loudly, and a variety of other desperate behaviors. In time, your headache will probably pass (temporarily), and the entire ritual then becomes an even stronger habit. The next time you have a headache, just guess what you'll do.

Your headache may have been trying to tell you, "Stay in bed a bit longer; you need more rest"—but you completely missed the message. Since an incidental part of your ritual included lying down, the headache passed after a while. But like the rat running from corner to corner, much of your behavior was unnecessary.

Another type of ritualistic behavior involves a totally passive response to discomfort. For example, do you respond to a headache by gritting your teeth and bearing it? Do you find yourself saying, "I suffer in silence"? Long ago, you may have learned (perhaps incorrectly) that *nothing* could help ease your discomfort. And so you stopped even trying.

This situation reminds me of the dramatic studies conducted by Martin E. P. Seligman, associate professor of psychology at the University of Pennsylvania, concerning "learned helplessness." To demonstrate this phenomenon, Seligman used a "shuttle box," an enclosed chamber with

SAMPLE

EXERCISE SEVEN: Are You Properly
Nourished?

DATE: _feb. 22_

TIME: _8:30 p.m._

	This specific source	Affects my discomfort because	To improve this situation, I need to
Food	processed and convenience foods	I may be allergic to one or more food additives	limit the number of additives I'm consuming
Water	tap water	I may react negatively to its contaminants	drink bottled water
Air	smog and cigarettes	the poisons in the air are harming my normal bodily processes	vacation for 2 weeks in the country & see if my condition improves, stop smoking
Sensory Impressions	sights, sounds, odors, tastes, touches	I'm not receiving enough positive energy from them	-redecorate my apartment - listen to beautiful music - get massaged - smell a rose
Electromagnetic Influences	power lines, microwave ovens	I may be overexposed to this radiation	be more cautious around sources of possible electro-magnetic radiation
Cosmic Influences	the sun and the moon	they may be causing subtle changes in my body temperature, pulse rate, etc.	be more aware of their possible influences
Life Energy	life-force and love	I am being oppressed by my own and other peoples' negativity	conscientiously try to fill my life with positive activities, emotions and people

NOTES

EXERCISE SEVEN: Are You Properly
Nourished?

DATE: _____

TIME: _____

	This specific source	Affects my discomfort because	To improve this situation, I need to
Food			
Water			
Air			
Sensory Impressions			
Electromagnetic Influences			
Cosmic Influences			
Life Energy			
NOTES			

two compartments separated by a small hurdle. Typically, when a dog is placed on one side of the box and subjected to shocks through the floor, he quickly learns to jump over the hurdle to the other compartment (which is shock-free) to escape from this unpleasant situation. He eventually adapts to jumping from side to side in order to avoid the shocks, and any anxiety he once felt soon gives way to an almost blasé indifference to the uncomfortable jolts.

However, Seligman's unique twist on this situation was to pretrain a dog before placing him in the shuttle box. He first strapped a dog into a hammock and subjected the animal to inescapable, random, moderately painful shocks. Initially, the dog howled sorrowfully with each shock, and became very anxious and agitated as he futilely attempted to avoid the noxious stimulation. Eventually, the dog gave up even trying to escape. When shocked, he became totally passive and immobilized.

Seligman then placed this dog into a shuttle box and again subjected him to shocks. Although the possibility for escape existed this time, the animal did not even attempt to do so. The dog had *learned to become helpless*. He had resigned himself to an inevitably painful existence and no longer even tried to take advantage of the obvious alternative available to him.

Does this sound familiar? Are you stuck in a rut of ritualistic behavior that may be unnecessarily prolonging or exacerbating your pain? Are there any alternatives that you haven't tried, because you've learned to feel helpless?

Like other ritualistic behaviors, learned helplessness often becomes a type of self-fulfilling prophecy. For example, one of my patients characteristically responded to stressful situations by anticipating the onset of a headache. Once, she told me: "Oh, my God, I'm so tense. I know my head's going to start hurting soon. I better go take a pain pill, lie down, and prepare myself to suffer."

With that attitude, it was not surprising that her fears often came true. Hurting had become her ritualistic response to stress. When she subsequently learned how to relax herself on command, she no longer experienced her "inevitable" headaches.

Conditioned (learned) Relaxation is one alternative that helps many people in pain. Later in the book, I'll fully describe it, as well as several other ways to break out of ritualistic habits.

But for now, let's briefly review some of the ways in which these ritualistic patterns begin. From the moment the nervous system first develops *in utero*, the way that it perceives and responds to pain can form habits that persist through an entire lifetime. Birth is generally thought of as the first pain experience that a human being endures, but I believe there may be painful prenatal times as well. An expectant mother is uncomfortable during much of her pregnancy: is the fetus any better off?

I can't remember what it was like being upside down in a closed, tight space (the uterus). But when you add that claustrophobic experience to all the other stimuli the fetus may be exposed to—like various violent motions, noises, and sudden hormonal changes—it's easy to see how pain might begin long before the baby is born.

The moment of birth itself can be a very unpleasant welcome to the world. Arthur Janov, Ph.D., director of the Primal Institute in Los Angeles, and E. Michael Holden, M.D., director of research at the Primal Research Laboratory, describe the birth experience thusly in their book *Primal Man*:

> *Everything* is too much and too sudden, and the infant suffers. The cry of the newborn child is not the lusty cry of vibrant life, it is the *cry of agony*. The room is too cold, too noisy, and the light is too bright. The eyedrops and the nasal suction catheter are suddenly applied. All this sudden input is experienced as agonizingly painful because the sensory windows of new-borns are extremely open. If obstetricians knew more of an infant's neurological status they would heed the advice of Dr. Frederick Leboyer in France and deliver children more gradually with none of the sudden overloading stimuli the American infant now encounters at birth.

Leboyer, author of *Birth Without Violence*, is highly critical of the "bright lights, cries and agitation that can only reinforce that *fantastic aggression* which is birth." As an alternative, he has developed a "nonviolent" approach to birth, which is conducted under dimmed lights in quiet surroundings. When the newborn baby emerges, he is placed on his mother's stomach and is tenderly massaged by his father or doctor. He is then gently lowered into a warm bath, and after washing, held softly in a swaddling blanket. Usually not a cry is heard from the baby; instead, his first grin often appears.

Some people believe that Leboyer's elaborate birth procedures are unnecessarily extravagant, but others cite Dr. David B. Cheek's reports of a possible correlation between trauma at birth and the development of illness later in life. Cheek used hypnosis to age-regress his patients back to the moment they were born. Some startling relationships emerged. In one case, for example, Cheek discovered that the experience of migraine headaches may have been related to the use of obstetrical forceps during that patient's delivery. In another case, severe angina pain was associated with emotional trauma at birth.

The hours immediately after birth may also be critically significant. Many research studies suggest that those first hours of life are an "imprinting" period during which it is important for a baby to be near his mother in order to experience her maternal warmth, hear her heartbeat, sense her gentle touch, and share her love. Imagine the helplessness that many infants must feel when they are taken from their mothers' arms after birth and placed alone in a crib for six to eight hours of observation in the newborn unit.

When my first child, Jennifer, was born, the hospital required this period of observation and isolation "as a matter of policy." Such callous indifference to my daughter's emotional needs so angered me that strange fantasies ran through my head. Should I handcuff the baby to my wife to keep them together? Should I tell the hospital nurses, "If you take this baby away, I'll call the police and have you arrested for kidnapping. This is *my* baby. Don't you dare touch her"?

It may sound absurd. But the evidence collected by Cheek and others suggests that we should reevaluate the way we now bring our children into the world. Although technological advances in obstetrics have certainly saved many lives, they might also be contributing to the development of physical and mental problems which may not surface until much later in life.

As James Fadiman has wryly stated, birth is more than a surgical solution to a nine-month-long disease. Babies are people, too. If you were pulled into the world with forceps, slapped on the behind, startled by bright lights and loud noises, and then deserted for eight hours (and quite possibly you were), wouldn't you feel pain and cry? Such a traumatic experience might well contribute to the way you experience pain later in life. It may teach you that the world is out to get you, and that at every new transition in life, someone will be waiting with bright lights, loud noises, and a slap! Worst of all, it may also teach you that there is absolutely nothing you can do about it!

During childhood, you learn to relate to pain based on how those around you—particularly your parents—react to it. Some parents, for instance, become overly disturbed and excited about minor scratches and bruises. By contrast, others show very little compassion or sympathy toward even serious injuries.

Let's suppose that, as a child, when you fell down and scraped your knee, your mother panicked, exclaiming, "Oh, my God, how horrible! What did you *do* to yourself? I'd better get you to the doctor right away!" With this type of parental reaction, your nervous system would learn to interpret the painful scrape and its consequences in one particular way. However, if your mom instead shouted, "Stop being such a crybaby; it's nothing but a little scratch. . . . Stop that crying or I'll send you to bed without dinner," your nervous system might interpret the same situation very differently. But if your mother had reacted with compassion, saying, "Oh, my poor baby; come here, let me kiss it, and it will feel much better," you would have learned to react to the painful knee in still another manner.

Think back to your own childhood. Were your scrapes, bruises, and cuts dealt with appropriately or inappropriately? To what extent did they teach you to feel helpless in the face of pain?

Our personalities are created very early in life (Freud said by the age of three). The way we learn to respond to pain during those early years may stay with us throughout the rest of our lives. One patient with severe headaches recalled that his father had suffered from headaches, too. "My dad used to be proud of the way he could cope with pain," he told me. "He used to say it proved he was a man." Did this patient subconsciously program himself to have headaches to prove his own manhood? Very possibly.

Let me share with you an incident from my own childhood. When I was in elementary school, there was a bully in my class who terrorized everyone, including me. One day I decided to taunt him, and as a result, he threatened to "tear my head off" if I showed up at school the following morning. Since he seemed strong enough to carry out his threat, I became quite frightened to put it mildly. I was too scared to tell my parents what had happened (they might have insisted that I go to school anyway, or even worse, they might have gone with me). Instead, I faked a cold so that I could stay home the next day. I simply pretended I was sick, and the more I told myself how ill I was, the sicker I actually began to feel. I was able to induce some shivering in my body, and I even raised my temperature a bit. In essence, I had told my nervous system that, by getting sick, I could avoid a potentially unpleasant situation.

More than twenty-five years later, I noticed that an interesting pattern had evolved in my life. I found that I tended to develop colds whenever I was faced with something unpleasant. It's amazing how long it took me to recognize the existence of this habit. Once I did, however, I sat down with myself and informed my nervous system, "I told you to do something many years ago that is no longer appropriate. There are no more bullies in my life. And even if there were, I think I could handle them now. So stop giving me colds." Thus far, it seems to be working.

Many other habits continue on into adulthood. Think back to the last time you visited the dentist. Quite likely you became anxious and uncomfortable before he even touched you. Deep inside, many of us remember the old-fashioned, bone-rattling, motor-driven drills that shook your brains as they ground away at your teeth. The horrifying discomfort they produced was so unique that it almost defied description.

But these old-fashioned tooth grinders were replaced long ago by high-speed, water-driven drills that produce little, if any, discomfort. Why is a visit to the dentist *still* aversive to you? Many of today's children have no fear of the dentist, for they were never exposed to the discomfort we experienced as children. Is your anxiety simply a bad habit?

Think about the many times in your life in which you've experienced pain as a result of injuries, accidents, and losses (such as the death of a loved one, separation from a spouse, or the loss of your health). What did these experiences teach you (consciously and subconsciously)?

Are you the victim of ritualistic behaviors, inappropriate habits, and self-fulfilling prophecies? Have you learned to believe that your own actions are ineffective in helping to relieve your pain? Have you prematurely given up trying?

Exercise Eight: Is Hurting a Bad Habit?

What is your reaction to the material I've presented in the last few pages? Could an inappropriate habit be partly responsible for the prolonged agony you're experiencing?

Although the subconscious remembers everything, the conscious mind often forgets many aspects of your childhood. Do you have any old photographs or letters from those days? You might want to review them, for the emotions you reexperience may help to identify inappropriate beliefs or ritualistic behaviors that started in your youth.

Was your birth difficult or easy? Were you held and comforted immediately after your birth?

How did your parents teach you to react to pain? How did they respond when you injured yourself?

Were your preschool years happy and fulfilling? Did you ever feel helpless or depressed for long periods of time? How well did you deal with pain? What inappropriate habits did you develop in relating to pain? How about during your nursery and elementary school years? Junior high and high-school years? All the years that followed, up to today?

How could all the above experiences be related to your current discomfort?

What inappropriate habits or ritualistic behaviors are you now engaged in that may be affecting your discomfort? What could you do to change them?

Do You Really Want to Get Better?

However unbelievable it may seem, many pain patients choose to keep hurting. These people typically reap certain benefits from their discomfort, and on either a conscious or subconscious level, it becomes advantageous for them to maintain their pain.

Many physicians and psychologists describe pain's benefits in terms of "gains." A typical "gain" occurs when a patient's pain helps him to manipulate others, or to avoid various situations that he finds undesirable.

If this benefit outweighs his discomfort, he may consciously or sub-consciously decide that the gain is worth the pain.

...r example, pain is one of the most effective ways to attract positive
... Each day, I see patients with their faces so contorted or their
...lk so disrupted that their discomfort is obvious to everyone
... they communicate the presence of this pain to others, it
...ersonal experience, but one that affects other people
...dvantage of the patient. Many individuals sub-
...nce they can attract positive attention and
...np, and grimace, the pain may be worth
...'t even know this decision was made.
...occupied with his job, or that he
... the daily newspaper. It is very
... the love and attention she
...ng to her pain as a way
...ching Steven work
...loved me," she

perfect
...ole-

SAMPLE

EXERCISE EIGHT: Is Hurting a Bad Habit?   **DATE:** _feb. 23_

TIME: _6 p.m._

| My birth was | normal as far as my mother can recall, but she says I was separated from her for almost fifteen hours after the delivery. |

My parents were | overly protective. They made too big a
out of minor "dangers." I remember having a lot of
They both had chronic headaches, and they complained
them a lot.

My preschool years were | spent at home with my
They were pretty happy, but my mom did te
overreact to everything that happened to w

My elementary-school years were | fun, but I
parents punishing me a lot. The punis
physical very much, but mostly emoti
a bit.

My junior-high and high-school years were
in a physical education class. I br
in a lot of pain. I also got my
for the first time, and it w

The years thereafter have been
after another - mostly
worst point when m
really haven't gotten

If this benefit outweighs his discomfort, he may consciously or sub-consciously decide that the gain is worth the pain.

For example, pain is one of the most effective ways to attract positive attention. Each day, I see patients with their faces so contorted or their ability to walk so disrupted that their discomfort is obvious to everyone they meet. Once they communicate the presence of this pain to others, it is no longer just a personal experience, but one that affects other people as well—often to the advantage of the patient. Many individuals sub-consciously decide that since they can attract positive attention and sympathy with every moan, limp, and grimace, the pain may be worth keeping. And consciously, they don't even know this decision was made.

Let's suppose that a husband is preoccupied with his job, or that he spends most of his time at home buried in the daily newspaper. It is very possible that his wife's pain may help her to get the love and attention she desires. One of my patients discovered that she clung to her pain as a way of proving that her husband really cared for her. "Watching Steven work so hard to pay my medical bills showed me that he still loved me," she concluded.

Pain can also be used to avoid human contact. It can provide the perfect excuse to postpone or cancel certain social engagements or entangle-ments. If your spouse or children demand that you spend most of your time with them, your subconscious may flare up your pain as a convenient justification for asking them not to interfere so much in your life. Pain is also frequently a means of avoiding unwanted sexual encounters with a spouse or other bed partner.

Pain fills other needs, including escape from existential problems. Several college-age patients have told me, "My pain keeps me from thinking about even deeper issues—like, 'Why am I here?' 'Is there any meaning to life?' or 'What's it all about?'" Sometimes these kinds of questions can become very intense or even overwhelming. In such instances, hurting may be preferable to dealing directly with these issues.

Often, clinging to one's pain provides financial advantages as well. For instance, let's assume an individual is receiving worker's compensation payments or other disability insurance payments related to his discomfort. Under such circumstances, he may be reluctant to relinquish the pain that provides him with such a regular income for not working. The *Wall Street Journal* recently published a report from the Emory University Pain Clinic, Atlanta, Georgia, in which its director, Dr. Steven F. Brena, stated that while 70 percent of all his pain-afflicted patients improve, only 43 percent of those receiving worker's compensation payments make any progress.

Some patients may want to return to work, but they are too insecure about their prospects for obtaining well-paying or respectable employ-

SAMPLE

EXERCISE EIGHT: Is Hurting a Bad Habit?   **DATE:** Feb. 23

                                                       TIME: 6 p.m.

My birth was	normal as far as my mother can recall; but she says I was separated from her for almost fifteen hours after the delivery.

My parents were	overly protective. They made too big a deal out of minor "dangers." I remember having a lot of fears. They both had chronic headaches, and they complained about them a lot.

My preschool years were	spent at home with my mother. They were pretty happy, but my mom did tend to overreact to everything that happened to me.

My elementary-school years were	fun, but I remember my parents punishing me a lot. The punishment was not physical very much, but mostly emotional. I felt guilty quite a bit.

My junior-high and high-school years were	marred by an accident in a physical education class. I broke both wrists, and was in a lot of pain. I also got my period in junior high school for the first time, and it was agonizing.

The years thereafter have been	filled with one painful experience after another — mostly headaches. They reached their worst point when my first marriage collapsed; they really haven't gotten too much better since then.

EXERCISE EIGHT: Is Hurting a Bad Habit?

DATE: _____

TIME: _____

My birth was

My parents were

My preschool years were

My elementary-school years were

My junior-high and high-school years were

The years thereafter have been

SAMPLE

EXERCISE EIGHT—*Continued*

These earlier experiences could affect my discomfort by

making me afraid of pain. I have also overreacted
to pain a lot. There's also been a lot of stress
in my adult life that may make me hurt more.

My current pain rituals are

I take too many pain pills – but
I don't really know what else to do. My doctor says they're
the best way he can treat me. Maybe they help a
little, but not much. I also spend too much time in
bed. And I feel sorry for myself because I hurt so much.

I could change them by

trying to figure out new ways of
making my pain stop. I want to try to learn how to
relax. I've even thought of psychotherapy, but right
now the idea of it scares me.

Notes

EXERCISE EIGHT—*Continued*

These earlier experiences could affect my discomfort by

My current pain rituals are

I could change them by

Notes

ment. For them, the pain (and its accompanying insurance payments) becomes the lesser of two evils.

One such patient, a divorcée in her mid-forties, had been plagued with pain in her lower back and hips for more than ten years. She had been treated by many doctors, been hospitalized several times, and operated on twice, but had never received any relief. After I had asked her to think seriously about any advantages that she might be deriving from her pain, she eventually declared, "Maybe I don't want to get better because I'm afraid I won't be able to get the job I want—and that would be murderous to whatever bit of ego and self-confidence I have left. The business world is very competitive, and my age isn't going to help any. But as long as I'm ill, I don't have to try to find work."

Your subconscious mind might also decide to cling to your pain if you have litigation pending. We all know that pain can be extremely costly in terms of doctor and hospital bills, surgical expenses, and medications. I have not encountered very many people with chronic illnesses who are not in debt. Thus, any legal settlements relating to your injury or illness can be extremely helpful to your financial predicament.

Our legal system is organized so that the more doctors you see who *fail*, the more money you'll receive. A medical history indicating that numerous doctors were unable to help you can be very advantageous when your case comes to court.

Of course, on a conscious level, few people would ever accept pain for money. In fact, most would gladly sacrifice any financial gain just to enjoy the luxury of a pain-free existence. But the subconscious mind may have other motives. It may be thinking, The only way I can solve my serious financial problems is to keep the pain alive until this litigation is settled. If this is the case, every positive treatment that's administered is simultaneously sabotaged by the subconscious. In support of this notion, several research reports indicate that many pain patients with litigation pending do not show improvement until their lawsuits are settled. For this reason, I typically encourage my patients to settle any pending litigation at the earliest possible opportunity.

Occasionally, a person's unwillingness to relinquish pain is based on fear of the unknown. For example, some chronic pain patients, who have lived with discomfort for many years, report, "I know what it's like to live with pain, but I've forgotten what it's like *not* to have it. I must admit that a part of me is afraid to see what would happen if my pain disappeared."

Finally, I have also met some people who have refused to relinquish their pain because they believe it is a justified punishment for something they have done. It may be no mere coincidence that the word "pain" is derived from the Latin word *poena*, meaning punishment. From early in our lives, pain is often interpreted as a chastisement for wrongdoing. The child learns that his misdeeds will lead to a painful spanking. And into adulthood, the relationship between pain and misconduct continues.

One of my former patients was a highly successful businessman in the entertainment industry. His rise from poverty to the vice-presidency of a major company is reminiscent of the Horatio Alger story. However, he admitted that in order to achieve his enormous good fortune, he deceived and cheated others all along the way. He destroyed the careers of many people, and each time he did so, he achieved more power, more fame and greater wealth.

Finally, at the age of forty-nine, he began to feel the effects of his strict Southern Baptist upbringing. Deep inside, some part of him held that his scheming was immoral, and that he should be punished for it. The only one left to punish him was himself—and his severe migraine headaches began shortly therafter.

Although he ultimately recognized what he was doing to himself, he still consciously refused to change. He told me that he would rather have pain than guilt, and that he did, in fact, deserve the severe, debilitating migraines that had afflicted him. He was content to live with them, preferring severe discomfort to a guilty conscience.

Do *you* stand to gain anything from your discomfort? Do you *really* want to get better?

Exercise Nine: Gaining from Pain

In Exercise Two, I asked you to list your goals for this program. In essence, I wanted you to note the reasons why you wanted to overcome your discomfort.

Now, after reading about the gains that pain may bring, I want you to look at your discomfort from a different perspective. As a learning experience, try to list some reasons why you *don't* want to overcome your pain problem.

Many patients have told me that, at least initially, they are unable to think of even a single reason why they might not want to overcome their pain. However, after they spend time really thinking about it, they begin to come up with some possibilities. I recall one patient who realized that he frequently used his headache pain to avoid uncomfortable situations, for his pain served as a convenient excuse when he needed one. He finally admitted, "It was much easier to tell people, 'I can't visit you because I'm hurting,' than to say, 'I can't visit you because I don't enjoy your company.' "

Once you begin to uncover some of the reasons why you may want to keep your pain, then you'll probably understand the real significance of this exercise. It's critical to recognize that while you're saying, "I want to overcome my discomfort" on a conscious level, your subconscious mind

SAMPLE

EXERCISE NINE: Gaining from Pain

DATE: feb. 27

TIME: 11 a.m.

	I don't want to overcome my discomfort because
1	My friends show me a lot of attention when I hurt.
2	I don't want to go to work *every* morning, but only when I want to.
3	I need my disability payments right now to make ends meet.
4	It's a good excuse to avoid social encounters.
5	It's a "legitimate" excuse to avoid having sex when I don't want it.
6	I have litigation pending.
7	My children won't bother me when I don't want them around.
8	The pain relieves my guilt of not working to help support my mother.
9	I need it to prove to my doctors that I'm really sick and not "a nut."
10	It gives me an opportunity to be alone when I want to.

EXERCISE NINE: Gaining from Pain

DATE: _____

TIME: _____

I don't want to overcome my discomfort because
1
2
3
4
5
6
7
8
9
10

may be saying, "Keep it!" It's very difficult to fight an invisible enemy, but once you're aware of the gains your pain provides, it will be much easier to make the changes necessary to rid yourself of your discomfort. You eventually must be able to change your behavior so that it's no longer necessary for your nervous system to want to hold onto your pain. This exercise will help you get started in that direction.

Did You Inherit Your Discomfort?

At about this time in the program, some patients tell me, "This psychological stuff is interesting, and I guess it can help the people who are crazy. But I'm not crazy; I'm sick. I have a *real* disease, for I'm certain that my pain is *genetic*. My grandmother had headaches, and my mother also had them. I inherited their bad genes, so that's why I have them, too."

There's probably some truth to the notion that heredity plays an important role in the pain experience. If your mother or father had a particular type of pain problem, perhaps you did inherit a genetic tendency for it. However, as I discussed earlier, it is also possible that, instead of inheriting the predisposition for pain, you *learned* to feel it by consciously and subconsciously observing and imitating the behavior of a parent.

Like the mind/body problem, the relationship between heredity and environment has long been a controversial subject for scientists and philosophers. To some extent, both may be factors that determine why you hurt. I've already discussed how acquired habits can affect your discomfort. Now, let's take a look at the other side of the coin.

Each of us inherits a unique combination of genes that predisposes us to certain inherent strengths and weaknesses. Depending on the parts of the body where those weaknesses lie, physical illnesses such as ulcers, asthma, and heart disease may develop, or perhaps psychological problems like anxiety and depression will occur.

For instance, if you inherited the gene responsible for your father's low back pain, you may be prone to a low back problem yourself. Or if you picked up the gene that precipitated your mother's chronic depression, you may be susceptible to depression, too.

Fortunately, your genetic endowment may also predispose you to certain unique strengths. For example, studies indicate that nearly 70 percent of all asbestos workers eventually die from lung cancer, falling prey to the tiny asbestos fibers that are inhaled on the job. Their tragically high death rate might seem to suggest that their lung cancer results from consuming a specific environmental carcinogen. But what about the other

30 percent? These workers were also exposed to asbestos fibers, yet they did not develop lung cancer.

Why not? Perhaps these "survivors" inherited a strong resistance to this type of cancer. The same may be true of people who smoke two or even three packs of cigarettes per day, yet never acquire the lung diseases that strike so many other heavy smokers. They may have inherited a strong resistance to the illnesses related to smoking.

I believe that there is essentially nothing you can do about the genes you have inherited. You were born with certain predispositions, both positive and negative, and you must adapt to them as best you can.

Why did you get your particular combination of genes? Some people might say that you *chose* them, for they believe that you are personally responsible for *everything* in your life (including "accidents" and your genetic predispositions).

To me, this premise is intuitively unsound. I find it difficult to believe, for example, that a one-week-old infant is personally responsible for his sickle-cell anemia or his Tay-Sachs disease. Such a premise is as nonsensical as contending that you control absolutely *nothing* in your life, and that everything you will ever experience is determined by your genes, or fate, or karma.

In short, if you hurt, you may or may not be responsible for the onset of your illness. That's open to debate. But you are certainly responsible for how you *deal* with your discomfort. Even if your actions and attitudes are not part of the problem, they certainly could be part of the solution.

Exercise Ten: Your Predispositions to Illness and Health

Heredity can be a major influence on the pain experience. It is therefore important for you to consider the role it may be playing in your discomfort.

In the first part of this exercise, I would like you to take a few moments to review what you know of your family's medical history. What kinds of physical and mental ailments have been prevalent throughout the past few generations? How could they be affecting your own discomfort?

For the second part of this exercise, I want you to shift your thinking from your weaknesses to your strengths. To the best of your knowledge, what types of illnesses have never occurred in your family history? What ailments does your own body seem to adapt to so naturally that they go almost unnoticed? How can your positive predispositions help you to overcome your discomfort?

SAMPLE

**EXERCISE TEN: My Predisposed
Weaknesses and Strengths**

DATE: March 1

TIME: 8 p.m.

My predisposed weaknesses make me

susceptible to pain in two major areas of my body —
my head and my back. In my family medical history,
there are cases of both of these ailments,
particularly headaches. Both of my parents had
long histories of headaches in their families.

DATE: March 1

TIME: 8 p.m.

My predisposed strengths make me

very resistant and adaptable to most other
pain-related problems. Nowhere in my family
medical history is there an indication of illnesses
like arthritis, ulcers, angina, neuritis or neuralgia.
My physical strength helps me deal with my
headaches, too.

**EXERCISE TEN: My Predisposed
Weaknesses and Strengths**

DATE: _____

TIME: _____

My predisposed weaknesses make me

DATE: _____

TIME: _____

My predisposed strengths make me

The Life Cycle

Change is fundamental to all of life. If you step back and examine how your own life changes, you'll see that it typically alternates between times of peace, contentment, and pleasure, and periods of pain and insecurity. Both are essential to life and health.

Life is filled with periods of dissolution in which old patterns are destroyed to let new ones develop. These transitional phases are painful, but without them you would never grow, advance, and progress. As Abraham Maslow used to say, "There is no growth without pain. If you're not hurting, you're not growing."

When I interview pain patients, I try to gain a full understanding of their life cycle—that is, the patterns of change that characterize their lives. Typically, I find that they consistently have difficulty moving from one of life's plateaus to the next. Again and again, they are unable to progress through life's transitional phases. They become stuck and immobilized, unwilling to let go of the old and make the hard but essential changes necessary for a meaningful life.

Some people think of the life cycle as a death/rebirth phenomenon. Whenever we reach a new plateau, something dies, but simultaneously, something new is born that replaces it. This death/rebirth process exists throughout the entire universe.

Take the human fetus, for instance. In a sense, it is more like a plant than an animal. It lives in water, and it sends roots into the uterus from which it receives nourishment. But at the moment of birth, the water is released, the stalk is cut, and the roots are ripped up. At this precise instant, as this "plant" ceases to exist, the infant is born. Something has died, but simultaneously, something else has begun to live. Isn't the "death" of the plant synonymous with the "birth" of the fetus? Aren't they two aspects of the same process?

The same phenomenon is found throughout nature. If you take a tree seed and plant it in the ground, it must grow through the fertilizer before it is exposed to the sunlight that nourishes it. As it grows to become a tree, it flourishes quickly, with trunk, branches, and leaves burgeoning. Finally, at the peak of its glory, the tree gives forth its flowers. But can the tree cling forever to those blossoms? No. The flowers must soon wither and die. But isn't the death of the flowers synonymous with the birth of the fruit—the real nourishment of the tree? After the fruit ripens and reaches its full maturity, it withers and dies, too. But in the process, it distributes its seeds, which provide for the real immortality of the tree, and the cycle begins once again.

The life cycle occurs in your personal life as well. For example, several years ago, I had an old 1966 Plymouth that I called Gertrude. I adored her. She was an extremely reliable car, and literally never spent a day in the repair shop. She never refused to start, never had a flat, never ran out of gas. But after nearly eight years, I was in a financial position to replace her, and since she had been driven so many miles, my wife and I decided to buy a new car. However, instead of being happy over the prospect of a new car, I found myself depressed. Terribly depressed. Although my wife was thrilled, I was stuck and didn't know why. Later, I realized that I was unwilling to let go of Gertrude—reluctant to give up my incredibly reliable, loyal car. It sounds silly, doesn't it? But I bet it's far more common than you might think. Eventually, I gave up Gertrude for a new car (named George).

In much the same way, many people with chronic illnesses and chronic pain are stuck. They are unwilling to let go of their old programming and proceed to a new place that may be less familiar.

However, others have had the courage to face their changing world. Although such people often must cope with horrendous injuries, they still manage to lead very good lives. Why? Because they have refused to allow themselves to be overwhelmed by their problems. They have admitted that their life is different now—their injury may have caused the loss of an ability or a function—and they have moved on to make the most of this new stage of life. Yes, they mourned and they grieved for a while, but then they stopped wishing for, say, the physical mobility they once had and set out to make the best of their new reality. If their back was severely injured, they accepted the fact that, although they could no longer work at their former job, other jobs could be just as rewarding. If they had crippling arthritis in their hands, they acknowledged that they could never play the piano with the fluid motions that they once did, but they could still play well enough to enjoy it. They changed, they survived, and they're living lives full of joys and rewards.

Pain is not the cause of your life stopping. It's the *result*. Pain has not brought a halt to your life, *you* have. Your pain is worse because you've allowed yourself to stop.

Your pain is a message that is telling you, "You're alive, but something is wrong." Although you, more than anyone else, can solve the dilemma you now find yourself in, other people may be able to help, too. In the following section, I'll introduce you to both conventional and unconventional sources for this assistance.

If you ultimately use your pain to help you grow, then the pain experience you've been through will not have been in vain.

SAMPLE

EXERCISE ELEVEN: How Are You Stuck?   DATE: <u>March 3</u>
                                            TIME: <u>6 p.m.</u>

I continue to return to situations that
involve searching for easy answers to my pain. I always want the "magic pill" to take away my pain.

I am stuck because
I'm not willing to work through the hard solution of trying to stop taking drugs. Even though I know better, pills are the easy way out.

I am unwilling to let go of
my fears. I'm frightened of what it might be like if I ever take responsibility for having my pain or not having it.

I need to change my
attitude and motivational level.

Notes
This is one of the most difficult exercises I've ever done. I don't know if my answers are the "right" ones, but I've sure thought a lot about them.

EXERCISE ELEVEN: How Are You Stuck?   DATE: _____

TIME: _____

I continue to return to situations that

I am stuck because

I am unwilling to let go of

I need to change my

Notes

Exercise Eleven: How Are You Stuck?

In the preceding section, I have discussed the concept of the life cycle and how it relates to the experience of chronic pain. For this exercise, I would like you to look at this process in terms of your own life. What unresolved situations do you continue to return to, time and time again? How are you stuck? What are you unwilling to let go of? What do you need to change?

Oasis

Time to stop again to rest for a while. Go back over your exercises and also feel free to reread any parts of the book if you'd like to do so.

When you're ready to move ahead, let's meet back on the next page to begin your search for help.

II

Seeking Help

4 *What Can Traditional Medicine Do?*

It is more important to know what kind of a person has a disease than what kind of a disease a person has.

—Sir William Osler

Everyone hurts.

From the physical pain of a headache or a stubbed toe to the mental anguish of depression, hardly a day passes when we don't feel pain of some kind.

Remember the last time you cut your finger in the kitchen or the workshop? If the injury wasn't too serious, you probably stopped cursing your clumsiness after a few minutes, and it's likely that the pain bothered you for no more than a day or two. Acute physical injuries like this generally heal on their own, and although you may swallow an aspirin or two to ease the pain temporarily, the problem will usually disappear in a short time.

The same is true with mental pain. Everyone feels depressed now and then. Following the death of a loved one, for example, depression can become so severe that we may wonder whether our own life is worth continuing. But time is a great healer, and even intense mental distress is usually short-lived. We soon bounce back to leading a normal life again.

Acute or short-term pain is a natural and healthy consequence of day-to-day living. If you listen to its message and take appropriate action, it will soon disappear by itself, for it is no longer needed.

But what happens if the physical or mental pain doesn't go away after a few days, weeks, or even months? What happens when pain lingers on and on, disrupting almost every aspect of your day-to-day life?

Often, when you're caught up in a chronic pain situation, the blame may lie with your own inability to decipher the message of your discomfort. Until you grasp its meaning and respond appropriately to its warning, the intensity of the pain will probably continue to increase, as if prompting you to try even harder to discover what's wrong in your life.

In the search for pain relief, most people first seek outside assistance from a physician. And why not? More than anyone else, he or she is assumed to have the most authoritative solutions to all of our bodily woes.

In the United States, we spend billions of dollars to educate our physicians, and billions more in providing them with support facilities (hospitals, research centers) and trained staffs (nurses, lab technicians). In a sense, the enormous amount of public money channeled into health care is like an insurance policy; we support the continued expansion and improvement of the health industry so that if we (or our families) ever need a competent doctor, one will always be available. This support also provides us with reassurance and peace of mind that someone, somewhere can help us when we hurt.

I grew up believing that physicians possessed powers somewhere between those of the U.S. President and God. When something was *really* wrong with me, a visit to the doctor was inevitable. How well I remember my kindly Welbyesque pediatrician. I was awed by his apparent magical powers to cure just about anything.

My parents' unquestioned acceptance of modern medicine was no different from that of millions of other Americans. For with the development of vaccinations, antibiotics, and other drugs, they saw the virtual elimination of diseases that once decimated entire civilizations. It seemed inevitable to them that science would someday overcome all ills, and their sense of trust was faithfully passed on to their children.

No wonder, then, that when people hurt, they turn first to their physicians. In fact, as many as 80 percent of all patients who consult physicians do so for pain-related problems.

The Search for a Diagnosis

When you see your physician, do you understand the diagnostic procedures he is utilizing? Why is he asking these particular questions? What is he looking for?

Actually, the diagnostic process is a simple one. Although there are probably as many different methods for reaching a diagnosis as there are physicians, a growing number of doctors have adopted a "problem oriented" approach. This system incorporates four distinct steps for each medical problem identified: (1) subjective information, (2) objective findings, (3) assessment of the problem, and (4) a plan of action.

Subjective Information

First, a doctor should take a complete medical history, including your family history, which may reveal a hereditary predisposition for your problem. A history of your present illness should also be carefully prepared. Your doctor should investigate when your pain started, what was happening in your life when it began, and the impact it has had upon your family and friends as well. A social history should also be taken, including drinking habits, recreational use of drugs, and cigarette smoking.

Your doctor may also find a vocational history valuable, particularly if your job(s)—either past or present—have exposed you to potential harm (remember the asbestos workers discussed in Chapter 3). And, of course, anything else you report that might relate in any way to your health problem should also be carefully considered.

Objective Findings

Once this subjective information has been compiled, your physician should then conduct a series of procedures designed to provide more concrete, objective information about your illness. These typically include a physical examination and laboratory tests (biopsies, blood and urine tests). If needed, other tests may also be ordered, such as X-rays, diagnostic nerve blocks, nerve conduction tests, psychological tests, an electroencephalogram (EEG), an electrocardiogram (EKG), an electromyogram (EMG), and other specialized procedures.

Assessment of the Problem

After your physician has collected this objective and subjective information, he will, it is hoped, arrive at a clear diagnosis of what's wrong. If not, he may order additional tests or send you for consultation with other medical specialists. An accurate diagnosis is essential for appropriate therapy.

A Plan of Action

Once a precise diagnosis has been established, your physician should then discuss his findings with you. He should carefully review the potential risks and benefits of each alternative available to you (including no therapy at all), and explain his reasons for any specific recommendations. Then a safe and effective therapeutic program can be developed that will help you to ease or eliminate your discomfort.

These four steps are the basis of a medical workup. But sometimes, despite your persuasive subjective complaints, your physician may remain unconvinced of a physical ailment, for dozens of tests and examinations may fail to uncover any objective evidence of disease or injury. In such a situation, your doctor may conclude, "There's nothing wrong with you." And consequently, his plan of action is to do nothing more.

Judging from the hundreds of people I have treated at the UCLA Pain Control Unit, patients are not very receptive to such a pronouncement. When they feel biting, pulsating pain in their shoulder, a grinding ache in their lower back, or an agonizing attack of depression, they are not agreeable to the suggestion that nothing is wrong with them. As one patient told me, "If anything, I think something's wrong with my doctor for telling me that I'm perfectly OK. If he had this pain, I'm sure he'd try harder to find out what's wrong."

Perhaps you've been in this dilemma—afflicted with an unyielding pain problem whose cause has not been pinpointed. Like other people in this predicament, you've probably left doctors' offices in a state of such utter frustration that you may feel even worse than you did when you walked in. Instead of relieving your anxiety, these physicians may have disturbed you even more by their declarations that "nothing is wrong."

Dan Greenburg, the brilliant humorist who authored *How to Make Yourself Miserable*, has aptly described how unsettled an individual can become when given a clean bill of health from his doctor. Writes Greenburg:

> [H]ow can you be sure there wasn't some fact you neglected to tell the doctor, something which you didn't even think was important enough to mention at the time, but which any medical man would have instantly recognized as the tipoff symptom?
>
> Or, even assuming there wasn't a single relevant fact you failed to tell him—how can you be absolutely certain he was competent enough to interpret correctly the information you gave him?
>
> Or even assuming he was competent, how can you be sure he gave you a *complete* physical examination? How complete *is* a complete physical examination? Couldn't there have been a test—perhaps the very one which would have revealed your illness—which he didn't consider worth giving you because the disease was too rare and the test too cumbersome?
>
> Did he, for example, give you a complete set of x-rays, including the so-called "G.I. series"? If not, that's probably the only thing which could have saved you.
>
> Or, let's say he *did* take x-rays but found no cause for concern. How can

you be sure you didn't move while the machine was on and the plate was being exposed, thereby blurring the image and covering up the subtle telltale characteristics of your affliction?

Or let's even say you're positive you didn't move while the plate was being exposed. How can you be sure that your x-rays weren't accidentally switched with those of a healthy person by some young intern in the darkroom who was simultaneously developing stag films?

In short, there is no situation that, with the application of a little creative Negative Thinking, cannot be turned into a true 3-Dimensional Worry.

.

Some of Greenburg's anxiety may be justified. If your discomfort has not been properly diagnosed, perhaps your doctor has failed to pursue a relevant technique that could provide the answers you're seeking.

For instance, one of the most unusual and potentially helpful techniques is auricular (ear) diagnosis—an ancient diagnostic method unfamiliar to most Western physicians. With a history dating back more than two thousand years, auricular diagnosis postulates that specific acupuncture points on the external ear are directly related to various internal organs. According to this system, disease can be analyzed by carefully examining these points, and treated by stimulating them in various ways.

As Figure 7 indicates, the points on the ear constitute a kind of microacupuncture system. More than two hundred points on the external ear have been identified, each of which corresponds to a different anatomical portion of the body.

Proponents of auricular diagnosis imagine the ear to represent the shape of a fetus *in utero*, with its head at the lobule. The points of the ear then correspond to the anatomical location of the various parts of the imaginary fetus. When there is illness or disease in specific areas of the body, the corresponding auricular points become increasingly tender, discolored, and electrically "active." Specialized electronic probes can be safely and painlessly passed over the ear to detect the presence of any active points. This complete auricular examination usually takes less than five minutes.

In studies at UCLA, Drs. Richard Kroening, Terrence Oleson, and I have found auricular diagnosis to be highly accurate in identifying a variety of pain-related problems. It is also helpful in treating infants who can't as yet speak and describe their pain. It may also have applications for comatose patients unable to talk. In emergency situations, auricular diagnosis is much faster than analyzing blood or taking X-rays, and it may offer even more important information.

Some other diagnostic techniques, although not quite as unusual, are still largely ignored by most members of the medical community. One of them—hair analysis—is a safe and effective means of detecting certain types of toxic poisoning. A striking example of the use of this technique

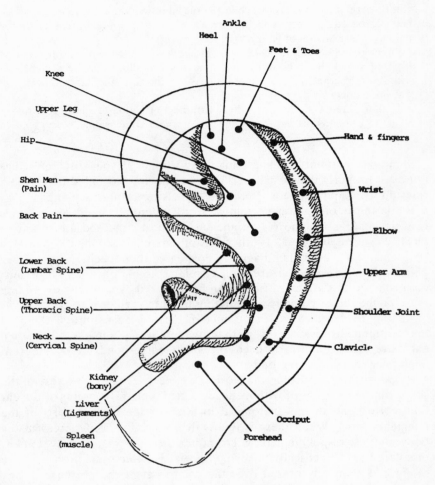

Fig. 7 *The somatotype of the ear.*

concerns a thirty-eight-year-old woman named Marilyn, who was referred to the UCLA Pain Control Unit for treatment of severe atypical head pain which she described as a "giant fist squeezing my brains into jelly." Marilyn considered each day to be a mini–horror story, with so little positive input that she came to dread most of her waking hours.

Like many other pain patients, Marilyn had been subjected to a "million-dollar workup," enduring many torturous months of endless tests. Based on the results of a pneumoencephalogram and brain scan studies, tumors were conclusively ruled out as the source of the problem. Other tests eliminated sinus and muscle contraction headaches as possible factors. All tests were essentially negative, and her personal physicians were starting to tell her that her pain was (no pun intended) all in her head.

When Marilyn arrived at the Pain Control Unit, we, too, had difficulty identifying her very mysterious problem. Although psychological factors are sometimes involved in disorders like hers, she seemed well-adjusted, and did not appear to be deriving any significant benefits from her illness.

We then conducted a complete nutritional workup, to ascertain whether a food allergy or an improper diet might be involved. Marilyn was given a chart and asked to write down everything she ate during the following week. This information was then analyzed by a computer, which provided us with a detailed nutritional breakdown, including her consumption of carbohydrates, proteins, and fats, as well as each of the major amino acids, vitamins, and minerals.

Unfortunately, no new clues surfaced. Marilyn's problem was baffling, and as we continued to pursue every reasonable method for diagnosing her ailment, my own frustration intensified.

Finally, to leave no stone unturned, we decided to have a small sample of Marilyn's hair analyzed. This procedure reveals important aspects of mineral and trace element consumption that often cannot be evaluated through blood or urine tests. When the results returned from the lab, they disclosed a startling fact—Marilyn's hair contained levels of lead that were five times greater than those generally accepted as safe. Initially, I thought the lab had made a mistake, for earlier blood samples had shown no signs of excessive lead levels. Nevertheless, I called Marilyn to inform her of the lab findings.

"I just received the results of your hair analysis. The lab has probably made an error, but have you had any direct contact with lead?"

"Well, about the only thing I can think of is that I make stained-glass windows as a hobby. Doesn't the metal solder contain some lead?"

"Yes, it does. Do you wash your hands thoroughly after working with the solder?"

"No. Should I?"

Diagnosis? Lead poisoning. Several highly specialized tests subsequently confirmed this finding. In Marilyn's case, we were lucky to stumble across the cause of her problem. After appropriate therapy to help remove the lead from her system, the headaches that had so devastated her life finally disappeared. All the therapies in the world would have been inappropriate in treating her except for the one designed to remove excess lead from her body. Yet until the hair analysis was performed, her ailment went misdiagnosed and mistreated for months.

Who knows what other diagnostic techniques, perhaps generally overlooked, could prove useful in explaining your own pain problem? For instance, I believe that one of the most important components of a complete diagnostic workup is a sexual history. But some physicians are reluctant to take one, for they regard it as improper or even superfluous.

However, I recall how important a sexual history was in the case of Mandy, a twenty-three-year-old student, who came to the Pain Control Unit with chronic pelvic inflammatory disease that had plagued her since her teens. Although her doctors had honestly tried what they thought was best, she was unfortunately subjected to horrendously inappropriate treatment.

An endless series of drugs and injections provided little more than temporary relief, and as a last resort, one of Mandy's doctors performed a total hysterectomy, removing her uterus and cervix. This major surgery was performed shortly before Mandy got married. After the operation, the pain still persisted. And she was referred to me.

In the process of taking a routine sexual history, I learned of a traumatic sexual experience Mandy had at the age of fourteen. After thoroughly discussing this problem with her, it became clear that the message behind her pain had an emotional, not a physical, basis. Still emotionally scarred by that early sexual episode, she was subconsciously clinging to her pain and using it as an excuse for avoiding sex. She had been in need of psychotherapy, not major surgery. And as she entered marriage, her ability to bear children had been unnecessarily taken away.

Such cases appall me. I think it's imperative for doctors to investigate all possible psychological, as well as somatic, sources of pain, particularly before something as drastic as surgery is performed. But for many physicians, psychological and sexual histories are too time-consuming, too complex, or, in their opinion, simply irrelevant for a proper diagnosis.

When doctors do refer patients to psychiatrists and psychologists, they often do so only as a last resort, after everything else has been tried without success. Because pain is a mind/body phenomenon, I think such therapists should often be involved in the diagnostic process from the beginning, *before* treatment is even prescribed.

Every avenue for arriving at a proper diagnosis must be explored until the message of pain is thoroughly understood. There are many simple procedures physicians can use to determine if psychiatrists or psychologists can help in the diagnostic process. If doctors, for example, were trained to ask their patients to draw a picture of their pain—as you did in Exercise Five—it might significantly affect their perspective of their patients' problems. These pictures often reveal information just as significant as the data that emerge from the most sophisticated laboratory tests.

Take a look at Figure 8. It was drawn by a patient who arrived at the Pain Control Unit with back pain. His artistic depiction of his discomfort is typical of the dramatic pictures drawn by many of my pain patients.

Examine it closely. There is a lot of important information there. On

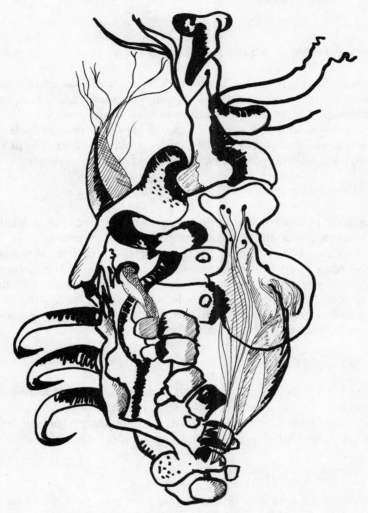

Fig. 8 *A patient's portrait of his back pain.*

the basis of this picture, it is easy to see why pain pills did little to cure the agony that this man felt—yet they were the only thing prescribed by his personal physician.

As I've said many times earlier in this book, if you hurt, something is wrong. And until the message of your pain is clearly identified, attempts to suppress it symptomatically will be successful only temporarily, if at all.

Exercise Twelve: What's the Diagnosis?

Although up to this point, you may have relied on physicians to diagnose and treat your pain problem, you have now acquired important new information of your own to add to the diagnostic process.

In this exercise, I'd like you to prepare your own "problem oriented" diagnosis, as outlined earlier in this chapter. Using this four-step process, summarize the most important aspects of your own pain problem:

Subjective Information

Refer back to some of the earlier exercises as a guide, then jot down your thoughts about the subjective information concerning your pain. Which aspects of your history are most relevant to your discomfort? Could hereditary and nutritional factors be playing a role? What about the effects of your own social habits, like cigarette smoking or liquor consumption? Also review your Comfort Log, your Life Chart, and the descriptions and drawings of your discomfort, and add any significant subjective information from them to this exercise.

Objective Findings

Record the major findings that your doctors and other specialists have told you about. For example, is there X-ray evidence of physical injury or disease? What were the overall results of the laboratory tests your doctors conducted? What did your physical examination reveal?

Assessment of the Problem

What are your own conclusions about your pain problem? Did your doctor perhaps overlook something in his evaluation of your ailment? What is your own assessment of the situation?

A Plan of Action

Given this assessment, what do you plan to do now in dealing with your pain problem? In order to reach your goals, what must you do—or stop doing?

Baseball, Apple Pie, and Pills

Whether or not your doctor arrives at a clear diagnosis of your pain problem, he will probably still choose to treat it in the same way—with pills. For decades, drugs have been the major therapeutic modality used by physicians. Patients themselves have become so accustomed to viewing drugs as a panacea that they often demand that their doctors prescribe them. As a result, nearly everyone has taken, is taking, or will take drugs for a pain-related problem.

When prescribed rationally and appropriately, drugs can be very helpful to people in pain. When you have an acute pain problem, like dental discomfort after a tooth extraction, a drug like aspirin with codeine may help to reduce your discomfort while the body heals itself.

However, chronic pain is a very different situation, yet doctors and patients still rely on drugs as the treatment of choice. As a result, drugs are frequently overprescribed by doctors and overused by chronic pain patients. The U.S. population gobbles up pills as if they were candy. Americans swallow more than 20,000 tons of aspirin alone each year. This averages out to more than 225 tablets annually for every man, woman, and child in the nation, at a total cost of well over $100 million.

Other drugs are taken with equal enthusiasm. The number of sleeping pills consumed by Americans is staggering—27 million prescriptions in 1976, equaling about one billion doses.

In 1971, the prescription drug industry spent more than a billion dollars to promote its wares. The largest share of these funds supported an estimated 25,000 detail men, who periodically call on physicians, pharmacists, and hospital purchasing agents. These detail men provide educational information concerning their companies' newest products and devices. But since most are paid at least in part on a commission basis, one could hardly expect them to be totally objective sources of data. Still, based on the information given to them, physicians write approximately 2.4 billion prescriptions each year, for an estimated 150 million people, averaging nearly 8000 prescriptions annually per practicing physician.

Drug companies also promote their nonprescription, over-the-counter (OTC) drugs with equal success directly to the public. For example, it is estimated that over $1.2 billion was spent in 1972 to promote OTC products through newspapers, magazines, radio, television, billboards, window displays, counter displays, pamphlets, and other media. Nearly $100 million of those funds were used solely to capture a share of the $500 million-per-year market for headache and other analgesic remedies. Promotional campaigns have even identified new "diseases" (such as "the

SAMPLE

EXERCISE TWELVE: What's the Diagnosis? DATE: _March 10_

TIME: _2:45 p.m._

Subjective information

I eat a lot of processed food, filled with additives. They may be harming me. My parents had severe headaches, so perhaps I inherited that tendency. I also smoke more cigarettes than I should.

Objective information

I have been to three physicians thus far, and none of them has been able to find any physical reason why I have headaches.

Assessment

I'm sure my headaches are real and that I'm not imagining them. So I'm disturbed that my doctors can't find anything physically wrong with me. Doctors can make mistakes; I think mine have.

Plan of action

I'm going to see another doctor, who I've heard specializes in nutrition. I want to start eating healthier and see if it reduces the severity of my headaches. I'm also going to try to be active as much as possible even with headaches.

Comments

EXERCISE TWELVE: What's the Diagnosis?   DATE: _____

TIME: _____

Subjective information

Objective information

Assessment

Plan of action

Comments

blahs") which allegedly respond instantly to the magic of modern chemistry.

As a result of living in our drug-oriented society, many people feel they need to swallow *something* to get through the day. Pain patients are no exception. Often they clutch their pill bottles as if they were sources of life-nourishing oxygen. Deep inside, they desperately hope that the answer to all their ills can be found in a laboratory-produced chemical that is swallowed four times a day.

Natalie, a fifty-one-year-old victim of severe back pain, is a typical example. I have never seen her when she wasn't carrying a purse large enough to pass for a small suitcase, for in it is an array of pills that might make the average small-town pharmacist envious. As she once told me, "When I hurt, I'll put anything round into my mouth!" I asked Natalie what her rainbow collection of pills consisted of, but she couldn't identify them by name or tell me their purpose. Still, she knew precisely what she was supposed to do with them.

"Every morning, I take two large greens, one white, one yellow, and two small oranges," she said. "In the afternoon, it's one small green, one yellow, and one large orange. At night, it's a purple, a white, a blue, and a yellow."

Natalie and other patients such as she have swallowed pills of every imaginable color, size, and description. They go nowhere without their medications, for they are convinced that drugs are essential to life. I have one such patient who jokes that his body is so full or medication that every time he sneezes, he cures somebody.

Take a good look at your own medicine cabinet, and you may be surprised to see how cluttered it is with plastic bottles of prescription and nonprescription pills. Do you *really* know what each of these bottles contains, what the pills are indicated for, what their side effects may be, when they should and should not be taken, and what combinations should be avoided? If not, let's briefly review some of the medications most widely used for treatment of pain.

Aspirin

Of all pain-relieving drugs, *aspirin* is certainly the most commonly used. When properly taken, it can often be effective in easing the mild pain from ailments like headaches, arthritis, other joint and muscle aches, and certain types of neuralgia. Essentially, all aspirin compounds are the same, although Madison Avenue would certainly like to have you believe differently. When the TV advertisements declare, "Brand X contains the ingredient that doctors recommend most for pain!" the chances are that Brand X contains aspirin.

Aspirin performs three functions: (1) it decreases inflammation when it is present, (2) reduces fever, and (3) relieves pain. To its credit, aspirin is rarely habit-forming, and its side effects are minimal when used according to directions.

But aspirin can be deadly, too. It is one of the leading causes of accidental poisoning in children, and is known to have potentially adverse effects on adults as well. According to a five-year study by the Food and Drug Administration, aspirin can produce stomach bleeding and abnormalities in liver and kidney function. Unless your physician specifically instructs you differently, you should probably not take aspirin if you have ulcers or iron deficiency anemia, or if you are taking blood-thinning drugs or medications for diabetes or gout. During pregnancy, aspirin (and all other drugs) should be avoided if possible.

Alternatives to aspirin, like Tylenol, have become very popular in recent years. But, unfortunately, they are not completely safe either. Tylenol's active analgesic agent is acetaminophen, and according to the FDA, "A large overdose of acetaminophen (Tylenol) can result in serious kidney damage which is not as amenable to therapy as salicylate (aspirin) intoxication."

Few over-the-counter drugs receive as much media promotion as aspirin and its alternatives. It is almost impossible to turn on the television set without seeing an actor or actress contorting in make-believe pain, and seconds later, making a miraculous, complete recovery, thanks to one brand of OTC drug or another.

Milton Silverman and Philip R. Lee, in their book *Pills, Profits, & Politics*, have indicted the drug companies for altering their products slightly to try to gain an advertising edge over the competition:

> More than half a billion dollars has been spent by the makers of Anacin, Bufferin, Excedrin, the various brands of aspirin, and other pain remedies to extol their products on the basis of what are mostly trivial formulation differences. For example, Anacin—a combination that now consists of approximately 6⅔ grains of aspirin and ⅓ grain of caffeine per tablet—has been held out to be vastly superior to 5 grain tablets of aspirin alone, although the value of caffeine in control of headache pain is reportedly without significant support.
>
> Another headache remedy, Excedrin PM—a combination of three traditional analgesics, aspirin, acetaminophen, and salicylamide, plus caffeine and an antihistamine, methapyrilene fumarate—made its bid in this field with a promotional campaign that will long be remembered. Based on what was reported to be a "major hospital study," the Excedrin PM story was related night after night in a dramatic, moving, and highly effective presentation by T.V. actor David Janssen. The manner in which Mr. Janssen spoke his lines cannot be faulted. The campaign itself came to a disastrous climax when the physician who directed the "major hospital study" demanded that his findings be disassociated from the promotion,

since he had tested the product only on postchildbirth pain. Soon afterward, the National Broadcasting Company refused to accept the advertising on its network, and eventually the campaign was dropped.

The effectiveness of advertising cannot be overestimated. Drug manufacturers spend well over a billion dollars each year promoting their OTC products, convinced of the influence of media exposure. Some of the claims in their ads are often highly exaggerated. But interestingly, those inflated promises may actually make the product work more effectively than it otherwise would.

When a patient asks me, "What type of aspirin compound should I take?" I often respond by saying, "Which one do *you* think will help you the most?" Although aspirin compounds contain similar ingredients, they may differ in their psychological impact, simply because of the way in which they have been promoted.

Mild Narcotics

When pain cannot be relieved with aspirin compounds, doctors often prescribe one of the weak narcotics. The one you're probably most familiar with is *codeine*. Although there is less danger of addiction with codeine than with more powerful drugs, the body does build up tolerance to it, and in time, larger doses must eventually be given. Codeine is actually a derivative of morphine, and resembles it in many of its actions, except that it is less potent and generates less of a euphoria or "high." However, like other narcotics, codeine is known to produce side effects such as nausea and constipation.

Propoxyphene (Darvon) is preferred by some doctors over codeine, since it is less prone to produce nausea and constipation. But it, too, has side effects, including stomach upset and dizziness.

For certain types of pain problems, other mild narcotics have been shown to be more effective analgesics (pain relievers) than either codeine or Darvon. These include *oxycodone* (Percodan) and *meperidine* (Demerol). But they also have side effects common to other narcotics.

Strong Narcotics

Some of the more potent narcotics used for pain alleviation include *hydromorphone* (Dilaudid) and *morphine*. While significantly curtailing an individual's perception of his pain, these agents also create an extraordinary feeling of well-being in the individual. As a result, addiction is a serious danger with both of these powerful drugs.

In addition, tolerance to morphine develops rapidly, so the dosage must be steadily increased to maintain pain relief. As the dosage is raised, the incidence of side effects such as nausea, vomiting, constipation, and mental clouding also grows. When consumed in excess, morphine can also depress respiration to the point of suffocation. This is why an overdose of heroin can be fatal, for it is converted to morphine by the central nervous system.

In short, the most effective analgesic agents also produce the most severe side effects, and possess the highest potential for abuse. In addition, recent findings suggest that the long-term use of narcotic analgesics may interfere with the body's own pain-suppression abilities. Therefore, many physicians have begun to rely more heavily on other types of drugs for pain control.

Antidepressants and Tranquilizers

Antidepressants, such as *imipramine* (Tofranil) and *amitriptyline* (Elavil), are sometimes indicated for certain patients in pain, when severe depression emerges as the most significant problem. Unfortunately, they often produce initial symptoms of drowsiness, dry mouth, blurred vision, and/or constipation for two or three weeks before their positive effects are apparent. Thus, patients frequently fail to complete an adequate trial of therapy. Even when careful instructions and a thorough explanation of the delay is given, many chronic pain patients will quickly stop taking a medication that produces no immediate results.

When properly utilized, tranquilizers such as diazepam (Valium) and chlordiazepoxide (Librium) may be helpful in the treatment of pain problems in which anxiety, agitation, and muscle spasm are prominent. Unfortunately, when used over an extended period of time, they can also produce side effects such as jaundice, blurred vision, changes in blood clotting, nausea, constipation, and hallucinations.

Diazepam, the most frequently prescribed drug in the United States, is also the most commonly misused. According to the Drug Enforcement Agency, diazepam causes more drug-related illnesses and deaths per year than any other drug—even alcohol. When taken in large doses over a long period of time, it can also produce or significantly increase depression. Chronic pain patients are usually already depressed enough *before* taking tranquilizers, so I don't generally recommend them except in small doses over a brief period.

Sleeping Pills

Most chronic pain patients take many other drugs or substances as well. For example, if you hurt, you probably have trouble sleeping. Consequently, you may have resorted to one of the more than sixty prescription sleeping pills on the market. Although these drugs promise quick deliverance from the misery of poor sleep, they typically lose their effectiveness after just a few nights of use.

Barbiturates are the most commonly prescribed sleeping pills, and more than a billion doses of them are consumed each year in the United States alone. The most widely used barbiturates are phenobarbital (Luminal), butabarbital (Butisol), pentobarbital (Nembutal), secobarbital (Seconal), and amobarbital with secobarbital (Tuinal).

When you find yourself tossing and turning on an isolated night or two, then perhaps barbiturates may be helpful in aiding sleep. But if you've ever taken them for an extended period of time, you know that they quickly lose their effectiveness as tolerance develops. One study revealed that secobarbital began to become ineffective after just four nights of use. In short, barbiturates are not the solution for sleep disorders.

To compound the barbiturate problem, these popular hypnotics suppress REM (rapid eye movement) sleep—that critical, active period during the night when most dreaming occurs. Thus, the quality of sleep is being reduced by the same drug that is prescribed to improve it.

Ironically, when barbiturate users attempt to reduce or withdraw completely from these drugs, the body makes up for the REM sleep previously lost with an onslaught of vivid dreaming. This REM "rebound," which typically lasts for a week or two, causes a barrage of nightmares so frightening that most people find them intolerable. Consequently, these individuals quickly return to taking the barbiturates in order to sleep. In effect, they have become addicted, and many authorities consider dependence on barbiturates to be a more serious habit than heroin use.

The greatest danger with barbiturates, as with many other drugs, is that they are potentially fatal when abused. In 1977, the National Institute on Drug Abuse announced that nearly five thousand deaths a year in the United States are either directly or indirectly related to barbiturates. Inappropriate use of barbiturates, according to the institute, results in about twenty-five thousand trips to hospital emergency wards each year.

Complications

There are safety problems with *all* drugs. Simply because a drug has received Food and Drug Administration approval is no guarantee that it is safe. *No* drug on the market is completely void of side effects, yet these potential dangers are rarely explained to the patients who most need to know about them.

Some drugs, particularly when improperly prescribed and consumed, badly disorient their users. According to Dr. K. Warner Schaie, director of the University of Southern California's Gerontology Research Institute, one of every four persons presumed senile, who is not institutionalized, is actually just disoriented because of misused drugs. On a national basis, about 600,000 to 700,000 people over age 65 would fall into this category. Of the so-called senile residents in nursing homes, nearly 50 percent of them—or about 300,000 people—are suffering drug-induced disorientation that could be reversed with the proper administration of drugs.

The ultimate drug-related tragedy—death caused by abuse, overdose, or drug interaction—is not limited to barbiturate use. In 1974, Dr. Robert Talley of the San Joaquin Foundation for Medical Care testified before a U.S. Senate subcommittee that an estimated "140,000 Americans die each year because of adverse reaction to one drug or interaction between combinations of drugs."

Unfortunately, medical science knows preciously little about the actions of drugs or what impact they have when taken in combination with other drugs. Equally disturbing is the phenomenon of patients simultaneously taking pain medications prescribed by different doctors. It's not unusual for a single patient to be taking a dozen or more different drugs prescribed by several doctors, each of whom are unaware that the patient is consulting other physicians as well.

Lawrence M. Halpern, of the Pain Clinic at the University of Washington, encountered a female patient who was taking twenty-four different drugs for her pain, prescribed by seven doctors. She was taking Valium under two separate but overlapping prescriptions. She was also taking separate, overlapping doses of Phenaphen and Compazine, again prescribed by different doctors. The other drugs that she consumed daily included Demerol, Benadryl, Combid, Temaril, Probanthine, Metreton, Darvon-N, Premarin, Talwin, Librium, Trilafon, Elavil, Azogantanol, Ampicillin, Wyamin Sulfate, Ducolax, Empirin, and Biphetamine.

The potential dangers of drugs cannot be overemphasized. Even when taken prudently under the careful observation of a physician, they can still cause problems. Dr. Kenneth L. Melmon, professor of medicine and pharmacology at the University of California in San Francisco, has studied the frequency of drug problems that occur in hospitals, and discovered:

—About 8.7 million hospital patients a year—or about 30 percent of all those individuals hospitalized—experience negative reactions to drugs.

—About 14 percent of all hospital days are devoted to caring for patients with drug reactions.

Senator Edward M. Kennedy, chairman of the U.S. Senate Health Subcommittee, has become concerned enough about drug use to warn, "Too many physicians are prescribing too many drugs on too little information. These adverse drug reactions cost the American people an estimated $2 billion per year. Most experts say 80 percent of these cases can be prevented."

The wholesale use of drugs, with all its risks, becomes even more questionable as researchers continue to find that many of modern medicine's most sophisticated drugs are no more effective than placebos ("sugar pills"). Although the placebo effect was a seldomly discussed phenomenon until the 1950s, its powers are now quite clear (as I shall review in the next chapter).

Despite all of these problems, many patients feel that drug-taking would be well worth its potential risks if it provided long-lasting pain relief. But usually, it only compounds the problem by producing serious side effects or addiction. For the chronic pain patient, who needs relief day after agonizing day, pills are therefore rarely, if ever, the long-range answer.

Occasionally, I will recommend pain medication for a very specific reason. For instance, it is extremely difficult, if not impossible, to learn stress reduction techniques when you are experiencing agonizing pain, so for a short period of time, drugs in small doses can help to "take the edge off." For some patients, supplemental use of antidepressant medication may also be helpful over the course of psychotherapy. Thus, drugs may occasionally become an aid to therapy, but I don't recommend their long-term use simply to suppress the symptoms of chronic pain.

If you are currently on a regimen of regular, chronic drug usage, talk to your doctor about the dangers these medications may present, and the advisability of reducing or eliminating their intake. I urge you never to cut back on your drug usage except under a physician's supervision, for there can be serious side effects during withdrawal from many drugs.

During drug withdrawal, your body may react violently. It has been my experience that most psychotropic (mind-altering) drugs will produce a "rebound" reaction when you stop taking them. For example, when sleeping pill usage is withdrawn, the user will sleep even more poorly than before he had ever started taking them. When stimulants are withdrawn, the user may become even more depressed. Somewhere along the way, your body is going to have to compensate for the temporary relief you may have experienced.

The Medical Merry-Go-Round

Drugs, then, are rarely, if ever, the ideal treatment for chronic pain, and at best they usually provide only temporary relief. Still, one combination of pills after another is tried, typically without success, as the pain lingers on and on. In the midst of their desperate search for relief, most patients soon find themselves caught up on what I call "The Medical Merry-Go-Round"—that endless and frustrating revolving door in which specialist after specialist is seen, each of whom may view the same ailment in an entirely different way.

Let me take you on an imaginary trip on this Medical Merry-Go-Round. For a moment, pretend that you awaken one morning with a dull, aching pain on the left side of your face. Initially, you think it is just a toothache, but over the next few days it becomes progressively worse. As the pain radiates to your left temple and eye, you soon become aware of a persistent ringing in your ear. Two aspirin do nothing to ease the discomfort, so you arrange to see your internist or family doctor for help. He examines you and uncovers no positive findings, but gives you some pills anyway in the hope that they might do some good.

Well, they don't. Nor does another combination of pills, or yet another. So now where do you go? Welcome aboard the Medical Merry-Go-Round!

Your dentist should have a look next, since the pain could be related to a problem tooth that needs to be extracted. While you're at it, you'd also better have your ophthalmologist check your eyes, your otolaryngologist examine your ears, nose, and throat, and don't forget your allergist as well. They may suggest other pills, nose, ear- or eyedrops, or even allergy tests.

If they can't help, perhaps consultation with your neurologist is indicated. He may recommend hospitalization in order to conduct certain sophisticated evaluations, including various blood analyses, EEGs, X-rays, brain scans, lumbar punctures, pneumoencephalograms, angiograms, tomograms, and other procedures. While in the hospital, your anesthesiologist may suggest a series of nerve blocks to provide temporary relief. If the blocks help, your neurosurgeon may consider cutting some nerves; if the blocks aren't effective, perhaps he will send you to a psychiatrist.

As you proceed on the Medical Merry-Go-Round, you may return once again to a dentist, who in turn may refer you to a gnathologist (jaw specialist) for a trial of dental splints. Meanwhile, your internist may have decided upon a new combination of drugs to try, or he may recommend electrical stimulation to see if that can help.

More tests, more drugs, more specialists. It's seemingly a never-ending ride of agony and frustration. After a while, you can barely remember which of your doctors recommended what.

Sound confusing? It is. Each of these health professionals will diagnose and treat your problem somewhat differently, depending on his or her own training and orientation. As is sometimes said, "When you're holding a hammer, you look for nails." Often, the therapeutic approaches your doctors favor depend more on their areas of specialization than on the unique aspects of your individual problem. Thus, many pain patients wander endlessly from doctor to doctor, hoping to find the one who has the answer to their problem.

While doctors frequently complain that some patients do not follow their recommendations, I am even more amazed to see how many patients *do* follow instructions exactly, without ever seriously questioning why such an approach was recommended, or what risks it may entail. As I mentioned earlier, Americans hold an almost spiritual respect for doctors, our nation's ministers of health. Thus, even when there are questions about our treatment that we'd like to ask, we don't. We remain silent and blindly follow instructions rather than risk insulting a doctor who we hope will be able to help. As patients, we must begin to accept personal responsibility for more thoroughly asking our physicians about the types of therapy being prescribed.

Bill Prensky, former director of the National Acupuncture Association, used to tell a story about a devoted priest who died in his sleep one night and was carried up to heaven. When he arrived at the Pearly Gates, the priest was surprised to see an almost endless line of people waiting to enter.

The man behind the desk must be Saint Peter, he thought. Perhaps if I talked with him, he could speed things up a bit.

Approaching Saint Peter, the priest introduced himself and said, "Down on earth, I was a devoted and faithful servant of God. Isn't there anything you can do to help me avoid this line? It must be at least five hundred years long!"

"I'm sorry," replied Saint Peter, "but up here, everyone is equal. Regardless of what you did down on earth, each person who made it here is treated exactly the same. I'm afraid you'll just have to wait in line like the others."

With a shrug, the priest returned to the end of the line.

One day, after he had waited nearly one hundred years, a taxicab pulled up and out stepped a man in a long white coat with a stethoscope in his pocket. Without even saying a word to Saint Peter, the man immediately walked right through the Pearly Gates into heaven. Leaving his place in line, the priest angrily walked up to Saint Peter's desk.

"I thought you told me that everyone is treated the same up here," he said.

"That is correct," Saint Peter replied.

"Well, I just saw a doctor get out of a taxicab, and without waiting at all, he just walked right through!"

"Shhh," whispered Saint Peter. "That wasn't a doctor, that was God. Every now and then he likes to dress up and *pretend* he's a doctor!"

Why do so many of us have such unwavering faith and trust in doctors? Perhaps because we need to. If my gallbladder were diseased, I'd want it removed by a surgeon who's a personal messenger from God, not just by a mere mortal human being.

Still, such reverence bestowed upon physicians is unrealistic, for modern medicine does not have a cure for all ills. Worse yet, when drugs fail, many people feel that all hope is gone. Some patients, unable to find an escape from their unbearable pain, decide that the only way to get off the Medical Merry-Go-Round is to commit suicide. There are no accurate statistics to indicate how many patients choose this way out. However, the majority of chronic pain patients continues to ride the Medical Merry-Go-Round, day after day, year after year, clinging to the hope that someday they will find someone who will deliver them from their agonizing existence.

Hospitalization

One way to free pain patients from the Medical Merry-Go-Round—at least temporarily—is to admit them to a hospital. I've always considered hospitals to be one of the more unpleasant places to spend time, whether as a doctor, patient, or visitor. Still, hardly a day goes by when I'm not meeting with patients or doctors in hospitals, which has made me very aware of the importance of these institutions.

Many people today owe their lives to modern and sophisticated hospital facilities. Hospital emergency rooms and intensive care units, for example, have kept many critically injured or ill patients alive, whereas they would certainly have died just a generation ago. Neonatal care units have dramatically reduced infant mortality, and coronary care units have resurrected heart attack victims. Operating rooms have witnessed organ and tissue transplants, reconstructive plastic surgery, the removal of tumors, and the routine repair of broken bones. Such "miracles" have become almost commonplace in today's hospitals.

Most chronic pain patients are not strangers to hospital care. People who hurt may be admitted as patients for any number of reasons. Diagnostic tests, for example, are often performed in the hospital, including X-rays, scans, the injection of test drugs and radioisotopes, and the analysis of various body fluids and tissues. Nerve blocks, electrostimulation, and physical therapy are also frequently administered in the hospital, as are certain types of psychotherapy such as behavior modification. Surgery, of course, is also performed on pain patients in hospitals.

I think almost everyone would argue that there are times when the modern-day hospital is indispensable. If I'm hit by a truck, don't tell me to meditate and don't stick acupuncture needles into me—take me to the Emergency Room!

However, I constantly meet chronic pain patients who say that they received little, if any, long-term benefits from the weeks or months spent in a hospital setting. Even worse, many report that the procedures used were often too invasive, too dangerous, and most of all, inappropriate or unnecessary. This viewpoint is vigorously argued by Norman Cousins, editor of the *Saturday Review*, who was seriously ill with ankylosing spondylitis in 1964 and was hospitalized by his physician.

"I had a fast-growing conviction that a hospital was no place for a person who was seriously ill," wrote Cousins in the *New England Journal of Medicine*. "The surprising lack of respect for basic sanitation, the rapidity with which staphylococci and other pathogenic organisms can run through an entire hospital, the extensive and sometimes promiscuous use of x-ray equipment, the seemingly indiscriminate administration of tranquilizers and powerful painkillers, more for the convenience of hospital staff in managing patients than for therapeutic needs, and the regularity with which hospital routine takes precedence over the rest requirements of the patient (slumber, when it comes for an ill person, is an uncommon blessing and is not to be wantonly interrupted)—all these and other practices seemed to me to be critical shortcomings of the modern hospital."

Cousins was also shocked by the poor quality of food served in the hospital. Despite the importance that nutrition can play in the healing process, hospitals are sometimes guilty of serving meals hardly fit for anyone, much less an ill patient.

"It was not just that the meals were poorly balanced; what seemed inexcusable to me was the profusion of processed foods, some of which contained preservatives or harmful dyes," wrote Cousins. "White bread with its chemical softeners and bleached flour was offered with every meal. Vegetables were often overcooked and thus deprived of much of their nutritional value. No wonder the 1969 White House Conference on Food, Nutrition, and Health made the melancholy observation that the great failure of medical schools is that they pay so little attention to the science of nutrition."

Cousins, who was ill with a rare disease, asked to be moved to a hotel room, which he felt would be more conducive to recovery. He may have been right. Although his doctors had given him only 1 chance in 500, Cousins made a slow, steady, and full recovery, surprising everyone but himself.

In recent years, I have learned of other cases of "miraculous" out-of-hospital recoveries, indicating that Cousins' dramatic improvement was not an isolated incident. Not only can people often get well outside a hospital environment, but occasionally the hospitalization may make the patient even *more ill*.

Dr. John Ruedy, chairman of the department of pharmacology at McGill University in Montreal, has concluded that many adverse drug reactions happen *after* patients are admitted to hospitals. Ruedy's study noted that of 731 patients observed at Montreal General Hospital, 132 suffered a total of 193 negative drug reactions. Ruedy blamed 18 patient deaths on causes directly attributable to adverse drug reactions.

Other research also indicates that hospitals may not always be conducive to good health. In 1974, a study in England revealed that the recovery rate of heart attack victims treated in coronary care units was no better than that of similarly-ill patients treated at home.

In a separate study conducted by Gordon Mather in Bristol, England, even more impressive findings surfaced. Of 450 heart attack patients studied, half were treated at home, while the other half spent forty-eight hours in a coronary care unit and then were transferred to regular hospital beds. Forty-five of the 225 patients who were sent home died there; however, 60 of the other 225 who were kept in the hospital to recuperate died. Thus, one-third more patients died while hospitalized than while at home.

How can the results of these studies be explained? Well, think what the hospital environment is like for a patient recovering from a heart attack in a coronary care unit. Typically, no visitors are allowed—they can be too stimulating. No television is permitted, either—it can be too upsetting. The patient is regulated to doing little else but staring in a pharmaceutical stupor at four bare walls, listening to the hurried sounds of doctors and nurses rushing to the bedsides of other patients whose hearts have stopped. It's a depressing and negative environment, devoid of much positive energy.

Now compare the hospital with a positive home environment. In his own home, the patient is in a familiar setting, surrounded by family and friends who support and nourish him with loving care that almost certainly facilitates the healing process. It's no wonder that many doctors are now thinking twice before hospitalizing their patients. If the results of the studies cited above are confirmed by other researchers, we may someday see signs in hospital lobbies reading: "Caution: the Surgeon General has concluded that the long-term use of hospitals may be hazardous to your health!"

While doctors must accept some of the blame for excessive hospitalization, so must the insurance industry. Health insurers write millions of policies that cover most hospital costs, but do not cover the same procedures when administered in a doctor's office. Thus, when you require treatment or even simple diagnostic tests, you will often be needlessly hospitalized because that is the only way in which your insurance will cover these expenses. Hospital costs, which have soared to $200 to $300 a day, totaled $110 billion in 1977.

Although we need hospitals for treating some illnesses, I believe that they should be "humanized" and used far more selectively. The home environment is the best place for healing, for even if patients are able to overcome pain in an artificial and temporary hospital setting, these positive results often don't last after returning to the outside environment in which the problem originated.

In my opinion, the hard work of regaining your health should be done in the most familiar environment possible. You can't live in a hospital forever, and if you want to maximize the benefits of therapy in the years ahead, effective treatment must be administered and experienced where you live.

Nerve Blocks

Whether you know it or not, you've probably experienced a nerve block. Essentially, this therapy involves injecting a local anesthetic into or around a nerve, which temporarily blocks its ability to communicate with the central nervous system. If you've ever sat in a dentist's chair to have a decayed tooth drilled or pulled, you've most likely had the area deadened with one of these blocks—usually an injection of Novocain.

Nerve blocks have revolutionized the practice of dentistry, and we should all be grateful for them. I recall the last time I was in my dentist's office, faced with having a cavity filled. My dentist knew that I was the director of the UCLA Pain Control Unit, so he asked, "Which technique do you want to use? Acupressure? Self-hypnosis? Guided imagery?"

"Well, it all depends. Just how painful do you think this procedure will be?"

"In my opinion," he replied, "about the only thing more painful might be to break apart your bones using a pair of pliers."

With that, I decided that a shot of Novocain was the best alternative.

For acute or short-term pain, nerve blocks are a blessing. They are frequently used in hospital emergency rooms to provide immediate pain relief for injuries. They also are administered regularly during minor surgical procedures for effective short-term anesthesia.

Nerve blocks can also play a role in the diagnosis and treatment of chronic pain. For patients with long-term pain, nerve blocks are used for three specific purposes:

Diagnostic blocks can help identify the specific nerve pathways that may be involved in the pain problem. In addition, by temporarily eliminating the somatic (physical) dimension of pain, they allow the physician to evaluate how the patient's overall level of discomfort is influenced by the absence of the physical component.

The results of *prognostic blocks* permit patients to experience temporarily how long-term interruption of nerve pathways will feel following neurosurgery or injection of neurolytic (nerve-destroying) agents. By experiencing the numbness and other side effects that often follow neurosurgical or neurolytic destruction, patients can determine in advance whether or not such procedures will be truly worthwhile.

Therapeutic blocks often provide immediate pain relief, but unfortunately their effects usually last for only a few hours. Thus, because of the impracticality of visiting a physician daily for repeated injections, blocks are not a satisfactory long-term treatment for most chronic pain patients.

Occasionally, however, a single therapeutic block provides improvement that far exceeds the duration of the anesthetic—perhaps because of the way it can change a patient's attitude. This was the case with Louise, a patient bothered by shoulder pain for nearly eight months before finally coming to UCLA for help. By her own description, she had been "miserable around the clock" since the onset of her pain, and had almost given up hope that her life would ever return to normal. She was, in a word, despondent.

But after receiving her first nerve block, Louise's attitude changed dramatically. Once she recognized that pain relief was at least possible, her hopelessness changed to optimism. For the first time in months, she began talking enthusiastically about her future. her spirits were raised and her anxiety was reduced, which in itself was enough to improve her condition.

For patients with certain musculoskeletal pain problems, repeated nerve blocks can sometimes produce longer and longer periods of pain alleviation. Thus, while the first nerve block may alleviate pain for only two to three hours, the second and subsequent blocks may provide relief for several days. Further, blocks may produce weeks, months, or even years of pain relief.

Although no definite explanation for this phenomenon exists, there is speculation that it may relate to an interaction between muscle tension and pain. Excessive muscle tension often leads to increased pain, which in turn causes more muscle tension, and so on. However, repeated blocks may somehow interfere with this "reverberatory pain circuit," gradually impeding the pain/muscle tension cycle, so that pain is alleviated for progressively longer periods of time.

There is a special category of nerve blocks—called *neurolytic blocks*—typically reserved for terminal cancer patients or for victims of severe and intractable pain. To provide even longer-lasting relief, they involve the injection of caustic agents such as alcohol and phenol, to deliberately damage the nerve pathways that may be involved.

Unfortunately, when neurolytic agents are injected directly into the nerve, or into the subarachnoid space (the fluid-filled area between the membranes that cover the brain and spinal cord), a post-injection inflammatory response may develop that can produce pain much more severe than the original complaint. Also, if a part of the nerve trunk blocked by these agents regulates muscle control in the body, a long-lasting motor paralysis can occur in the area being blocked. In addition, even if the neurolytic block works properly, it may cause a numbness in the affected area that some patients find more uncomfortable than the original pain itself.

In summary, nerve blocks can provide your physician with critically important diagnostic and prognostic information. But in your search for long-term relief, therapeutic blocks are rarely the ultimate answer. Although they may provide temporary improvement, they affect primarily the sensation of pain. As I discussed in Chapter 2, pain is more than just a sensation, and removal of its physical component won't necessarily terminate the entire pain experience. Some individuals continue to feel pain even when the area of their discomfort has been totally anesthetized. Thus, although nerve blocks can be helpful, other approaches are also needed for most chronic pain patients.

Surgery

There are few moments in life more terrifying than being wheeled into an operating room, knowing that for the next few minutes or hours, parts of your own body will be cut and sewn. Although surgery is one of modern medicine's most frightening experiences, many chronic pain patients readily consent to it if it holds the promise of pain relief.

Surgery has become so widely utilized and acceptable that one out of every thirteen Americans will go under the surgeon's scalpel this year alone. As with pharmaceutical agents, surgical advances have saved millions of lives, and the surgeons who perform these operations can rightly be proud of their skills.

Some of the surgical procedures used to treat chronic pain are rather staggering in their names alone—from peripheral neurectomies and percutaneous cordotomies to medullary tractotomies and commissural myelotomies.

In certain situations, surgery may be the only appropriate mode of therapy. For example, if a foreign object becomes deeply imbedded into a major nerve trunk or the spinal cord, surgical removal of the object might be the treatment of choice. But in other situations, less invasive types of treatment may be preferable. The dangers inherent in surgery have been well documented, and any benefits that might be gained must be carefully weighed against the known risks.

Over a hundred thousand deaths occur each year related to complications of surgery. Particularly hazardous are neurosurgical procedures involving deliberate destruction of nerve pathways. For example, the mortality (death) rate following unilateral cordotomy (surgical division of the nerve fibers on one side of the spinal cord) is about 10 percent, and increases up to 30 percent following bilateral cervical cordotomy (surgical division of the nerve fibers on both sides of the spinal cord). Short of death, other problems can occur with cordotomies, including motor paralysis, development of palsies, bladder and bowel dysfunction, impotence, mental aberrations, and formation of scar tissue, all of which can produce problems far worse than the original complaint.

Even when pain is surgically eliminated by severing a nerve, the numbness associated with sensory deprivation may become more intolerable than the original pain problem. Even worse, pain often returns within six months to a year. In such cases, patients generally feel that the short-lived relief they obtained was hardly worth the trauma of the operating table and the potentially dangerous side effects of surgery.

Each time I see postsurgical pain patients who suffer from complications related to their operations, it both saddens and angers me. For in many cases, surgery was neither appropriate nor necessary.

Too many surgeons have the attitude, "If it doesn't work properly, cut it out." My philosophy is quite different. I believe that you may need your nervous system intact in order to overcome your discomfort, for the nervous system has its own pain-inhibiting network which could be disrupted by surgery. This may explain why alternative healing approaches such as acupuncture are less effective in patients who have undergone pain-related operations.

Make certain you exercise extreme caution before agreeing to any surgical procedure. Throughout the history of medicine, various surgeries have been performed that were so limited in effectiveness that their eventual disappearance came as no surprise. These operations included ice irrigation of the stomach (for peptic ulcers), sympathectomy (for high blood pressure), and internal mammary artery ligation (for angina pain).

There are many surgical procedures still being done today that are hard to justify. Some authorities report that laminectomies (removal of the vertebrae's posterior arch) are performed as many times when it is medically imprudent as when it is medically sound. The same is true with tonsillectomies and hysterectomies.

Even when a patient is fortunate enough to obtain pain relief following surgery, the psychological factors associated with the operation may play a more significant role than the surgical procedure per se. Consider, for example, the internal mammary ligation technique used to treat angina pain twenty years ago. This procedure involved tying off the internal mammary artery, with the hope that it would improve circulation to the heart. Following the ligation, many patients reported a disappearance of pain and a significant improvement in the quality of their lives. Even EKG tests demonstrated increased cardiac function following exertion. However, Dr. H. K. Beecher found that identical results were obtained in angina patients who underwent a mock procedure, in which the artery was not touched.

This apparent placebo effect may be important in other surgical procedures as well. Coronary bypass surgery, for instance, is now a common treatment for angina pain. It was performed on about a hundred thousand patients in 1977, and at an average cost of $12,000 each, it generated over $1 billion in surgeons' fees and hospital costs. Although many patients have received immediate postsurgical relief, the power of the mind may be largely responsible. As Dr. Jerome Frank, professor of psychiatry at the Johns Hopkins University School of Medicine, wrote in the *Johns Hopkins Medical Journal*:

> The patient suffering from a life-threatening symptom approaches the treatment with a mixture of apprehension and hope that renders him especially susceptible to psychological influences. His expectant faith is enhanced by the surgeon's explanation of procedure, which is based on a belief system both share, and which is reinforced by elaborate preparatory examinations utilizing impressive scientific gadgetry. This builds up to the climax, a dramatic, expensive and impressive operation in which the surgeon stops the patient's heart, repairs it and starts it up again. The surgeon literally kills the patient and then resurrects him. Few faith healers can make an equally impressive demonstration of healing power.

With the benefits of surgery often so questionable, and with its risks so clear, it is not surprising that many authorities are claiming that millions of operations now being performed are both unnecessary and dangerous. Herbert Denenberg, who dealt continuously with hospitals and health insurers as insurance commissioner of Pennsylvania, estimates that there are two million unnecessary operations performed annually. In his consumers' booklet, *14 Rules on How to Avoid Unnecessary Surgery*, Denenberg advises the public to submit to surgery "only as a last resort." According to Denenberg, "Most surgeons are competent, conscientious, careful and conservative." But, he adds, "There is a tendency for surgeons to do their own thing—which is to perform surgery."

A U.S. House subcommittee agreed with Denenberg's statistics. A report entitled "Cost and Quality of Health Care: Unnecessary Surgery"—released by the Subcommittee on Oversight Investigations of the Committee on Interstate and Foreign Commerce—alleged that 2.38 million unnecessary operations were performed in the United States in 1974. These surgeries, proclaimed the report, resulted in 11,900 deaths, at a cost of $3.92 billion.

Dr. Lawrence P. Williams, a pseudonym of a West Coast surgeon and author of *How to Avoid Unnecessary Surgery*, contends that almost one-fifth of all the surgeries performed are senseless—including 50 percent of the tonsillectomies and adenoidectomies, 30 percent of the hysterectomies, and 20 percent of the appendectomies.

Testimony before a House subcommittee in 1977 revealed that a sizable number of the nation's 796,000 hysterectomies performed each year provide no benefit at all for the patients.

Even some surgeons themselves admit that there are operations being performed that may be unnecessary. An American College of Surgeons survey released in December 1971 revealed that 11 percent of the surgeons responding believed that "operations of questionable value" occur in their hospitals "once a week or more."

Well, you may be asking, if there is agreement over the rampant abuse of surgical procedures, then why are unnecessary operations continuing? Dr. Sidney M. Wolfe, of the Health Research Group of Washington, D.C., blames these unnecessary surgeries on "too many surgeons, greed, fee-for-service, outmoded ideas and training, and lack of proper training."

Probably the most important of these causes is the fee-for-service plan of paying surgeons. Under this system, the more surgeries a doctor performs, the more money he will make. Forty years ago, Dr. Richard Cabot, professor of medicine at Harvard University, wrote these words which are still valid today:

> We would never put a judge on the bench under conditions such that he might be influenced by pecuniary considerations. Suppose that if the judge were to hand down one decision, he got $5,000, and if he decided the other way he got nothing. But we allow the private practitioner to face this sort of temptation.
>
> The greatest single curse in medicine is the curse of unnecessary operations, and there would be fewer of them, if the doctor got the same salary whether he operated or not.
>
> I am not accusing the medical profession of dishonesty, but I am saying that we should be defended from unfair temptation. I maintain that to have doctors working on salary would be better for doctors as well as for patients.

For the past several years, I have tried to encourage my colleagues in the medical profession to consider using approaches other than surgery for controlling pain. In my opinion, only when every other appropriate technique has failed, and there is a clear indication that surgery may help, can it be justified.

Dr. C. Norman Shealy, an internationally respected neurosurgeon, recommends that before you submit to any surgical procedure, your doctor should answer these questions to your satisfaction:

1. Why is this operation "necessary"?
2. What are the risks of death and complications?

3. What are the risks if surgery is *not* performed? Are there other methods of treatment that don't involve surgery?

4. What are the chances that the surgery will do what it is intended to do?

If your doctor has prescribed surgery for your pain problem, I strongly recommend that you obtain a second opinion. Use every safeguard to ensure that you are not being unnecessarily subjected to the surgeon's scalpel. Although surgery may be warranted in some circumstances, it should generally be considered a treatment of last resort for pain control.

Electrostimulation

According to the medical history books, a Roman physician named Scribonius Largus used electricity to relieve pain in A.D. 46. Sound a little crazy? After all, electricity did not come into common use until relatively recent times, and it seems a bit farfetched to presume that it was used as a therapeutic tool in the Roman Empire.

But despite the apparent illogic of it all, Largus did, in fact, use electricity—an electric ray or "torpedo fish," to be exact—to ease the pain of migraine headaches and gout. The fish was apparently placed directly on the area of discomfort, and the resulting jolt often provided temporary pain relief. However, in the process, some of the patients were shocked to death—a very serious side effect by anyone's standards.

Today, electrical stimulation is being used again for pain patients, but in a far more sophisticated manner. One approach that is still highly experimental involves the implantation of tiny electrodes into the pain-inhibiting areas of the brain. These electrodes are wired to a small, portable electronic stimulator outside the body, which can be activated whenever a patient's pain reaches intolerable levels.

Although it would have seemed like science fiction a decade or two ago, two-thirds of the first thirty implants performed at Stanford University produced significant pain relief. However, this procedure carries all the serious risks associated with neurosurgery, thus diminishing its potential value for widespread use in pain control.

Electrical stimulation is also being utilized in other ways for pain patients. Drs. C. Norman Shealy and Blaine S. Nashville have developed the "dorsal column stimulator" (DCS), which has been used in treating discomfort associated with disorders ranging from spinal-disk disease to cancer. The DCS device is composed of two tiny electrodes attached to a small radio receiver. The entire device is surgically placed under the skin adjacent to the spinal cord, and its electrodes are implanted into the dorsal (posterior) column areas of the spinal cord. Whenever pain occurs, the patient holds a small antenna near the skin's surface, directly over the area where the DCS has been placed. This antenna is connected to a battery-powered transmitter worn on the belt, and when it dispatches the signal to the DCS, the patient feels a slight tingling sensation.

Although no one fully understands how and why the DCS is capable of alleviating discomfort, it has been found to be helpful for a small group of patients with certain types of pain. Still, because it involves a surgical procedure, it should be used very cautiously, and probably only as a last resort.

Still another device, called a transcutaneous nerve stimulator (TNS), was widely publicized in the early 1970s when Governor George Wallace of Alabama used one for the severe pain that resulted from injuries he sustained during an assassination attempt. With TNS, small electrodes are taped directly on the skin's surface above the area of discomfort. These electrodes are connected to a portable electronic unit which generates a pulsating electrical stimulus, specially calibrated to reduce discomfort.

An early study of TNS was conducted by Dr. Shealy, in which 136 patients were treated. According to his report, moderate pain relief was received by 102 of them, and 30 more were helped so significantly that they required no further pain alleviation therapy. I have also found TNS to be particularly useful for individuals with musculoskeletal pain in the neck, shoulder, or back.

TNS is available to patients twenty-four hours a day, because they can carry the small unit with them wherever they go. As a result, it may help to ease patients' feelings of helplessness, for it provides them with some degree of personal control over their discomfort instead of a dependence on doctors for drugs or surgery. It is also relatively inexpensive when compared to the costs of surgery, and seems to be generally safe when properly utilized.

Many variables in the use of TNS are still being studied. For example, there are some indications which suggest that the level of pain relief can be doubled or tripled by placing the electrodes directly on the acupuncture points corresponding to the area of discomfort.

Meanwhile, because TNS is a relatively new approach, there has not yet been a thorough evaluation of possible side effects and limitations. For instance, certain patients receive only temporary relief, since they apparently develop tolerance to the treatment. Also, a few of the TNS units now on the market utilize a wave form that can produce skin burns if the patient is overexposed to the electrical stimulation. In addition, TNS is similar to other pain-alleviation approaches (like nerve blocks) that primarily treat only the physical component of pain. When this physical dimension is only one aspect of the pain experience, other therapeutic support will also be needed.

I expect that in the next few years, electrical stimulation will be increasingly used for pain control. There's an old saying regarding new medical miracles—"Doctor, use that medicine while it still works." Well, electrical stimulation seems to have some benefits now. Whether or not it becomes more than just a medical fad will depend upon its performance in the upcoming years.

Psychotherapy

"My psychiatrist is a very religious man. Every morning he gives thanks to God that all of his patients are crazy."

It sounds like a line from the act of a nightclub comedian. But I've heard my patients say almost the same thing. People with chronic pain often end up in a psychiatrist's office after a series of physicians has been unsuccessful in discovering any physical explanation for their pain.

In many cases, psychotherapists can play a helpful role in a pain-alleviation program. After all, pain is a psychophysiological phenomenon—involving not only the body, but the mind as well. Anxiety and depression are usually as much a part of the pain experience as the physical discomfort itself. Also, each individual's reaction to painful stimuli may be related to personality factors and past life experiences, which psychiatrists and psychologists are trained to investigate and identify.

A well-trained, competent psychotherapist can probably help all pain patients to some degree. He may, for instance, be able to help an individual deal with the everyday stresses of modern living which can strongly contribute to the pain experience. He may also help a patient through the "mourning" period often associated with chronic pain, an experience similar to the mourning period that follows the death of a loved one. It's natural for an individual to grieve after the loss of a loved one, but if that heartbreaking mourning continues unabated for years, then psychotherapy may be indicated. Similarly, when an illness or injury has caused a person to lose many of life's pleasures, it's understandable to be depressed for a while. But if this loss is mourned for months or even years, then psychotherapy will be helpful, if not essential.

Incredibly, some people become so accustomed to their painful lifestyle that they are actually reluctant to get better. As I discussed in Chapter 3, hurting provides them with certain benefits or "gains" that would disappear if they stopped feeling pain. So they are content to hurt rather than heal. Psychotherapy can often help such people to realize the self-destructive nature of this situation.

As pain evolves from an acute phenomenon into chronic discomfort, a pain patient's personality may begin to significantly reflect his medical dilemma. Too often, his entire life may begin revolving around his discomfort. He becomes, as Dr. Thomas Szasz of the State University of

New York says, an *homme douloureux*—that is, a pain person. He literally makes a career of his pain, for he does little else beside think and talk about it, and consult doctors because of it. Without pain, his life would lose its focus, for the pain experience has become as important as any profession.

Until the *homme douloureux* is extricated from his plight, he will usually avoid tackling the problem directly, perhaps by playing "pain games." Pain games are one way to sidestep any meaningful therapy that doctors may be able to provide. Physicians have now begun to recognize many of these games, but unfortunately this has also made some doctors suspicious and cynical of *all* their pain patients, and thus less sensitive to their real needs.

One of the most familiar pain games might be called "The Addict" or "Cut Me." When played well, the dialogue between patient and physician goes something like this:

Patient: Doctor, those pain pills you gave me last month just aren't helping me at all. Can't you cut a nerve or something?

Doctor: Oh, let's not do anything that drastic. Why don't we try some stronger pills instead?

In fact, the patient's sole intention in the first place had been to obtain more potent medication. And the doctor unknowingly satisfied that wish. If the physician had been more aware of this game, the dialogue might have gone quite differently.

Patient: Doctor, those pain pills you gave me last month haven't helped me at all. Can't you cut a nerve or something?

Doctor: No, there's really no indication that cutting a nerve is appropriate. If the pain pills I've already given you haven't helped, I'm going to stop prescribing medication altogether. Why don't we try some other alternatives?

With this second approach, the game has been successfully frustrated, and it is hoped, patient and doctor can begin communicating in a more candid manner about both the pain problem and a possible dependence on drugs.

Another common pain game might be called "You Do It." Usually it is played by a patient who has already been examined and treated by many doctors, some of whom are particularly well-known and respected. Now, as he moves on to a new specialist, the scenario may develop thusly:

Doctor: I see by your medical history that you've been to the Mayo Clinic, the Scripps Institute, the City of Hope, and several other major medical centers throughout the nation. You've seen some very knowledgeable doctors, and none of them has been able to help you. How do you feel about that?

Patient: Yes, I've been to all those places, and not a single one of those so-called "experts" had a cure for my problem. What have *you* got for me?

The implicit message that the patient is attempting to communicate is, "It's up to you to fix me." This kind of patient is not willing to take any responsibility for his own treatment program, for he expects someday to find a miracle worker to do it all for him. Lots of luck!

Other common pain games include "Love Me or Leave Me." In this game, the pain patient will be as unpleasant and uncooperative as possible in relating to doctors, as a way of testing to what extent they really care. Is the doctor willing to put up with brash and surly remarks by the patient? Or will he instead be so "insensitive" as to oust such an immature patient from his office?

It might be justified to feel anger toward pain patients who play such games, except that doctors also sometimes play games of their own. One of the games very prevalent in the medical profession has been called "You're Just Too Dumb," which can be played in many types of situations. For instance, when a patient asks a question like "Why do I have arthritis?" some doctors refuse to spend the time on a lengthy explanation, or are unwilling to admit that they simply don't know. Instead, they may respond, "The medical literature is too complex for a layman to understand. Trust me. I'm doing everything possible to make you feel better."

Some doctors also indulge in a game called "You're Imagining the Whole Thing," in which they are unwilling to work extensively with the patient, to spend the time needed to get to know him, or to truly empathize with his plight. Instead, they will briefly encourage him to deny his own experience, and to accept the belief that the pain is not real. The patient knows otherwise, and as a result, the credibility of all doctors is diminished in the patient's eyes.

Certainly, pain games are inexcusable, whether engaged in by one or both parties in the doctor-patient relationship. A competent psychotherapist can often help pain patients to confront the games they may be playing, and eventually to reverse such counterproductive behavior.

Of course, without a patient's full cooperation, the potential benefits of any type of psychotherapy are limited. And too often, patients display strong resistance to psychotherapy because of fear. Some are frightened by the possibility that hidden, insidious mental factors may be involved in their chronic pain. Others fear that seeing a psychotherapist is a sign of mental weakness. Still others, like the businessman described in Chapter

3, are frightened to probe into the haunting guilt they might feel for some wrongdoing, having chosen instead to accept pain as a preferable form of punishment.

Other patients resist therapy in reaction to a subconscious fear instilled in them by their own physician. When a doctor is unable to help a patient, he may state, "I've tried everything to help your pain, and nothing has worked; you're just going to have to learn to live with it." Dr. David Cheek has suggested that when your doctor concludes that you must learn to "live with pain," your subconscious might interpret that to also mean, "You will be free of pain only when you are dead." It's no wonder that many patients subconsciously give up even trying to overcome pain.

Even when a patient overcomes his resistance and enters psychotherapy, there still may be limitations to this type of treatment. Much like the Medical Merry-Go-Round, psychotherapy is often a miniature merry-go-round of its own. You can receive widely differing types of therapy for the identical problem, depending on the type of psychotherapist who treats you. The approach utilized could be Freudian, Jungian, Adlerian, Rogerian, Gestalt, Reichian, or any number of other orientations. Each of these approaches is radically different, and most patients fail to even ask their therapists which type of therapy they favor until they are well into therapy.

New types of psychological techniques are constantly being added to the psychotherapeutic merry-go-round. One of these newer approaches is called "operant conditioning," or "behavior modification." With this technique, patients are rewarded for activities incompatible with pain behavior, and nonreinforced, or even punished for activities that perpetuate pain behavior. The administration of narcotic drugs, for example, is conducted on a "time contingent" rather than a "symptom contingent" basis—that is, medications are given, say, every four hours, regardless of an individual's pain level, rather than only when he hurts. Under "symptom contingent" conditions, the patient would receive narcotics every time he says, "I hurt," thus reinforcing each recurrence of his discomfort. Whenever he wants or needs more narcotics, his pain will flare up. But under "time contingency," his receipt of medications does not hinge in any way upon the intensity of his discomfort; thus, it reduces any drug-related incentive for him to hurt.

I find three major drawbacks to operant conditioning. First, the environment has to be very carefully controlled, which usually means that the patient must be hospitalized. Even if operant conditioning is successful in the hospital, once the patient moves back to his old, pain-reinforcing environment, his pain behavior can quickly return as if the operant conditioning had never even occurred.

Second, the goal of operant conditioning is to modify pain *behavior*, not necessarily the pain *experience*. As a result, it may produce changes in a

SAMPLE

EXERCISE THIRTEEN: **DATE:** March 11

What Can Traditional Medicine Do?   **TIME:** 8:30 p.m.

	EXPERIENCE			OVERALL RESULTS					CURRENT EXPECTATIONS				
	Have Tried Before	Wish to Try Now	Refuse to Try Now	Condition Worsened	No Relief	Temporary Relief	Substantial Relief	Complete Relief	Will Definitely Help	Probably Will Help	Probably Won't Help	Will Definitely Not Help	Don't Know
Analgesics	X					X						X	
Weak Narcotics	X					X					X		
Strong Narcotics			X									X	
Tranquilizers	X					X					X		
Sleeping Pills	X					X						X	
Antidepressants				X								X	
Other Medications		X											X
Surgery	X					X						X	
Nerve Blocks	X					X				X			
Neurolytic Blocks			X								X		
Transcutaneous Nerve Stimulation (TNS)	X			X								X	
Operant Conditioning			X									X	
Electroconvulsive Shock			X									X	
Individual Psychotherapy		X											X
Group Psychotherapy			X									X	

EXERCISE THIRTEEN:

What Can Traditional Medicine Do?

DATE: _____

TIME: _____

	EXPERIENCE			OVERALL RESULTS					CURRENT EXPECTATIONS				
	Have Tried Before	Wish to Try Now	Refuse to Try Now	Condition Worsened	No Relief	Temporary Relief	Substantial Relief	Complete Relief	Will Definitely Help	Probably Will Help	Probably Won't Help	Will Definitely Not Help	Don't Know
Analgesics													
Weak Narcotics													
Strong Narcotics													
Tranquilizers													
Sleeping Pills													
Antidepressants													
Other Medications													
Surgery													
Nerve Blocks													
Neurolytic Blocks													
Transcutaneous Nerve Stimulation (TNS)													
Operant Conditioning													
Electroconvulsive Shock													
Individual Psychotherapy													
Group Psychotherapy													

patient's willingness to verbalize or demonstrate pain, but not necessarily any changes in his subjective amount of suffering and discomfort.

The third disadvantage to this approach is that the contingencies must be constantly and carefully scrutinized. I have seen some instances of operant conditioning in which it is unclear who's manipulating whom for what. Although a change in pain behavior has occurred, it merely reflects the patient's realization that he can get what he wants by "pretending" to be better. In a sense, the patient is conditioning the doctor, not vice versa.

Some psychiatrists and psychologists, when unable to obtain positive results with psychotherapy, rely on extreme treatments like electroconvulsive shock therapy (ECT). In my opinion, ECT is a terribly invasive approach that should be considered only as a last resort. Although its advocates point to studies indicating that ECT can alleviate painful symptoms in some patients, it can also have devastating effects upon memory and other important mental functions.

Even at its best, psychotherapy is usually extremely expensive and time-consuming. At $60 to $80 an hour, many chronic pain patients literally spend thousands of dollars over a period of months or years to obtain only minimal relief.

One of my patients, a gentle, sensitive woman who suffered from severe headaches, offered one of the most fitting descriptions of her own years on a psychiatrist's couch. "I talked to my psychoanalyst for eleven years," she told me, "and it gave me a very good understanding of my childhood, my relationship with my family, and all the other things that you talk about in a psychiatrist's office. But I still have pain.

"So now I know that knowledge of my problems isn't enough. I also have to do something to try to change the situation I've been in all these years."

She's right. Knowledge in itself is not enough to change anything. Only when you combine that knowledge with personal experience will you achieve understanding and change. It takes more than lying on a psychoanalyst's couch to help ease your pain; you also have to make what you've learned a part of your everyday life experience.

Exercise Thirteen: What Can Traditional Medicine Do?

Exercise Thirteen is designed to help you summarize the different types of medical treatment you have received from your physicians. Please indicate: (1) your experience with each of the therapeutic approaches listed, (2) how successful they have been, and (3) your expectations as to whether or not each therapy might be of help.

And If You Still Hurt? . . .

So what if you've tried everything? What if you've seen dozens of doctors, consumed countless combinations of pills, wallowed in hospital beds, and submitted to nerve blocks, surgery, psychotherapy, and everything else under the medical umbrella? Thousands of dollars and many months later, what if you still hurt?

Although your doctors may say, "Learn to live with it," I believe that you should continue your search for relief. Keep in mind that painful symptoms are your friends, telling you that something is wrong. When you finally decipher pain's message and take appropriate action, your discomfort will be significantly reduced if not eliminated altogether. In the meantime, your body is telling you to keep looking and not to give up.

Even if you've exhausted all the therapies described in this chapter, there's still a world of other possibilities. In the next chapter, I'll discuss some of these less conventional, more controversial alternatives.

5   What About
Unconventional Therapies?

The doctor of the future will give no drugs, but will interest his patients in the care of the human frame, in diet, and in the cause and prevention of human disease.

—Thomas A. Edison

"I've tried everything, Doctor. Drugs, surgery, nerve blocks, electrical stimulation, even psychotherapy. But I still hurt. Isn't there anything else that can help me?"

Those desperate words are frequently recited by patients with pain. Perhaps you've spoken them yourself. After enduring the physical and mental anguish of having tried every conventional treatment suggested by your doctors, you may have nothing to show for it but utter frustration, continued pain, and a stack of oppressive medical bills.

Chronic pain is often poorly controlled by traditional medical approaches. Consequently, amid their growing despondency, people in pain can become prime targets for charlatans and exploiters. I have heard many horrifying stories about fraudulent pain-control medications and devices that some of my patients have tried, including "miracle ointments," "ethereal healing instruments," and other expensive and ineffective gimmicks.

Frankly, it upsets me to see how easily pain patients can be victimized by greedy and unethical promoters of worthless devices. For not only are the patients being unfairly cheated, but as a result, many have become skeptical about *all* nontraditional approaches to pain control. Even so, many alternative therapies can be truly helpful when properly utilized, and thus, they should be more carefully considered before a doctor proclaims "nothing more can be done."

How can you determine which techniques may be valuable for you? Perhaps a good place to start is by identifying the criteria that an "ideal" analgesic (pain-reliever) should meet. Admittedly, these criteria, listed below, are quite rigorous, but they provide solid standards against which alternative approaches can be compared:

1. The ideal analgesic should be highly efficient and reliable in its ability to alleviate pain. It should not only eliminate all pain, but it should do so every time it is used.

2. Its analgesic effects should be immediate and long-lasting. Unless pain relief occurs shortly after administration, its value is limited. And, of course, the longer your pain is eased, the better.

3. It should be safe to administer. It shouldn't make the patient more ill, and it certainly shouldn't kill him. (Unfortunately, patients occasionally *do* die from many medically accepted pain-alleviation treatments, including surgical procedures and drug administration.)

4. It should be simple to use with a minimum of expensive equipment. If a treatment is beyond the financial reach of a patient, it is worthless to him. At some of the interdisciplinary pain clinics treating individuals on an inpatient basis, the fees are prohibitively high; thus, the care is beneficial to only the very few who can afford it.

5. It should not adversely affect the patient's personality or cognitive ability. Diazepam (Valium), for instance, often causes depression at high dosage levels—hardly an attractive side effect. Other drugs make people sleepy, irritable, or even paranoid. Still others disrupt learning, memory, and basic thinking processes.

6. It should not be habit-forming. Patients frequently become addicted to or dependent upon many of the currently available analgesics; thus, in addition to their pain, they must now also deal with a drug abuse problem.

7. It should not destroy normal neural tissue. Contemporary medicine's understanding of the neurophysiology of the pain experience is still relatively primitive, but it appears that neural tissue may be involved in turning *off* pain as well as turning it *on*. Thus, therapy should not interfere in any way with the body's own pain-suppressing mechanisms.

8. It should not produce other long-term adverse effects, ranging from the possibility of infection to emotional dependence on the therapy or therapist.

9. Finally, while providing relief from discomfort, it should not suppress or mask any critical, survival-oriented message that the pain is trying to communicate.

When you examine these criteria carefully, it is clear that none of Western medicine's most commonly utilized approaches fares particularly well. Certainly, neither drugs, surgery, nerve blocks, nor any of the other traditional techniques discussed in Chapter 4 can qualify as an "ideal analgesic." As a growing number of Western physicians have begun to recognize the shortcomings of traditional therapy, they have become increasingly receptive to a variety of alternatives that they once considered "eccentric" or "esoteric," but which now are receiving some degree of scientific validation.

Several of these alternative approaches—like acupuncture and hypnosis—are centuries old. But in this modern era of explosive advances in medical technology, they have been largely overlooked. Others, like biofeedback and guided imagery, have been developed only quite recently.

In addition, considerable attention is now being given to the subtle social and psychological factors associated with all types of illness. The stress of modern living is now recognized as a major factor in the development of many chronic diseases, and special programs incorporating techniques like relaxation training and family therapy are being more widely utilized.

Let's now take a closer look at some of these nontraditional alternative approaches to pain control.

Physical Therapies

Physical therapies are perhaps the oldest form of treatment for pain. From the beginning of time, when man hurt, he instinctively rubbed or massaged the area of his discomfort. The caveman who stubbed his toe while fleeing from an unfriendly beast probably used his hands to provide the initial (and perhaps the only) relief to the painful area. Later, he may have learned to put some icy snow on it, or to apply heat by pressing hot stones against it. If he was lucky, his mate tenderly kissed the painful area, providing not only physical therapy, but emotional support as well.

Such ancient techniques are still valuable today. Thus, I strongly encourage my patients to experiment with these and the newer types of physical therapy now available.

Heat and Cold

When you hurt, how does heat—a hot shower, a hot bath, a visit to a steam room or sauna—affect your discomfort? Does it intensify the pain, or does it provide soothing relief? Does heat administered through diathermy, infrared, or hot packs affect your pain positively or negatively? You'll never find out unless you try it.

Many patients with chronic pain experience significant relief with heat.

It also helps to induce sleep and to soothe jangled nerves. A hot bath often provides immediate relief from tension and anxiety, and is one of the simplest ways to promote muscle relaxation.

However, certain pain sufferers should use heat cautiously. For instance, if you're severely depressed and despondent, it may tend to make you feel even more sorrowful. Heat should also be avoided by individuals with certain allergies, clotting defects in their blood systems, and by those with certain types of malignancies, since heat may stimulate the growth of cancerous cells.

While heat is often helpful for *chronic* pain, cold is more often the treatment of choice for *acute* discomfort. For best results, cold is typically applied directly to the painful area, since it usually provides an immediate feeling of "numbness" in the nerves that innervate that region of the body.

Richard J. Kroening, M.D., a pain specialist in the UCLA Department of Anesthesiology, has developed a simple technique for applying cold directly to a painful area of the body. Dr. Kroening recommends taking an empty frozen orange juice can, filling it with water, and putting it in the freezer. Once the water is frozen, remove the ice from the can, and place it directly on the area of your discomfort. Rub the ice briskly over the area, until the skin is beyond the sensation of numbness and begins to feel warm and stingy. Once this condition is achieved, remove the ice, for if you continue too much longer, you could actually cause the skin to become frostbitten.

Cold can also be applied to the entire body rather than just specific parts. A cold shower or a brisk swim can be stimulating and invigorating, and very beneficial when you're feeling depressed or lethargic.

As I discussed in Chapter 2, the distinction between pleasure and pain is often uncertain. A cold shower can be a very unpleasant experience. But when it is over, you will probably enjoy its aftereffects and be very glad that you took it. Yes, it's both pleasurable and painful, but for the person feeling depressed and listless, the benefits of a cold shower may be worth the unpleasantness that accompanies it.

As with heat, there are certain situations in which prolonged cold should probably be avoided. For example, if you suffer from rheumatoid arthritis, cold may make your joints stiffer and even more uncomfortable. Nor is cold appropriate if you have certain types of allergies such as those that produce hives. Also, some people develop blood clotting abnormalities when exposed to extreme cold.

For physiological reasons, both heat and cold have a definite impact upon the neural transmitters that regulate pleasure and pain. So don't underestimate the powerful effects they can have on how you feel.

Pressure

The application of pressure can be successful in treating both chronic and acute pain. Therapeutic massage, for example, whether applied in a specific area of discomfort or throughout the entire body, can create both physical relaxation and psychological peace of mind.

Unfortunately, the word "massage" has been discredited in recent years. In cities across the country, so-called "massage parlors" have offered just about every type of physical stimulation imaginable except for an authentic therapeutic massage. Consequently, people who might have benefited from the treatment of a licensed masseur have shied away from this very legitimate type of therapy.

Massage is almost always helpful for muscle-spasm pain. A skilled masseur can also provide an amazing degree of comfort for the patient who is tense, anxious, or depressed.

When a trained masseur is not available, a massage by a caring friend or loved one can be just as rewarding. Let's face it—massage is like sex; you can do it to yourself, but it's much more fun when you do it with someone else.

Pain relief can also be produced by applying pressure to a part of the body distant from the area that hurts. For example, not long ago I developed a terrible toothache. To ease the pain, I applied deep pressure to a point located between my thumb and index finger. This point is called "Ho-ku" by acupuncturists, who frequently use it to treat dental pain. Acupressure, *Shiatsu*, *Jin Shin Do*, and other techniques which utilize pressure applied to acupuncture points will be discussed in the acupuncture section of this chapter.

Chiropractic

Some people with pain turn to chiropractors for relief from their discomfort. In fact, eight million Americans are treated each year by chiropractors, or doctors of chiropractic, as they prefer to be called. Although chiropractors are licensed to practice in all fifty states, they are under constant attack from the American Medical Association, which has labeled chiropractic "an unscientific cult whose practitioners lack the necessary training and background to diagnose and treat human disease."

The basic theory of chiropractic is that many, if not most, ailments and pains are caused by "spinal subluxations" (dislocations of the vertebrae). A shift in the vertebrae as small as one millimeter is said to apply enough pressure to the spinal nerves to produce illness. Chiropractors physically manipulate the vertebrae in an attempt to correct the subluxations so as to cure disease and eliminate pain.

Unfortunately, in-depth studies of chiropractic by unbiased investigators are rare. The greatest body of research has been conducted in England, Germany, France, and Denmark. At a conference held at the National Institutes of Health in Bethesda, Maryland, in 1975, James Henry Cyriax, M.D., of St. Thomas Hospital in London, reported that two-thirds of all cases of back pain treated at St. Thomas responded favorably to manipulation (chiropractic). He stated that because physicians are not taught this technique in medical school, they generally do not use or recommend manipulation; but, he added, manipulators probably use it *too* often. He believes the wisest approach lies somewhere between these two extremes.

Why is chiropractic so popular? A study conducted at the University of Utah Medical School perhaps best describes an important part of chiropractic's appeal. Robert L. Kane, M.D., who participated in the research, summarized a portion of the report as follows:

"On the basis of our study and others, it appears the chiropractor may be more attuned to the total needs of the patient than is his medical counterpart. The chiropractor does not seem hurried. He uses language patients can understand. He gives them sympathy and he is patient with them. He does not take a superior attitude. He has an egalitarian relationship rather than a superordinate-subordinate relationship."

Despite the AMA's negative pronouncements, there are many physicians who work closely with chiropractors. In a survey published in *Medical Economics*, more than 25 percent of a thousand physicians questioned stated that they receive referrals from chiropractors. Almost 5 percent of the M.D.s reported that they send patients to chiropractors.

Hippocrates once said, "In case of illness, look to the spine first." More than two thousand years later, many people still agree with him.

Orgone Therapy and Bioenergetics

The Science of Orgonomy was developed by Dr. Wilhelm Reich, an associate of Freud, who believed that whatever happens in the mind is simultaneously reflected in the body. Thus, every unresolved emotional conflict and every undischarged emotional need was thought to be reflected by muscle tightness, inhibited breathing, constrained movement, and "character armoring" as a defense against external and internal changes.

Reich claimed that "nearly everyone by maturity has developed not only a few—or many—neurotic traits, but a way of standing, looking, holding the mouth and jaw, speaking, of breathing and holding up the chest and perhaps pulling in the pelvis, that is characteristic and set—if not rigid and unyielding." These visible, analyzable muscular traits were thought to represent the character structure in its physical form. Thus, if one could break down muscular armoring, one could change the neurotic character structure to the same degree. Reich believed that treatment focused on the body was far more effective than "talking-out therapy" such as psychoanalysis.

Practitioners of orgone therapy use various types of physical manipulations, all designed to increase freedom of breathing and movement and thereby bring repressed emotions into the foreground to be consciously dealt with. One type of orgone therapy, called bioenergetics, was developed by Alexander Lowen, a student of Reich, who combined strenuous breathing exercises with stretching techniques and deep massages to achieve emotional discharge. The goal of bioenergetic therapy is to achieve greater physical vitality, more spontaneous emotional responses, and a release of muscular tension.

Although there are few studies in the medical literature concerning the use of orgone therapy for chronic pain, Arthur Nelson, M.D., has reported success in its use to treat chronic tension headaches. One of Dr. Nelson's patients, a twenty-six-year-old social worker, had suffered very painful tension headaches daily for six years. After being treated unsuccessfully with everything from drugs to chiropractic manipulation, orgone therapy was attempted. In the *American Journal of Psychotherapy* (January 1976), Dr. Nelson wrote, "I compressed the temporomandibular [jaw] joints bilaterally with one hand, and the occiput [back part of head] with the other, while having her hit and scream at the same time. This was extremely painful but endured. I also had her push her jaw against my hand in a defiant manner. This brought out anger, which was followed by crying."

Dr. Nelson conducted twenty-five sessions with this patient, during which her headaches gradually declined in frequency and intensity. Eventually, she was headache free.

Rolfing—Structural Integration

Structural integration is another technique which is sometimes used to treat pain patients. Developed by Ida P. Rolf, an organic chemist, it is a method of reordering the body structure with carefully planned physical manipulations and deep tissue massage, taking place during ten sessions of about one hour each. Considerable force and pressure are involved, designed to release excessive tensions and to realign body weight in order for the body to move more naturally with gravity.

Before participating in a rolfing session, be aware that it hurts. I mean, it *really* hurts. True, the pain is short-lived, but don't go into the rolfing experience expecting it to be a particularly pleasant one. However, many people who have been rolfed have claimed that their bodies feel much more relaxed and natural after the sessions are completed, and that their original pain has diminished.

Movement and Exercise Therapy

Movement and exercise are other, very positive forms of physical therapy that can help to relieve tension and reduce pain. Unfortunately, according to a recent Gallup poll, only 4 percent of adult Americans exercise enough to make any significant difference in combating chronic degenerative diseases. With pain patients, that percentage is probably even lower.

If you have chronic pain, sitting motionless most of the day probably retards the healing process. That doesn't mean that you necessarily have to jog through the neighborhood each afternoon or plunge into the community touch football game. But neither should you be satisfied with the other end of the physical exertion scale. I've seen pain patients (and "healthy" people, too) who think they've done their daily exercise by walking to the television set to turn on the baseball game. They're wrong. Even something so simple as a long walk every day could significantly improve the health of their bodies and minds.

Western researchers have only recently begun to explore the value of exercise systems like yoga. Yoga is a three-thousand-year-old system that combines both physical and spiritual training. Many disciples of yoga claim its various postures help relax them, and energize both the body and the mind.

Two of the better known modern movement therapies are the Alexander and the Feldenkrais techniques. Frederick Alexander was a young actor in Melbourne who began losing his voice during performances. Medical treatment brought only temporary relief. But Alexander started observing himself carefully in the mirror and concluded that his malady was due to a tendency to pull his head backward and downward when he talked. This discovery led him to postulate that how we move our bodies critically affects the total physical, emotional, and mental state of the organism, and that by eliminating negative, habitual patterns of movement, the natural functioning of the organism can be restored.

The Alexander technique is designed to help the individual to develop a "sensory appreciation" of movements which originate from the "primary control" center of the head and neck. Using everyday movements like walking, standing, and sitting, a new awareness of "natural" movement is facilitated, and old habitual patterns or "sets" are inhibited.

The Feldenkrais technique (also called Functional Integration), developed by physicist Moshe Feldenkrais, is a system of movements designed to eliminate patterns of stress and tension that have been programmed into the body. Using light touch and manipulation, the instructor helps to move muscles in more "natural" ways, thereby releasing mental and emotional tension, and restoring "harmony" to the "integrated self."

Many other systems of movement and exercise have been developed, and in Chapter 9, I'll describe several specific techniques that I have found helpful for patients with chronic pain and/or depression.

Therapeutic Touch

There is now increasing evidence which suggests that merely touching an ill person can have very positive therapeutic effects. For centuries, the laying on of hands, particularly by religious or spiritual healers, has occupied a central role in many societies. For example, Biblical stories about healings by Jesus, Peter, John, and others helped make the laying on of hands a common phenomenon in Christianity.

In your own life, haven't there been times when a simple human touch has had a very positive physical and mental impact? When you were a child, wasn't a hug or even a pat on the head from your mother or father very comforting? And as an adult, isn't the touch of another human hand soothing and consoling?

No one knows for certain why touching is so therapeutic. But whatever the explanation, some physicians are now closely examining the physical and mental changes produced by merely touching patients.

Robert Swearingen, M.D., an orthopedic surgeon at the University of Colorado School of Medicine, treats hundreds of patients each winter who have suffered serious injuries on the Colorado ski slopes. It's a particularly unpleasant job, since most of the people he treats are in excruciating pain. But he recently told me that he has begun to teach the ski patrol rescue teams laying on of hands as a means of limiting traumatic discomfort.

To reduce anxiety and discomfort, Dr. Swearingen instructs the rescue team members to remove their gloves immediately upon reaching an injured skier, and to place one bare hand behind his neck to make skin-to-skin contact. The rescue team member then gently strokes his face with the other hand and calmly says, "Everything's going to be OK. You've hurt yourself, but we're here to take care of you now. Just relax and take it easy, and you're going to be fine." Dr. Swearingen tells me that these simple acts, like touching and soothing conversation, have worked miracles on the Colorado slopes.

Impressed with these results, Dr. Swearingen has also begun using similar techniques in treating patients with dislocated shoulders once they arrive at the hospital. If you've ever dislocated your shoulder, you know how very, very painful that can be. Normally, a patient is heavily anesthetized before his shoulder is put back in place; otherwise, the pain is unbearable.

However, Dr. Swearingen uses a different approach. As he gently talks to the patient, he uses his hands to locate areas of tension in the individual's shoulder muscles. While he lightly runs his hands over the shoulder, he simultaneously leads the patient through some breathing exercises to relax him as much as possible. "Try to relax this muscle," he will say. "Ah, that's better . . . let it relax completely . . . very good . . . let yourself relax as much as you ever have before."

When the patient is as comfortable as possible, Swearingen prepares to adjust the shoulder back in place. "You might feel a little pop as your shoulder comes back in," Swearingen tells his patient, "but because these muscles are completely relaxed, it won't hurt." And it doesn't.

Surprised? Most of Swearingen's patients are. After all, how is it possible that laying on of hands, combined with simple breathing exercises, could be just as effective as medicine's most potent anesthetics?

We still know relatively little about the role that laying on of hands can play in medical care. Nowadays, very few doctors touch their patients, except during a physical examination. Yes, doctors talk to patients endlessly. And they prescribe drugs for them. But most medical procedures, often with the very best intentions, are antitouching. During surgery, for example, the doctor never directly touches his patient. Instead, he is sterilized, gowned, and gloved, as skin-to-skin contact is intentionally avoided. Perhaps some direct doctor-patient touching—say, before the operation begins—could help ease the patient's anxiety by making him feel closer and more intimate with the surgeon operating on him.

My own feeling is that two processes may be occurring during a laying-on-of-hands experience. First, pain may be alleviated because the hand is stimulating the neural receptors in the skin at one or more acupuncture points. These are the areas of the body which, when stimulated by touch or by a needle, can potentially ease or eliminate pain in specific regions of the body. Even a physician unfamiliar with these acupuncture points may instinctively place his hands on these areas, since they are generally the most tender parts of the body.

But another phenomenon may be at work, too, unrelated to where the hands are placed. I think that when physical contact is made with another person, some psychological, energetic, or other subtle "life-force" may be operating that is highly therapeutic in nature. Think back to the last time someone placed his or her hand on your arm. Didn't you feel more than the mere physical sensation of the palm and fingers on you? Most people experience a psychological warmth as well, much more meaningful than the physical sensation.

Kissing can be interpreted the same way. A kiss is much more than just the stimulation of the lips. It has psychological and emotional components to it, and often sensual ones, too. In the same way, the laying on of hands may be a multidimensional phenomenon whose scientific basis is yet to be understood.

Dolores Krieger, a registered nurse at New York University Medical Center, has perhaps described this phenomenon best. Writing about her own experiences using therapeutic touch on patients, she said, "I soon realized that the touch in which I was interested was not simple physiological touch, but rather a humanized touch which conveyed an intent to help or to heal, and which was indeed suffused with this motivation. Moreover, the touch was that of a fairly healthy person whose ego structure was oriented towards serving the patient's needs, rather than bolstering his own needs."

Most nurses recognize the important therapeutic value of laying on of hands, for as a patient once told Dolores Krieger, "A patient will remember your touch long after he has forgotten your face." Yet, surprisingly, it has not generally been included as a formal part of training in most nursing schools. Fortunately, this is beginning to change. For example, therapeutic touch is now incorporated into the nursing curriculum at New York University Medical Center, particularly in the master's program. In-service hospital programs and continuing education workshops at universities are also instructing medical service personnel about this simple technique.

Laying on of hands is vital to many new approaches aimed at achieving muscle balance. The Touch for Health program developed by Dr. John Thie of Pasadena, California, uses the techniques of touch, acupressure, massage, and applied kinesiology to detect and correct muscle imbalance and to relieve tension, anxiety, and pain resulting from physical, emotional, and mental stress. Although the therapeutic potential of Dr. Thie's program for treating chronic pain and depression has not yet been thoroughly documented in the medical literature, many pain patients have reported to me that they have found it to be extremely helpful.

In the upcoming years, I believe that laying on of hands, movement, exercise, and other physical therapies will become more recognized as invaluable therapeutic tools. Comparing them with the "ideal analgesic" described earlier, they fare well, for they are generally safe, simple, nonaddicting, natural, and often highly effective. In Chapter 9, I'll discuss some of the specific physical techniques that are used with positive results by my patients with pain-related problems.

Acupuncture

"You know, Dr. Bresler, maybe I'm just imagining this. But sometimes my pain seems to get better when I rub certain areas of my body. It's kind of weird, because although these areas are tender when I push them, they don't seem to be related to my pain problem. Yet after I massage them for a while, my pain really feels better."

This patient was not imagining his pain relief. Like many other people with pain, he discovered—perhaps accidentally—that when pressure is applied to specific points on the body, pain often decreases and, in some cases, even disappears.

Although pressing these points can often be helpful, even better results can be obtained by stimulating the points by inserting tiny needles into the skin. This technique, called acupuncture, is the oldest system of medicine known to contemporary man.

Acupuncture originated in China at least five thousand years ago. That's about the same time that the Great Pyramid was being built in Egypt. Although some American physicians still consider acupuncture to be "experimental," more people have probably been treated with it than all other systems of medicine combined.

Most Westerners had not even heard of acupuncture until 1971, when a team of American table tennis players was invited to match strokes with their counterparts in the Republic of China. They were the first group of U.S. citizens to visit China in twenty-five years. When they returned to the United States, they told about a Chinese medical system in which needles are inserted to treat various illnesses, achieving similar or even better results than some of Western medicine's most sophisticated techniques. Everything from arthritis to headaches was reported to respond successfully to acupuncture treatment. It was hard to believe. Many American physicians still don't.

Probably the most publicized acupuncture story was told by *New York Times* editor James Reston. During his own visit to China in 1971, he became very ill and underwent an appendectomy at a hospital in Peking. Conventional anesthesia was used during the surgery, but when he began experiencing severe postoperative gas pain, Chinese doctors recommended acupuncture. Reston agreed, and needles were inserted into the skin below both knees and at his right elbow. The pain in his abdomen was relieved almost immediately.

"I remember thinking that it was rather a complicated way to get rid of gas on the stomach, but there was a noticeable relaxation of the pressure and distension within an hour and no recurrence of the problem thereafter," Reston later wrote.

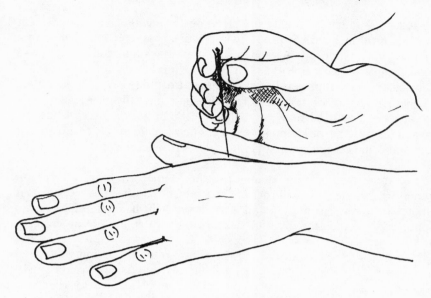

Fig. 9   *The insertion of an acupuncture needle.*

The following year, the Acupuncture Research Project (now a division of the Pain Control Unit) was established at UCLA. Since then, we have administered nearly eighty thousand acupuncture treatments. Our experience indicates that acupuncture is frequently very effective for a wide variety of ills—including acute and chronic pain.

Let's assume that you were to come to the UCLA Pain Control Unit for an acupuncture treatment. After undergoing a thorough medical workup, one of our staff acupuncturists would discuss with you the potential benefits and risks of this therapy. He or she would then determine which of the more than five hundred points would be used for treatment, based on a variety of factors including the results of specialized diagnostic techniques (such as pulse diagnosis, tongue diagnosis, and auricular diagnosis), the nature of the problem being treated, the duration of illness, and nutritional considerations. Typically, ten to fifteen needles are inserted during each treatment.

Many people are unnecessarily frightened by the prospect of receiving acupuncture, for they incorrectly equate acupuncture needles with the type of needles used for hypodermic injections. Hypodermic needles are large and hollow with a razor-sharp beveled point for piercing through tissue. Acupuncture needles, on the other hand, are extremely thin— often no thicker than a human hair. They are made of solid stainless steel with a rounded pencil-tip point that pushes the tissue aside without cutting it. As a result, only a slight pinprick sensation is felt when they are inserted, and there is usually no bleeding during the entire treatment process. Once the needle is properly in place, a characteristic tingling or a heaviness is experienced. Although this sometimes may feel strange and unusual, most patients report that it is not painful.

To achieve maximum results, the acupuncturist may decide to stimulate the needles in one of several ways. He may carefully rotate them for several seconds. Or he may gradually heat them with a stick of burning moxa, a Chinese herb. He might even connect an electronic stimulator to the needles in order to pass a gentle, painless electrical current through them.

After about twenty to thirty minutes, the needles are removed without discomfort. A brief rest will then be recommended after the treatment is completed, because some patients experience light-headedness and even euphoria. Most patients describe a characteristic feeling of contentment and relaxation.

The number of sessions required varies according to the individual and the problem being treated. For acute ailments, only a few treatments— sometimes just one—are necessary. Chronic problems usually require a greater number.

You may be fortunate, experiencing improvement in your condition immediately. However, you may instead feel even worse after the initial treatments, and then begin making profound improvement later. If acupuncture is capable of helping you, progress is usually noticeable by the tenth treatment. But for certain chronic ailments, fifteen to twenty treatments may be necessary. Typically, about two treatments are given per week.

In this era of nuclear energy, trips to the moon and miracle drugs, it is difficult to accept a technique that seems so primitive and bizarre. Contemporary Western physicians stare in disbelief when they see a needle inserted into the ear to treat knee pain. But ancient healers would certainly have been equally baffled by the modern doctor placing a compressed white powder tablet (aspirin) into their patients' mouths. We, of course, know that the aspirin dissolves in the stomach, enters the bloodstream, and quickly reaches the area of the knee. As we learn more about acupuncture and the way it works, I believe it, too, will become as acceptable and ordinary as our most commonplace treatments.

Most of us tend to think that the West is much more scientifically sophisticated than the East, and that if acupuncture had any validity, it would have been incorporated into our medical system long ago. But we are now discovering that the ancient Chinese were far more advanced than we had ever assumed. Although we give them credit for discovering porcelain, paper, silk, and gunpowder, their insights into the field of medicine are even more astounding.

In a book called *Nei Ching (The Yellow Emperor's Classic of Internal*

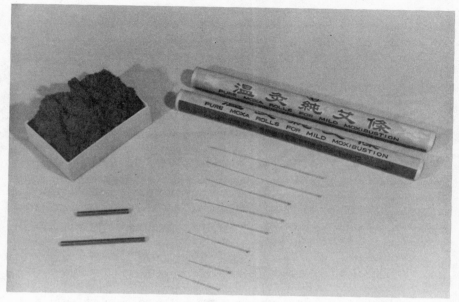

Fig. 10 *Various types of acupuncture needles and moxa.*

Medicine), the world's oldest known medical treatise dating back to the second century B.C., there is an explanation of blood circulation in the body—centuries before the English physiologist Sir William Harvey "discovered" how blood circulates. In the same book, vaccination against smallpox is described in detail—long before the English physician Edward Jenner devised his own smallpox immunization in the eighteenth century. The Chinese would scrape the pox off an infected person, grind it into a powder, and blow it through a tiny tube into the nostrils of anyone who came into contact with the victim. Smallpox was virtually unknown in ancient China, while it had devastating effects on Western civilization.

The ancient Chinese distinguished five levels of the healing arts. The lowest was practiced by the veterinarian, or animal doctor. Next came the acupuncturist and herbalist who treated minor symptomatic problems. The third level was the surgeon who treated more serious, life-threatening injuries. Second highest was the nutritionist who taught people what to eat; his was the science of longevity and preventive medicine. But highest of all was the philosopher-sage who taught the "laws of the universe." He was the only practitioner who could effect a genuine cure, for he went directly to the heart of the problem: the patient's inability to live harmoniously with nature. (Interestingly, this notion is similar to the modern concept of integral medicine, which will be discussed later in this chapter.)

The ancient Chinese system of medicine was also sophisticated in its heavy emphasis on prevention. One traditional aphorism states, "The superior physician cures before the illness is manifested; it is the inferior physician who can only treat the illness he was unable to prevent." Traditionally, people paid their doctors to keep them well. If a person got sick, it was then his doctor's responsibility not only to care for him, but also to provide support for his family. If too many people got sick, the doctor was banned from the village. Can you imagine how health care in America would change if such a policy were enacted today?

To determine the state of a person's health before the symptoms of disease were manifested, four types of diagnostic procedures were used:

1. *Looking* at the vessels of the eyes, the ears, the tongue, the hair, as well as subtle changes in skin color, posture, walk, and body language.

2. *Listening* to the patient's breathing, and the emotion in his voice.

3. *Questioning* the patient about his medical history, including every factor that could affect his health, like his family, diet, sleep habits, job, etc.

4. *Taking of the pulse* with three fingers along the radial artery of each wrist. According to Chinese doctrine, a sophisticated pulse reader—by pressing lightly or deeply at certain points on the wrist—could determine with incredible accuracy whether problems existed in the lungs, large intestine, stomach, spleen, heart, liver, kidney, gallbladder, or other organ systems.

Unlike Western medicine, the ancient Chinese healing arts were not based on a knowledge of human anatomy. The Chinese worshiped their ancestors, so gross dissection of a cadaver was unthinkable. Instead, the Chinese system of medicine was based on an energetic concept of the body rather than a material one. In a sense, the early Chinese philosophers antedated Einstein's theory of relativity, for they recognized that matter and energy are just two different manifestations of the same thing. Rather than focusing on the material aspects of the body (muscles, nerves, organs, bones, and so forth), they concentrated on the vital life energy that creates and animates the physical body. This life energy, called "Ch'i," is conceptually similar to the "orgone energy" described by Reich, or "prana" in the Hindu theosophical tradition. The term "Ch'i" is perhaps best translated as "breath." Thus, all things that respire have Ch'i, including invertebrates and plants.

According to classical Chinese theory, Ch'i moves through the body along specific pathways, called "meridians." Ch'i controls the blood, nerves, and all organs, and must flow freely for good health to be maintained. When this energy flow becomes blocked or impaired—because of trauma, poor diet, excessive emotions, cold, stress, or any number of other factors—the individual becomes susceptible to illness. Consistent with this notion, pain is nothing more than an excess accumulation of energy that occurs when the flow of Ch'i becomes

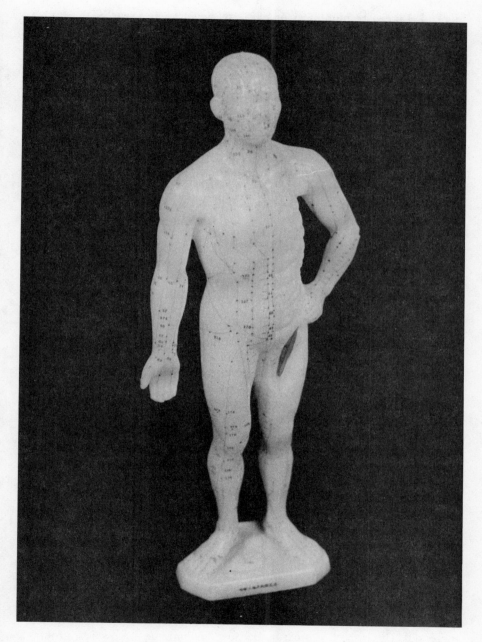

Fig. 11 *The acupuncture points and meridians.*

blocked. Likewise, numbness or paralysis develops in areas of the body with insufficient Ch'i flow.

With this in mind, I have found it fascinating that many patients with pain in the upper part of the body often report a weakness in the lower part. Typically, a patient with neck or shoulder pain will say, "My legs feel very tired in the afternoon and I have to sit down to rest for a while." I've also observed the opposite relationship as well.

By selectively stimulating the acupuncture points that lie along the meridians, the ancient Chinese believed that the flow of Ch'i in specific organ systems could be rebalanced, thus alleviating pain and strengthening the body's ability to combat disease. (In addition to acupuncture, the Chinese utilized a variety of herbs, which were taken as broths, teas, or applied directly to the skin. Western medicine has not yet recognized the value of herbal therapy, but I believe that someday herbs will become an even more valuable therapeutic tool than acupuncture.)

The traditional Chinese theory of Ch'i flow has generally not been accepted in the West. Instead, many research studies conducted in the United States, Canada, France, Germany, Austria, England, Italy, the Soviet Union, and China have indicated that acupuncture points represent different types of neural receptors. These points possess unique electrical, chemical, and thermal properties, and when stimulated, they are known to produce various bodily reactions, including change in heart rate, brain activity, blood flow, endocrine function, and immune/inflammatory responses. Exactly how these neural receptors affect the central nervous system is not yet known. However, studies suggest that acupuncture's pain-relieving properties may be due to the release of naturally occurring, morphine-like substances (endorphins) in the brain. Thus, rather than having a direct effect on pain, acupuncture may stimulate the body's own ability to turn pain off.

Many "authorities" who are unfamiliar with these reports or with acupuncture's demonstrated clinical effectiveness still maintain that it is nothing more than hypnosis. When I was first exposed to acupuncture, I, too, was very skeptical, believing that its pain-alleviating properties probably represented nothing more than an effective use of hypnotic or suggestive procedures. My introduction to acupuncture occurred in the late 1960s, years before former Secretary of State Henry Kissinger "rediscovered" China in 1972. One afternoon, at the urging of two adventurous friends, I agreed to observe the treatment of several patients in the office of Master Ju Gim Shek, an acupuncturist practicing very quietly in the Chinatown community of Los Angeles. If Master Ju is at all successful, I reasoned, it must be because his patients are a select group. After all, only those people who already believe that acupuncture will help would bother to search Chinatown for an acupuncturist. In Southern California, it's easy to find people who believe in pyramids, flying saucers, astral traveling, exotic drugs, wife-swapping, and faith healing—so why not acupuncture? The disbelievers, I assumed, would never end up in Master Ju's office.

I also reasoned that the aura and mystique of the Orient could be mobilized to create positive expectations in pain patients, even when the best Western doctors had reached a verdict of "hopeless." This is what is called the "placebo effect." Also, I recognized that well-known phenomena such as distraction and counterirritation could explain why placing needles into an area of the body distant from the painful area might give relief. If your hand hurts and needles are put into your back, ears, and feet, now your back, ears, and feet hurt and you forget about your hand, at least temporarily.

One of the first patients I saw Master Ju treat was a man in his late sixties who had been afflicted with severe osteoarthritis in both hands. His knuckles were swollen to the size of walnuts, and he complained of such agonizing pain that it was difficult even to examine him. Master Ju went to work, placing needles not only in the patient's hands, but also in his back, ears, and feet. The specific locations didn't seem to be related to the hands in any neurological manner.

About two minutes after the last needle had been inserted, the man began to move his fingers slowly. His eyes opened wide as he exclaimed, "My God, the pain is gone! It's a miracle!" With tears streaming down his cheeks, he began to enthusiastically thank Master Ju, his "angel of mercy."

I smiled.

"Tell me, how do those needles in your back, ears, and feet feel?" I asked.

"Why, I don't feel them at all!" the patient exclaimed through his tears. "I feel wonderful all over! This is the first time in fifteen years that I don't have pain!"

I was stunned. This guy must be a nut, I thought to myself. He's crazy. He still has pain; he just *thinks* he doesn't have pain.

But later that day, I reflected back upon the dramatic event I had witnessed. If that same patient had been treated for osteoarthritis by a Western doctor, he would have been told, "Get the largest jar of aspirin you can find and eat one every four hours"; or worse, "Nothing can be done; you'll just have to learn to live with it." Master Ju's acupuncture treatment made the patient think he no longer had pain. What more could Western medicine hope to offer such a patient?

If the results were due solely to hypnosis or suggestion, acupuncture was certainly the fastest and most effective form of hypnosis I'd ever seen. Patient after patient seemed to respond miraculously to Master Ju's needles, and soon my interest deepened. Over the next several years, I conducted many research studies that explored the physiological nature of the acupuncture points, the use of acupuncture as a surgical anesthetic, and the effectiveness of acupuncture in treating pain, bronchial asthma, obesity, cigarette smoking, sensorineural hearing loss, and drug addiction (see articles listed in the reference notes).

Clearly, something more than hypnosis was involved, for when careful controls were used, subjects responded quite differently to stimulation of real acupuncture points as opposed to sham (placebo) points, even when both the acupuncturist and the subject did not know how the points differed. How could "hypnosis" explain these findings?

In addition, acupuncture was effective in treating animals as well as humans. Long before most Americans had even heard of acupuncture, I met a young veterinarian named Richard Glassberg, who had also become interested in the subject. While collecting all the literature I could find, I had come across some very ancient charts showing the location of acupuncture points in donkeys, cows, and horses. When I showed them to Dr. Glassberg, he agreed to contact Alice DeGroot, a highly respected veterinarian who worked with thoroughbreds, to ask if we could use her horses as subjects. Because thoroughbreds are such valuable animals, I was skeptical about her cooperation. Dr. Glassberg later told me that the conversation went something like this:

Glassberg: Alice, I've met somebody from UCLA who's interested in acupuncture. We'd like to come out and give it a try on your horses.
DeGroot: Sure, come on out.
Glassberg: Alice, perhaps you didn't understand. I said we'd like to do some acupuncture on your horses.
DeGroot: Sure, come out anytime. The last nut who was here tried to treat laminitis [inflammation of the hoof] by playing Tchaikovsky through a rectal probe!

Though initially skeptical, Dr. DeGroot discovered that acupuncture significantly helped a variety of animal problems previously thought to be "hopeless." As a result, the National Association of Veterinary Acupuncture was established to train veterinarians in the use of acupuncture. Many carefully conducted studies have now been published in respected veterinary journals, and it seems unlikely that "hypnosis" can explain them all.

The debate may continue for years over precisely how and why acupuncture works. But for you—the patient with pain—does it really matter? Many of my own patients tell me that they frankly aren't interested in an explanation of the phenomenon. They're just delighted that they finally have relief from their discomfort. To them, that's all that's important. No one fully understands how aspirin, morphine,

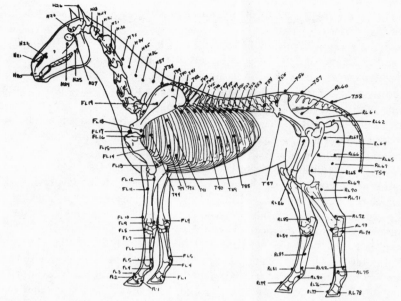

Fig. 12 *Chart showing acupuncture points on the horse.* (Courtesy of the National Association for Veterinary Acupuncture)

physical therapy, or hypnosis work either, but we use them because they help to alleviate pain. The same should be true for acupuncture.

Certainly, acupuncture is no panacea. But often, when other types of therapy have failed, acupuncture can help. On the basis of my experience with it over the last eight years, I have found it particularly effective in treating a variety of chronic pain problems, including:

—Musculoskeletal pain (for example, low back, neck and shoulder, hip, and knee pain). As a rough guideline, areas close to the trunk seem to respond better than those in the extremities.

—Osteoarthritis localized in specific joints. (Rheumatoid arthritis, a systemic illness affecting the entire body, does not appear to respond as well.)

—Muscle contraction and migraine headaches. (There is no conclusive data yet available as to its effectiveness in treating allergic headaches.)

—Various neuralgias (e.g., trigeminal neuralgia, postherpetic neuralgia, etc.) and pain related to nerve injury.

Acupuncture may also be effective in treating psychological as well as physical pain. I have cared for many patients suffering from anxiety and severe depression, some of whom have been helped by acupuncture when accompanied by appropriate psychotherapeutic care.

One of my patients was a psychotherapist named Sharon. I first treated her several years ago when, at age thirty-five, she found herself very despondent over the breakup of a relationship which she was convinced was her last chance for marriage.

In our first session together, I learned that Sharon had been chronically depressed since childhood. She had even attempted suicide three times, desperately trying to escape her unhappiness. Although Sharon had received extensive psychotherapeutic help throughout her life, plus many different types of drugs, several hospitalizations, and even electroshock therapy, nothing seemed to help. She was finally referred to me by a psychiatrist who thought that maybe, just maybe, acupuncture might improve her state of mind.

Sharon herself told me that she "couldn't care less." As she said, "I'm a psychotherapist myself, and I've read up on my condition. Everything's been tried and I don't think anything else can help me."

Then she added, "Do what you want. But you're wasting your time. Life just isn't worth it anymore, not one bit."

Frankly, I was doubtful whether I could help Sharon either. But I decided to try. I utilized the acupuncture points that the Chinese claim are helpful for "excessive sadness." Amazingly, she responded almost immediately, showing not just subjective changes, but many functional changes as well, like improved sleep and appetite, and increased motivation to deal with her problem. According to her psychiatrist, the change was unprecedented.

How can this transformation be explained? Some people might say that acupuncture gave Sharon an excuse to get better, or perhaps that she "spontaneously remitted." But I tend to think that the acupuncture had a direct physiological effect on her nervous and endocrine systems.

Sharon is still one of my patients. I've treated her five additional times with acupuncture over the past five years, when small bouts of depression have recurred. But in general, she's leading a very productive life and has her own private practice in Northern California. Overall, she's doing just fine.

Since that initial attempt at treating depression with acupuncture, I have treated approximately twenty-five severely depressed patients in a similar manner. Almost all of them have shown at least some degree of improvement. But the recovery has been short-lasting unless the acupuncture was accompanied by appropriate psychotherapeutic care.

Although acupuncture is helpful in the treatment of a variety of chronic pain problems, it is still far from qualifying as the "ideal analgesic" discussed at the beginning of this chapter. Foremost among the failings of acupuncture are the following:

—Acupuncture is not readily available in most parts of the country. Although there might be many people in your community sticking needles into people, very few may be formally trained and experienced in traditional acupuncture. Those who are just poking needles into the body may be doing physical therapy, but acupuncture is much more than that. For example, if your lower back hurts, and if a therapist is placing needles only into the area of your discomfort, they're not doing traditional acupuncture. But if the needles are being placed behind your knee or by your ankle, then you are probably being properly treated.

—Acupuncture is an invasive technique. It involves inserting a foreign object into the body, and for that reason, the possibility of infection or nerve, vessel, or organ damage, though minimal, always exists.

—You need a trained therapist to administer acupuncture. It is not a procedure that can be self-administered by the patient. Thus, if you hurt at 2:00 A.M., it's unlikely that you'll find an acupuncturist who will treat you at that time.

—Acupuncture therapy can be expensive. Depending on the practitioner, fees can range from $25 to $75 per treatment. Thus, if you were to undergo a typical therapeutic sequence—a consultation and eight to twelve treatments—the cost would be from $200 to as much as $900. Although Medicare does not yet cover acupuncture expenses, many private insurance companies will reimburse their policyholders in part or in full for this therapy.

Despite these shortcomings, acupuncture is an extremely safe technique when administered by a skillful, trained professional. At UCLA, after tens of thousands of acupuncture treatments, there has not been a single case of infection, broken needle, or nerve or organ damage.

However, it is essential to find a competent therapist. So many poorly trained acupuncturists have surfaced in recent years that an editor for the *Washington Star* once coined his own description of them—"quackupuncturists." *Newsweek* magazine recently reported a $1650 correspondence course in acupuncture, which, according to the magazine, attracted two hundred students. Many states now certify acupuncturists, and if possible, you should try to find a practitioner with this status. I would also suggest that you contact your local medical association, hospital, or medical school for a referral. If you have friends who have been helped by acupuncture treatment, you might find a competent therapist through their recommendation.

Until the American Medical Association reverses its opposition to acupuncture and begins encouraging medical schools to teach it, it may not be easy for you to find a competent therapist. It seems ludicrous to me that this therapeutic system, which has been in continuous use for thousands of years, is still viewed with such disdain by the medical establishment. But that is the cold, sad fact. In too many cities across the country, an individual seeking professional acupuncture treatment tragically has nowhere to turn.

My own feeling is that in ten to fifteen years, acupuncture will become an accepted, commonly utilized medical modality. Gradually, respected physicians are being won over. When surgeon Sam Rosen, M.D., emeritus professor at Mount Sinai School of Medicine in New York City, returned from a visit to China, he wrote a glowing article about the ancient art of acupuncture in *The New York Times* titled "I Have Seen the Past and It Works." As Rosen said, "We had to make a choice between what we thought and what we saw, and we had to stay with what we saw."

One last note of interest. Often, when a trial of acupuncture proves helpful, I will teach my patients how to massage their own acupuncture points so that they can assume greater responsibility for their own care. Although there are several systems of "acupressure," all are based on the same system of points. *Shiatsu* (which literally means "finger pressure") is a Japanese acupressure-massage technique in which the thumbs are used to apply deep stimulation to points along the traditional acupuncture meridians. It often produces profound muscle relaxation, coupled with a feeling of being "energized."

Do-In ("The Soft Way") has been popularized by Jacques de Langre, and involves gentle rubbing, pressing, and pounding techniques. *Jin Shin Do* ("The Way of the Compassionate Spirit") is derived from traditional Oriental practices and also involves meditative and breathing exercises. The therapist applies deep pressure to one or more of thirty basic acupuncture points until tension is "released," and replaced by a pleasurable sensation. Tsubo Therapy ("Acupoint Therapy") is a similar acupressure technique which is widely used in Japan for treating chronic pain and other problems.

In my opinion, nearly every person in pain can significantly benefit by learning a few simple acupressure techniques. When you hurt at 2 A.M., pressing the appropriate acupuncture points can often provide immediate relief. Several books on acupressure are listed in the reference notes. Shouldn't you consider giving it a try?

Hypnosis

Have you ever been hypnotized? Yes or no?

You probably answered no. Most people do, because they have a misconception of what hypnosis is all about. For instance, when someone mentions hypnosis, do you immediately think of the comic book advertisements you read when you were a kid, showing a hypnotist emitting magical waves from his fingertips, putting a mysterious spell over a beautiful girl? Or do you think of the stage hypnotists who can seemingly make their subjects do just about anything ("Whenever I tug my right earlobe, you will cluck like a chicken")?

Most people know very little about hypnosis. In essence, hypnosis is a state of attentive, responsive concentration in which there is a heightened degree of suggestibility. Contrary to popular belief, it is not sleep. In fact, it is exactly the opposite of sleep. You are awake, very alert, with your attention so highly focused that minor distractions are minimized.

Let's see how attentive you are right now. At the count of three, I want you to raise your right hand. OK . . . one, two, three—raise your right hand. Come on. Really do it as you read this. Raise your right hand high up in the air. . . .

OK, now raise your right arm. . . .

What's that? You say that you had already raised your right arm? So does everyone else. Everyone, that is, except those who are hypnotized when the commands are given. Under hypnosis, your attention would have been so focused that, when asked to raise your right hand, your arm would have remained stationary as only your hand flipped up.

Although you are probably not under hypnosis now, hardly a day goes by when you fail to enter a type of hypnotic state. For instance, how about when you drive a car? When you are paying close attention to the road, are you even aware of all your activities at the time—like shifting gears, or applying pressure to the brake and gas pedals?

Or think back to the last time you used a typewriter. As your attention was focused on the copy in front of you, were you aware of depressing one typewriter key after another? Probably not. That was a state of hypnosis, too.

Next time you go to a movie theater, sit near the front. During a particularly dramatic moment of the film, turn around and look at the people near you. They'll probably be sitting with their mouths open and their eyes intensely riveted to the action on the screen. Try talking to the person sitting next to you—"Would you like some buttered popcorn?"— and he may not even hear you. Although *you* may think he's in the audience, he doesn't. He's up on that screen, as much a part of the movie as the actors themselves. Not until those final credits have been run, when he licks his lips and takes a deep breath, does his own identity return. Yes, he had been hypnotized, and was highly suggestible to the actions in the movie.

What does all this mean to the person with pain? If you have severe headaches, or lower back pain, or terrible aches in your shoulder, what can hypnosis do for you? Perhaps quite a lot. Although medical hypnosis is still in its infancy, a variety of hypnotic techniques have been used effectively in treating pain.

For instance, while in a state of hypnosis, a patient can be given the suggestions that "sensations typically interpreted as painful will now be experienced in a different, more positive way . . . perhaps as warm, tingly, itchy, or tickly . . . whatever way is most comfortable for you." This technique is called "symptom suppression." And because the patient is in a state of focused attention and quite suggestible, he is highly receptive to the possibility that the part of his body that once felt "painful" now feels reasonably comfortable and relaxed. As J. A. Hadfield said, "Suggestion does not consist of making an individual believe what is not true; suggestion consists of making something come true by making a person believe in its possibility."

Of course, symptom suppression is not a "cure" for the pain problem. After all, it doesn't deal with the cause of the pain, nor the psychological trauma that may be associated with it. But there are still at least two reasons why I have found it useful for some of my patients:

—Symptom suppression takes the edge off the pain. When an individual is in agonizing discomfort, it's difficult, if not impossible, for him to gain insight into his pain problem. But if some degree of relief can be provided, he may then be able to detach himself enough from his pain to try to understand its causes and effects.

—As with other pain-management techniques, symptom suppression can sometimes be used to prove to a patient that it is possible for his pain to be controlled. Once he no longer feels completely helpless and hopeless, he can then begin to approach his pain problem with a more positive attitude.

"Symptom substitution" is another hypnotic technique that has been applied successfully with chronic pain patients. While not necessarily relieving pain, it involves moving that discomfort from one area of the body where it has been incapacitating to another where it is less disruptive. For instance, when you feel a severe headache coming on, wouldn't you rather experience that intense pain in your little finger instead of your head? You're not asking your nervous system to stop experiencing pain or to mask the message it may be trying to communicate. The pain is still there, but it has moved to a part of the body where you can work better to overcome it.

One of my patients, a forty-five-year-old executive named Henry, suffered from severe back pain, but through symptom substitution, he was able to move that pain from his back down to the bottoms of his feet. The displaced pain was equal in intensity to what he had experienced in his back. But he found that when the discomfort was located in his feet, life was significantly more bearable.

Henry continued to work with symptom substitution techniques, and eventually he was able to rid himself completely of his pain whenever it recurred by "walking it away." With the discomfort focused in his feet, he imagined the pain leaving his body and scattering on the ground as he walked along. Weeks earlier, when his back ached, he usually had to lie down for a while. He couldn't stand, much less walk. But with this new technique, whenever his back hurt, he transferred that pain to his feet, walked a block or two, and felt much better.

The advantages of symptom substitution are similar to those of symptom suppression. It makes the pain more tolerable, thus allowing the patient to deal with it more effectively, and helps relieve the oppressive feeling of helplessness and hopelessness. Once an individual recognizes that he can move his pain from, say, his head to his little finger or his big toe, he gains a profoundly clear sense of the extent to which he can control his own experiences.

I have also used a hypnotic technique called "time distortion" with pain patients. Think about your own problem for a moment: Do the times of excruciating discomfort seem to drag on forever, while the periods when you're relatively pain-free seem very fleeting? Well, what if you could reverse that situation? What if the terribly painful times could be made to seem like they lasted for only a moment? And what if your times of comfort could appear to last forever?

Sound too good to be true? Well, it's possible using time-distortion hypnosis. Time is a relative phenomenon. As Einstein once said, in explaining his theory of relativity, "When you sit with a nice girl for two hours, it seems like a minute; but when you sit on a hot stove for a minute, it seems like two hours. That's relativity!"

You can be hypnotized to experience time as being much slower or faster than it is objectively. This technique has been used successfully with terminal cancer patients for whom narcotics no longer provided relief. Under hypnosis, their painful times flash by, so that hours seem like seconds; when they feel comfortable, however, the time moves so slowly that seconds seem like hours.

No matter what hypnotic technique is used, one feature they all have in common is anxiety reduction. It is well known that for most chronic pain patients, a reduction of anxiety usually eases the level of pain. For some terminal cancer patients, the anxiety-reducing properties of hypnosis have been more effective in controlling discomfort than even morphine.

Not only can pain patients achieve a remarkable degree of comfort and relaxation under hypnosis, but with the assistance of posthypnotic suggestions, they can continue to feel that way long after the session is over. While you were under hypnosis, if your hypnotherapist were to tell you, "Every day in every way, you will feel better and better," you may just find your pain becoming more and more bearable.

"Age regression" is also possible under hypnosis, and it can often be an indispensable therapeutic tool. Regression techniques can help an individual arrive at the basic causes of his pain by putting him in touch with earlier traumatic events that may have been repressed or forgotten.

Very often, when a person's chronic pain is the outgrowth of an accident or injury, his ongoing discomfort may be primarily a reflection of the fears, anxieties, and threats of bodily damage that accompanied the original trauma. By hypnotically regressing the individual back to the time of the incident, and thus allowing him finally to confront and deal with the situation, the pain can often be significantly eased.

I recall a forty-four-year-old patient named Stanley, who began experiencing intense neck pain following a minor whiplash injury. He was subjected to dozens of tests, including brain scans, EMGs and myelograms, but they were all negative. He was treated with nerve blocks, but his pain remained. His personal physicians concluded that there was simply nothing physically wrong with him, despite his excruciating discomfort.

When Stanley arrived at the UCLA Pain Control Unit, he could barely move his neck in any direction without experiencing agonizing pain. While taking a routine medical history, I asked him if he had ever had neck problems earlier in his life. He replied, "I vaguely remember injuring my neck when I was a kid. But I can't really remember too much about what exactly happened."

Under hypnosis, Stanley's memory improved dramatically. He recalled injuring his neck in a fall at age six, which led to endless hospital tests, weeks of painful traction, a cumbersome neck brace that he had to wear, and deep concern on the part of his parents. He also remembered how his schoolmates ridiculed him for wearing a brace. In short, it was an extremely traumatic childhood event that he had effectively repressed. But when he reexperienced a problem with his neck later in life, his repressed fears resurfaced, causing his current pain problem.

While he was under hypnosis, I suggested to Stanley that although his childhood injury had been serious, the present one was not. The extensive diagnostic tests indicated that nothing was physically wrong with him. His current pain was primarily a reflection of the misery caused by the incident early in his life. When he emerged from the hypnotic state, he said, "I feel like a tremendous weight has been taken off my shoulders; my neck feels incredibly better now." More and more, I find that childhood experiences—often forgotten on a conscious level—play a crucially important role in pain problems that develop later in life.

There are other applications of hypnosis, some of which will be discussed later in this book. For now, just be aware that hypnosis may be helpful in dealing with your own pain experience—if you are hypnotizable. Almost everyone can be hypnotized, although some people respond to it much more easily than others.

If you're willing to try a simple exercise, you may receive a good indication of how susceptible you are to hypnosis. In this exercise, we will use a hypnotic technique to see if we can briefly stick your hands together using "magnetic glue." Shall we try?

Sit comfortably in a chair and take a few moments to let yourself relax as much as possible.

Pay careful attention to your breathing. Inhale . . . exhale . . . inhale . . . exhale. Let your breathing move more slowly and rhythmically, going deep down in your abdomen. Slowly . . . comfortably . . .

Now, I'm going to give you a chance to see how hypnotizable you are. As you continue to be aware of your breathing, raise your arms and extend them out in front of you, parallel to the floor. Your palms should face upward. . . .

Soon, you may be surprised to notice a tingling sensation developing in the center of your palms—or even at the tips of your fingers. Perhaps this sensation is stingy or itchy. Or maybe your hands feel numb. Just let it happen. . . . This is a good way to prepare yourself to receive "magnetic glue." . . .

For the purpose of this exercise, the ink on the pages of this book has been "magnetized." So place your hands briefly on the pages, and then raise them into the same position as before, palms upward. Can you feel the magnetic glue starting to work on your hands? . . . Your palms might really be tingling . . . or they might feel warm. . . . However you experience it is fine.

Magnetic glue works for only a short period of time, so to be certain that you fully experience its effects, lock your elbows, keeping your arms straight out in front of you. Now turn your hands so that the palms face each other. Can you sense a magnetic feeling between your hands? Now bring your palms together and interlock your fingers, pressing as hard as you can to let the glue set.

As you continue applying this pressure, you may notice a warm, sticky feeling developing in your hands. Your fingers may have become quite rigid and immovable. But that's fine. . . . The magnetic glue only lasts a very short period of time. . . .

Well, if you have been squeezing together very hard, I think the glue has probably set by now. Why not see how firmly set it is by gently trying to pull your hands apart? Let's see how well the glue has affixed them together.

You may be surprised to see how much trouble you have separating them. The glue seems to have really worked. . . . But don't worry. Releasing the magnetic glue is simple. In fact, it will release by itself in a few seconds. But if you'd like to break it even before then, simply bend your elbows so your hands come in toward your chest, and relax your fingers. As you do so, the glue will just drain away, and you will be very easily able to pull your hands apart. Briskly rub your hands together, and they will immediately return as they were before the exercise began.

Now are you willing to say you've never been hypnotized? If the magnetic glue worked for you, you are probably an excellent candidate for medical hypnosis.

Hypnosis has progressed considerably since the eighteenth century, when Western scientists first began to accept its therapeutic possibilities.

Friedrich Anton Mesmer, an Austrian physician, hypothesized that all men were living magnets, and that some people ("magnetic animals") were able to affect the magnetic fluids of others. Sick people suffering from "an imbalance of magnetic fluid" were thought by Mesmer to be susceptible to help from these "magnetic animals." From this point of view, if "magnetic glue" worked for you, you were quite literally "mesmerized."

For a time, Mesmer treated ill people from all over Europe in his Paris clinic. He wore flowing silk robes, and held an iron wand in his hand as he cared for patients. But he was eventually castigated by a royal commission in 1784. Mesmer left France and died in obscurity in Switzerland.

"Mesmerism" was a precursor of hypnotism. Others borrowed some of his ideas, adapted them, and eventually a more sophisticated approach to the technique surfaced in the nineteenth century. Still, until 1958, hypnosis did not have the sanction of the American Medical Association as a subject to be taught in U.S. medical schools. Now, more and more medical practitioners have begun to recognize its therapeutic value.

If you're interested in finding out whether hypnosis can help alleviate your pain problem, be sure that you see a well-trained, professional hypnotherapist. You may end up paying $50 to $60 per session, but it's worth it, for hypnosis in the hands of amateurs can be dangerous. If hypnosis is used inappropriately, the following problems could possibly occur:

—Hypnosis could lead to "traumatic insight"—that is, the sudden recollection of earlier traumatic events that the patient is unable to deal with on a conscious level. If an individual is in a prepsychotic state, the inappropriate use of hypnosis could break down his safeguards and defenses, thereby triggering a full-blown psychosis.

—While hypnosis can mask the symptoms of an ailment, it usually does not affect the underlying cause. Assuming that pain is a message that something is wrong, the hypnotic suppression of painful symptoms may cause the patient to ignore seeking appropriate help for the basic problem. To my knowledge, there is no evidence in the literature to support this possibility, but it should be kept in mind. Be sure you have been thoroughly evaluated by an appropriate health professional before using *any* symptom-suppression technique for severe pain.

—When age-regression techniques are used, some patients react with panic. If, for example, a person is regressed back to the time of an automobile accident, he can reexperience the horror and terror of it all over again. Thus, regressive techniques must be used carefully, and if a panic situation arises, competent psychotherapeutic support may be essential.

—If conflicting or inappropriate posthypnotic suggestions are given, they can produce many disturbing effects, including anxiety, agitation, or even increased physical discomfort. Even the most innocent suggestions can have traumatic consequences if, unknown to the therapist, they are associated with earlier traumatic events.

—When hypnosis is effective, the patient may credit the hypnotherapist for the improvement, and become excessively dependent upon him for solving the problems associated with pain. A patient must be made aware that all hypnosis is essentially self-hypnosis, and that his improvement is due to his own actions and responses, not the therapist's. In my opinion, a patient's best interest is served when he assumes responsibility for his own care, rather than being continually dependent on a therapist.

Factors such as these keep hypnosis from qualifying as the "ideal analgesic" defined earlier in the chapter. Still, in the hands of a well-trained, experienced hypnotherapist, it can be one of the most useful, safe, and successful modalities available for treatment of chronic pain.

Guided Imagery

Many of the most successful hypnotic procedures—including symptom suppression and age regression—can be utilized more easily with the help of another technique called guided imagery. By creating and utilizing personalized mental images, guided imagery enables an individual to make contact with the deepest levels of his body, psyche, and soul. Images are the language of the unconscious mind, and when properly programmed, they are able to mobilize, to a remarkable degree, the body's intrinsic ability to heal itself.

Guided imagery does not require the formal, trancelike state characteristic of hypnosis to produce heightened suggestibility and its ensuing benefits. All that's needed is for the individual to become as relaxed and comfortable as possible. Thus, guided imagery is available to a larger number of people, since it can be used on people who tend to be resistant to hypnosis.

Although guided imagery is a newer technique than hypnosis, I believe that both modalities operate through a similar mechanism—that is, guided imagery is really just a highly permissive, hypnotic procedure, which utilizes the patient's images as the focus of its activity. Or conversely, hypnosis is just a highly authoritative guided imagery procedure, which utilizes the therapist's suggestions as the focus of its activity. Pay your money, and take your choice.

Despite guided imagery's recent emergence as a therapeutic tool, the importance of images and symbols has been known through the ages. The roots of this new technique may date back to the ancient Hebrew mystics, who recognized the relationship of images to events that went beyond normal experience. In more recent times, psychotherapists have utilized a variety of imagery techniques to tap the content of the subconscious mind. For example, Hermann Rorschach, the Swiss psychiatrist, used standardized ink-blot designs to assess the psychological relevance of various images and emotions to his patients' mental states.

Freud developed a technique he called "free association" as a way of reading the unconscious. He believed that the unconscious was the storehouse of instinctual and forbidden desires and fears that were outside of conscious awareness, and through the images produced in free association, much of this rich information could be evaluated.

Carl Jung contended that the unconscious held more than just our forbidden desires and fears, but also was the repository of our deepest, most positive hopes for fulfillment and self-actualization. He developed several innovative imagery techniques designed to explore these aspects of the unconscious.

Most recently, O. Carl Simonton, M.D., and Stephanie Matthews-Simonton have used guided imagery as an adjunct to conventional methods of treating cancer. As one aspect of their program, they teach their patients to imagine their white blood cells attacking and destroying their malignancies. Irving Oyle, D.O., author of *The Healing Mind,* utilizes a variety of guided imagery techniques to treat many different kinds of medical problems. He believes that we are normally in contact with only 10 percent of our brain, and that guided imagery is a way to find out what the other 90 percent thinks about.

As a growing number of therapists acknowledge the potential benefits of guided imagery, new techniques are constantly being developed. One basic approach involves having the patient draw a symbolic picture of his or her ailment (which is what I asked you to do in Exercise Five). Such a picture can provide a more comprehensive perspective of the illness or pain than any verbal description can. Compare your picture with one of how your body might look if it were healed and healthy. Guided imagery can then be used to try to change your reality from the "ill" image to the "healthy" one.

One of my patients visualized her facial pain as her mouth "being on fire." With this image in mind, I asked her to devise ways to put out the flames. The innovative ways available for extinguishing a fire are limited only by the patient's imagination, and she eventually began visualizing herself absorbing those flames into cool, floating clouds of imaginary water. As she continued to practice this guided imagery exercise, her pain gradually subsided.

In Chapter 10, I'll teach you several guided imagery techniques which are designed to help you deal more effectively with your own personal pain problem. One of the most powerful approaches I utilize involves the creation of an "adviser," a "counselor," an "inner doctor," or a "spirit guide." During a session of guided imagery, the patient is taught to relax, and then is instructed on how to locate an imaginary living creature in his unconscious, who thereafter serves as his adviser. These advisers have taken the form of everything from dogs and frogs to religious figures— but, of course, they are just a reflection of the person who is creating the image.

By definition, the adviser has access to the entire realm of our unconscious—that "90 percent of the brain" normally outside our awareness. Our unconscious is a valuable storehouse of insights, suggestions, and desires, and through regular communication with our advisers, critically important information about our inner world often emerges. Advisers frequently provide insights into past experiences that may have contributed to pain. They can offer advice on specific ways to relieve discomfort, and sometimes they can even alleviate pain completely in an instant.

One of my patients, a fifty-two-year-old cardiologist named John, was suffering from excruciating low back pain following treatment for rectal cancer. Although surgery and radiation therapy had apparently eradicated the cancer, the pain that remained in its aftermath was "unbearable." Because the area had been so heavily irradiated, neither repeated nerve blocks nor further surgery could be used to help relieve his terrible discomfort, and he had long ago developed tolerance to his pain medications.

When John came to the UCLA Pain Control Unit, he had already narrowed down his personal alternatives to three: (a) successful treatment at the Pain Control Unit, (b) voluntary commitment to a mental institution, or (c) suicide.

John was convinced that under no circumstances could he continue to live with pain and at the same time keep his sanity.

In reviewing his medical records, I noticed that during a psychiatric workup, John had described his pain as "a dog chewing on my spine." This image was so vivid that I suggested we make contact with the dog, using guided imagery. With his training in traditional medicine, he thought the idea was silly, but he was willing to give it a try. (In Chapter 11, I'll describe the techniques I use to help establish such contact.)

In John's case, our goal was to get the dog to stop chewing on his spine. Over the next few sessions, the dog began to reveal critically important information. According to the dog, John had never wanted to be a doctor—his own career choice was architecture—but he had been pressured into medical school by his mother. Consequently, he felt resentment not only toward his mother, but also toward his patients and colleagues. The dog suggested that this hostility had in turn contributed to the development of his cancer and to the subsequent pain problem as well.

The dog told John, "You're a damn good doctor. It may not be the career you wanted, but it's time you recognized how good you are at what you do. When you stop being so resentful and start accepting yourself, I'll stop chewing on your spine." These insights were accompanied by an immediate alleviation of the pain, and in only a few weeks' time, John became a new person as his pain progressively subsided.

No one really fully understands the physiological basis of how guided imagery works. My own theory is that part of the answer may lie in the two fundamentally different ways the nervous system communicates with itself. One higher-order communication system uses verbal language. This system is your "conscious mind," that little voice in your head that talks to you constantly. It has control over your *somatic* nervous system, the part of your nervous system that controls your muscles and mediates voluntary movement.

If you'd like a quick demonstration of how this particular part of your nervous system works, try the following:

First, raise your arm high into the air. Go ahead. Do it right now. Raise your arm as high as you can.

Now, *how* did you do that? . . . Did you have to tell your body how to go about raising your arm? Did you have to say, "Deltoids—contract! Latissimus dorsi—relax!"?

No, your body knew exactly what to do. When your mind gives certain verbal commands—"I'm going to raise my arm"—you just do it. Verbal commands or thoughts have immediate access to functions controlled by your somatic nervous system.

Now that you've raised your arm, tell your body to raise your blood pressure. Go ahead. Raise your blood pressure.

What's that? You're not having much success? Well, it worked when you raised your arm, didn't it? Then why can't you raise your blood pressure? My explanation is that the autonomic nervous system, the part of your nervous system which regulates your blood pressure, doesn't respond to the same language you used to raise your arm. To raise your blood pressure, a second type of communication system is involved—one that uses the language of imagery.

Do you want to see how easy it is to use imagery to raise your blood pressure? Just try the following exercise. *(Note:* if you already have high blood pressure, your nervous system apparently knows too well how to raise your blood pressure; don't give it further encouragement here!):

Sitting quietly and comfortably in a chair, imagine finding yourself in the deepest, darkest woods of Africa, alone on a cold, wet night, naked and shivering. . . . You don't know how you got there or what you're doing there. But you're lost and terribly frightened. . . .

Then, suddenly, you realize that you're not alone! Off in the distance, you hear a crashing, pounding noise that is quickly becoming louder and louder. . . . closer and closer. Your heart begins to beat faster, and as the sounds become even louder, you panic and begin to run. . . . You run slowly at first, but then desperately faster as this "thing" in the woods comes even closer. And closer still.

It is now clear that this beast is chasing *you*. As you race through the forest, faster and faster, with the brush tearing at your flesh, the beast is coming closer and closer, until you can feel its hot breath burning down on the back of your neck. . . . As it reaches out to grab you, you scream more loudly than you ever have in your life. . . .

Well, what happened? If you really were able to involve yourself in the scene described above, your mind almost certainly caused your blood pressure to rise. How did it do so? In the same way you were able to raise your arm—by having an appropriate thought. But in this case, the language you used was not one of words but images. Imagery is the way we access what was once called the "involuntary" *(autonomic)* nervous system. This term is really incorrect, for when the proper language is used, many of the functions regulated by the autonomic nervous system (including heart rate, blood pressure, skin temperature, and so forth) *can* be voluntarily controlled. Sexual arousal, for example, is much more easily affected by your imagination than by any attempt to control it through verbal commands.

The language of imagery may be the most fundamental way that animals communicate with themselves and with each other. Man, on the other hand, relies on a language of words, which in many ways overshadows his more primitive, instinctual ability to protect himself against illness and danger. Verbal language is thus a curse as well as a blessing, for although it has helped us to survive in the outside world, it has disconnected us from the powerful systems of self-control and self-healing that lie within.

If you hurt and are unable to help yourself, perhaps you are speaking the wrong language to your body. Commands like, "Headache, go away!" or "Arthritis, go away!" have probably done little to help. But if you can learn to use your imagination to access the nonverbal part of your nervous system, there is a great deal more you can do to stop hurting.

I always encourage my patients to describe their pain as symbolically as possible, using vivid images that they'll later be able to work with. But it's usually only after lengthy prompting and trial and error that they understand how to communicate in images rather than in the precise, verbal language to which they're accustomed. I recall a dialogue I recently had with Sandy, a thirty-five-year-old woman with back pain. She had seen at least three dozen doctors, and although she had received a wide variety of drugs, nerve blocks, and several laminectomies, all she had to show for it was increased pain, surgical scars, and a sophisticated medical understanding of her problem.

Doctor: How do you see your discomfort?
Sandy: Well, I've got spinal fusions at L2-L3 and L3-L4, and I have these radiating dysesthesias that . . .
Doctor: Wait, wait. I know all that. But tell me how you *see* your discomfort. How do you experience it? What does it *feel* like?
Sandy: Well . . . it feels like there is this charcoal broiler filled with burning hot coals placed up against my back that is searing the flesh and muscle away.

Now, that's a picture that can be worked with. Sandy can say from now until forever, "Radiating dysesthesias—go away!" but it probably won't communicate any meaningful message to her autonomic nervous system. However, in a relaxed state, she might imagine a cool, refreshing mountain stream, flowing gently through a magnificent wooded forest. As she sees herself carefully enter the water, she might experience the shock of the water on the hot charcoal broiler, and as the burning coals suddenly cool, she might sense the eruption of steam vapor from her back. As the entire back area gradually cools down in Sandy's imagination, her discomfort may cool down as well.

Sound farfetched? It did to me, too, at least initially. But this technique helped Sandy to stop hurting for the first time, and I have seen the proper application of imagery work effectively for hundreds of other pain patients as well.

Think for a moment of how you envision your problem. Although a positive picture may significantly facilitate the healing process, most pain patients use self-imagery to their detriment. For instance, if you see yourself as a helpless, hopeless victim of an incurable illness, that kind of negative image tells your nervous system, "Don't even try to get me better."

Or how about the patient so distraught by pain that he sees his own body as an enemy. Each time his pain flares up, he wants to cut it out, kill it, exterminate it, destroy it. When you have an image of destroying a part of your own body, your nervous system may react accordingly. But if you see your area of discomfort becoming healed and regenerated, perhaps a "spontaneous remission" can occur.

In my experience, guided imagery has proven to be a safe and effective means of reprogramming the nervous system to maximize self-healing. It has some of the same advantages as hypnosis, but it is easier and safer to use in many ways. For example, when the adviser technique is properly employed, the problem of traumatic insight is easily avoided. If there is danger in breaking down a particular safeguard or defense, the adviser will usually refuse to pursue the matter until the patient is able to deal with it more effectively.

One of my patients, a young woman named Susan, suffered from chronic shoulder pain that appeared to be related to a traumatic event that had occurred in her life. Using guided imagery, she found an adviser—an owl named Jerry. During one of our sessions, I began talking with Jerry through Susan, who reported his responses:

Doctor:	Jerry, do you know the details of the incident that happened to Susan many years ago?
Jerry:	Of course.
Doctor:	Would you be willing to tell her about it?
Jerry:	No.
Doctor:	Why not?
Jerry:	I don't think she's ready to hear it yet.
Doctor:	What does she have to do to be ready?
Jerry:	First, she has to learn to accept herself and to love herself more.

It's my belief that, when properly utilized, advisers will never tell people something they're not psychologically equipped to handle. Even more important, advisers can often tell exactly what must first be done in order to make this information safely available.

My experience with guided imagery also indicates that, unlike hypnosis, it tends to decrease dependency on the therapist. After all, it is clearly the adviser, not the therapist, who is providing the insights that facilitate healing.

To the best of my knowledge, there are no proven complications resulting from guided imagery therapy, but because it has not yet been thoroughly explored, the following factors should be kept in mind:

—I don't recommend guided imagery for people who are emotionally hysterical, mentally unstable, schizophrenic, or prepsychotic. For these individuals, guided imagery may prove to be as effective, or even more so, than conventional psychotherapy. But until more research has been conducted, I think it should be used with great discretion for such individuals.

—Theoretically, guided imagery could mask the symptoms of an underlying disease that are trying to communicate an important message. Although this possibility exists, I doubt that the risks are as great as with traditional analgesic techniques. We know that symptoms can be suppressed by modalities that artificially affect the body, such as drugs or surgery. But if pain's message remains unanswered, I believe that it will eventually break through when attempts to smother it are made with techniques (like guided imagery, hypnosis, acupuncture) that require the body to suppress its own discomfort.

—Guided imagery may be addicting, in the sense that anything that reduces or terminates pain is strongly reinforcing. However, I'm not at all alarmed when people depend on advisers and communicate with them on a regular basis. William Glasser, a Los Angeles psychiatrist, has coined the phrase "positive addiction" in reference to beneficial activities (like exercising, meditating, eating properly) that people get hooked on. From this point of view, I believe that getting in touch with yourself (with the help of an adviser) is certainly a positive experience, and a beneficial one to those who become positively addicted to it.

Despite the success that many of my patients have had with guided imagery, a part of me is still a bit uncomfortable. After all, I'm teaching people to do what I would have had them committed for ten years ago. ("Doctor, I have this frog named Henry, who told me what to do about my pain . . .") At the same time, patients report that they're getting relief using guided imagery, and it does appear to be totally safe when properly used. In the final analysis, that's all my patients (and their families and friends) really want.

Relaxation and Meditation

Like sockets with too many plugs, people with pain are often victims of overloaded circuits. With all the publicity about the devastating effects of stress, you might think we would conscientiously limit the tension-producing activities in our lives. After all, since stress has been directly linked to ailments like hypertension, heart attacks, strokes, ulcers, asthma, diabetes, cancer—and pain—it seems self-destructive to allow uncontrolled anxiety and tension into our lives. But almost all of us do anyway.

Modern society encourages us to lead active, hectic lives. We're usually well aware of the stress this produces, but we accept the rat race as a product of our times. And even though we know it can cause us to become ill, we only get serious about sickness when it actually comes.

Unfortunately, for many of you reading these words, illness has finally struck. And the continued stress that has accumulated for years may be making the situation even worse.

Many patients with musculoskeletal pain soon find themselves trapped in a vicious cycle. Their discomfort causes them to become anxious and tense, and this tension causes their muscles to tighten. This, in turn, produces more pain, which causes more tension, and so on. It's a devastating cycle from which some people never escape.

Hans Selye, the world's foremost expert on stress, believes that we must take preventive measures to cushion ourselves against stress's potential damage. That makes sense. But what preventive measures are effective? Well, as a starting point, something as simple as a relaxation exercise can often serve as an important stress reducer.

When I tell my patients that they need to relax, a typical reply is, "Oh, I relax all the time, Doctor. I watch television, I walk the dog, I go to picnics, and I even go on vacations. And every night before dinner, I spend at least half an hour reading the newspaper."

But as helpful as these types of activities may seem, they primarily distract you rather than relax you. If you're watching an exciting television drama, for example, it may in fact *increase* your muscular tension, and thus cause more pain. Or simply listening to the evening news can be a pretty grim experience, and hardly a relaxing one. Even a vacation, with its fast pace and unpredictability, can increase rather than alleviate anxiety and tension.

The type of relaxation I recommend requires an absolutely minimal amount of neuromuscular activity; in other words, a passive type of rest as valuable in its own way as sleep itself.

Theoretically, relaxation should be an easy state for you and everyone else to achieve. After all, relaxation is the body's natural condition, for unless muscles are specifically tensed—either consciously or unconsciously—the body is always relaxed.

But most people have to do more in order to relax than just allow it to happen. Our inability to deal with the excessive tensions and pressure of everyday life has forced us to rely on specialized techniques designed to help us return to this natural state of being. In other words, modern man has to relearn how to relax.

Unfortunately, although doctors often advise their chronically ill patients to relax, they seldom teach them *how* to do it. Given what is known about the harmful effects of excessive stress, it seems amazing to me that Americans are not systematically taught how to relax. Neither my parents nor my friends ever taught me. I went to school for a long time, and none of my teachers ever taught me. Nor did any doctors.

A relaxation exercise is so important and yet so simple that I believe it should be introduced into the public schools in the first grade. I think this might be the most significant way possible to reduce spiraling health care costs in the United States.

The art of relaxation is a prerequisite for working with some of the pain-alleviation techniques discussed earlier, like hypnosis and guided imagery. But it is also beneficial in its own right, producing a pleasant, comfortable state of well-being. Relaxation is also a way of helping your body to balance itself—that is, allowing it a rest period in which it can maximize its healing, restorative, and disease-preventing abilities.

One of the most popular means of achieving a state of relaxation is through meditation. There are dozens of popular meditative techniques taught by yogis, Zen masters, religious leaders, and secular philosophers. In clinical tests conducted by respected medical researchers, some of these relaxation procedures have clearly produced significant physiological changes that appear to contribute to the organism's overall well-being. The yogis themselves, like Indian physician and yoga instructor Rammurti

Mishra, often describe the benefits of meditation quite poetically. In *Fundamentals of Yoga,* Mishra writes, "The conscious mind can transform poison into nectar and nectar into poison; hell into heaven and heaven into hell; life into death and death into life."

Several research studies indicate that meditators may be better able to cope with life's stresses than nonmeditators. Jessica Jo Lahr, while a graduate student at Ohio State University, compared groups of meditators and nonmeditators, and discovered that although the meditators underwent more life-change stress than nonmeditators, they had less illness. Experienced meditators had more changes than beginning meditators, but had even less illness, suggesting that the ability to cope with stress improves with the increased practice of meditation.

Transcendental Meditation, or TM, is currently the most widely known meditative technique in the United States. The technique, which can be learned in just a few hours, involves sitting comfortably in a chair with your eyes closed, and then silently repeating a mantra (a specific but meaningless sound) over and over for twenty minutes.

Although TM was initially introduced here in 1959 by Indian teacher Maharishi Mahesh Yogi, it did not begin attracting large numbers of followers until its ranks of disciples included some well-known celebrities (like the Beatles, the Beach Boys, and Mia Farrow). TM flourished for a year or two in the mid-1960s, but seemed to be going the way of other fads as its popularity temporarily waned. However, interest in TM resurfaced in 1969 and 1970, and for good reason: Scientists conducting laboratory tests on TM practitioners discovered that the technique had a dramatic and beneficial impact on the human body.

In studies by Robert Keith Wallace and Herbert Benson, M.D., TM was found to cause declines in heart rate, respiratory rate, cardiac output, oxygen consumption, and carbon dioxide elimination. Simultaneously, there was a rise in skin resistance, indicating a reduction of stress.

Wallace found that people who regularly practiced TM simply felt healthier. In a survey of 394 meditators, 67 percent said that their physical health had improved, and 84 percent reported an improvement in their mental well-being.

The scientific evidence supporting TM is impressive, and many of my patients with pain have told me they feel better after meditating. But keep in mind that although TM is well-known, it is not the only relaxation technique with proven results.

Another effective approach to relaxation is autogenic training, a system developed more than forty years ago by German psychiatrist Johannes H. Schultz. This technique is used to induce various positive physical states in your body by passively concentrating on specific commands ("My heartbeat is calm and regular," or "My right arm is heavy"). Silently repeating these phrases tends to induce deep relaxation, which in turn often eases pain and discomfort. Some investigators report that it is particularly effective in treating migraine headaches.

A detailed explanation of autogenic training, including its exercises, could fill a chapter or more of this book. Instead, let me refer you to an excellent explanation of the technique in *Mind as Healer, Mind as Slayer,* written by Kenneth R. Pelletier, Ph.D., a research psychologist at the Langley Porter Neuropsychiatric Institute of the University of California.

In Chapter 7, I will teach you still another technique called Conditioned Relaxation, which I developed with the specific goal of helping people who have pain. With diligent practice, nearly every patient who has learned this technique has experienced at least some pain relief. But no matter what relaxation technique you finally decide upon, it's important that you practice it regularly—at least twice a day.

Anyone can learn to relax. In a sense it's like learning to play the piano—some people can learn more quickly than others. While certain people may play Tchaikovsky after just a few weeks of practice, others are still playing "Chopsticks" after months. The same is true with relaxation. But if you make a commitment to learn how to relax, no matter how long it takes, you will certainly be able to accomplish it.

Does relaxation meet the criterion of the "ideal analgesic"? Not entirely. Although it's often effective almost immediately, its impact is usually not long-lasting. Typically, it has to be repeated at least twice daily for maximum results.

However, relaxation is very safe, simple to administer, and is free of any known adverse effects on personality and cognitive abilities. And although this technique is habit-forming, it, too, is a positive addiction.

Biofeedback Training

From early childhood, most of us have been taught that certain bodily functions are beyond human control. Our heart rate, we were told, is impossible to control. So is our blood pressure, and our body temperature.

True, we have all heard about yogis able to accelerate or retard their own heartbeat, or change their blood pressure upon command. But to most people, these claims are a bit suspicious and certainly beyond explanation.

However, in the last few years, the use of a technique called biofeedback has shown that the body *is* capable of such control. Essentially, biofeedback devices provide personal, objective information about the body's silent activities immediately as they occur. Using these devices, you can "tune in" to your body's own inner processes, and when they deviate from a healthy pattern, you can redirect them onto a more positive path.

If you were to come to UCLA for biofeedback training, you would be seated in front of a special device with a panel of dials, instruments, and lights. Electrodes from this biofeedback machine would be attached to various parts of your body in order to record levels of nervous activity. This information would be communicated back to you via either a visible or audible signal—a dial or a tone so that you would instantaneously know exactly what was happening inside you.

During a series of biofeedback sessions, patients learn how to alter that nervous activity through experimenting with different mental strategies. By systematically observing how the gauges are affected by these strategies, people quickly learn to control their muscle tension, blood pressure, heartbeat, skin temperature, and other biological functions. Eventually, after the technique has been mastered, most patients achieve the same degree of control without the assistance of the machine.

It sounds like something out of a science fiction novel—hooked up to a machine, with multicolored wires attached to your hands and head, and bright lights flashing in front of you. But it works. Seated comfortably, you might begin to imagine the coldest day you've ever experienced. In your mind, you can visualize your extremities becoming numb in the freezing cold air, and bone-chilling coldness beginning to spread throughout your body. As you imagine becoming colder and colder, a dial in front of you measuring your body temperature has suddenly started to move downward . . . 98 . . . 97 . . . 96 . . .

It really happens. But in order for you to learn this technique properly, you need the guidance of a trained biofeedback professional (that's why it's called biofeedback *training*). The biofeedback machine itself is like an acupuncture needle; it's what you do with it that makes the difference. The machine is just a tool; how it is used determines whether it will be helpful.

With proper training, people can achieve a remarkable degree of self-control. For instance, many individuals can learn to regulate the finger temperature dramatically with the assistance of a thermistor (an electronic temperature sensor). If thermistors are placed on two fingers of an individual, and he is asked to raise the temperature of one finger and to lower the other, he can often develop a temperature differential between the two fingers of several degrees. Differences as great as 13 degrees Fahrenheit have been reported.

When I talk with some physicians, I am surprised at their resistance to biofeedback (not to mention most of the other techniques described in this chapter). Often, their opposition is due to nothing more than their lack of familiarity with the studies that have been published. Most professionals who have used clinical biofeedback believe that it is a safe technique that has clearly helped many patients with pain.

Not long ago, Melvyn Werbach, M.D., director of clinical biofeedback at the Pain Control Unit, treated a middle-aged man suffering terrible pain in his back due to muscle spasticity. Dr. Werbach placed a biofeedback electrode on the troubled muscle, and was able to demonstrate to the patient just how tight that muscle was. Over a number of sessions, the patient gradually learned how to reduce tension in that muscle. Today, he has mastered the coping strategies learned in biofeedback so well that he can now execute them at home without the use of a biofeedback machine as an aid. Whenever he feels spasticity in his back, he is now capable of easing it on command.

Some headache victims have also been helped by biofeedback, although this is still a subject of controversy, even among biofeedback advocates. According to a popular but disputed theory, some types of migraine headaches may be caused by an expansion of blood vessels in the head. When these blood vessels become distended, they cause pain.

Here's the way biofeedback could help in such cases. While holding a temperature probe with your fingers, you would be taught to warm your hands. To do this, the blood vessels in the hands would become dilated, thus altering the pattern of blood volume in the body, shifting some of the blood from the head to the hands. This, in turn, would allow the distended blood vessels in the head to contract back to a normal level. And the headache would disappear.

At the University of Colorado Medical School, Thomas Budzynski, M.D., and Johann Stoyva, M.D., have effectively trained tension headache sufferers to relax the muscles which generate their discomfort. For instance, they successfully treated a twenty-nine-year-old woman whose headaches had afflicted her for two decades. With electrodes attached to her forehead, and earphones placed on her head, she listened to a tone which would become higher or lower as her muscle tension changed. After nearly half a year of practicing with this biofeedback technique, she learned how to relax the muscles in her forehead at will. Her headaches subsequently disappeared.

In a study by Jose L. Medina, M.D., Seymour Diamond, M.D., and Mary A. Franklin, M.S., twenty-seven patients with chronic migraine and muscle contraction headaches were evaluated. The patients were trained in biofeedback, and then observed for six months following the training. In thirteen of the twenty-seven patients, the number and severity of the headaches were reduced significantly.

There's at least one other way that biofeedback can help people with pain. As I will emphasize throughout this book, relaxation is one of the most important techniques a patient who hurts can learn. However, what about the person who doesn't know what it feels like to relax? (In today's fast-paced society, such individuals are not rare.) If he can't be taught to relax through a method like Conditioned Relaxation, then I recommend biofeedback training to help him get started. With electrodes attached to his body, he can receive instantaneous information about when he's doing the right thing. Unintentionally, he may initially make the muscles tighter instead of more relaxed; in such cases, I'll tell him, "You're doing exactly the right thing but in the wrong direction. It's clear that you have the ability to control muscular tension, so whatever you were doing that increased it, now do the opposite." Before long, he is relaxing—possibly for the first time in his life.

Typically, once an individual masters the biofeedback technique, he also acquires renewed confidence and self-control, which can help extricate him from his desperate feelings of helplessness and depression. For biofeedback provides him with irrefutable, objective evidence that he can, in fact, control his own body.

And does biofeedback qualify as an "ideal analgesic?" The answer is yet unclear, for research is still under way on many aspects of the training. When long-term clinical trials are completed, perhaps we will have a better impression of how long-lasting the benefits of biofeedback can be. We also don't understand to what extent the technique may mask symptoms.

One obvious disadvantage to biofeedback training is that it requires expensive equipment, and as a result, each individual training session can cost from $40 to $65. But aside from the cost, no other major drawbacks have yet been discovered. Because it requires the active participation of the patient, it is an extremely desirable approach to pain relief. Biofeedback is another important way that patients can be taught to heal themselves.

Nutrition

In earlier times, man ate his food very close to its natural source. Either he grew food for himself and his family on his own land, or he bought it from nearby farmers. Eaten just hours after it was picked or harvested, it was extremely nutritious.

But times have changed. And from a nutritional point of view, that change has been for the worse in many respects. Although we need essentially the same nourishment as our forefathers did, we're eating a far different diet today. Most food production is now controlled by major corporations, and the food we eat is often far removed from its original source.

Frankly, "progress" has been cruel to our bodies. Nutritionist Adelle Davis called many of the products on our supermarket shelves "trash foods." Other nutrition experts haven't been much kinder, and for good reason. If reading the labels on the foodstuffs in your cupboards doesn't make you ill, then eating the food might.

Breakfast cereals, for example, may look delicious on TV commercials, but don't expect to be well-nourished by them. Dr. William Caster, professor of nutrition at the University of Georgia, analyzed the value of breakfast cereals in 1970 by feeding them to rats. Simultaneously, a second group of rats was fed a diet of the cardboard boxes in which the cereals were sold. Both were ground up and served with nonfat milk and raisins. According to Caster's findings, the cardboard diet was more nourishing than 92 percent of the breakfast cereals tested. No wonder Ralph Nader once proclaimed, "Food, when it comes in breakfast cereal form, is part entertainment, part diversion, part fraud, part air, and part food. You go through a breakfast cereal plant and you think it's a paper mill."

Many of the other foods we eat aren't much better. In 1968, the U.S. Department of Agriculture published a three-year national dietary study, concluding that 50 percent of the 7500 households surveyed ate diets that fell below the recommended dietary allowances for one or more nutrients. Although more poor families were malnourished than rich ones, people from all economic groups were eating inadequately.

So what does all this have to do with your pain? If pain is a message that something is wrong, then perhaps an improper diet may be part of the message being communicated. No one really knows to what extent food may be related to pain, but the evidence is mounting that there is at least some relationship. For instance, many people have food allergies that may contribute to their chronic pain. If you have headaches with no apparent basis, have you considered your diet as a possible factor?

One of the great unexplored areas of nutrition is the various additives that are put into our foods—preservatives, stabilizers, emulsifiers, coloring agents, and flavoring agents. Yes, the Food and Drug Administration can tell you the short-term effects of large doses of these additives. But *no one* knows the impact these chemicals have when consumed in small quantities over a long period of time. And just as significant, there has been little, if any, research into how these various agents interact with each other or with the drugs you may be taking. What happens when a stabilizer, coloring agent, and an emulsifier encounter one another in your body? Or a preservative and a pain pill? Can they cause long-term harm? Can they make pain worse? No one knows for sure.

Michael Volen, M.D., formerly the clinic medical director at the UCLA Pain Control Unit, has said, "If you eat processed food, you may be eating a little poison every day." But he and other nutritional researchers are convinced that if the proper foods are chosen, your diet can work *with* your body rather than *against* it. A poor diet can contribute to the pain experience, but a good one may help your body to heal itself.

In Chapter 8, I'll discuss my own recommendations as to how you can best nourish yourself. In addition, there will be specific and detailed dietary suggestions that can help ease your pain. But to whet your appetite, let me relate a story told by Dr. Volen. In the backyard of his home, he has a large apple tree, and at sundown he often goes out and gently tugs at each apple until one just falls off right into his hand. When he bites into that apple, there's something in that fruit that's still alive. Dr. Volen believes that a "life-force" exists within that apple that becomes part of the experience of eating it. According to him, you won't find this "life-force" in supermarket food that's been picked green prematurely, artificially ripened, and then shipped to the supermarket where it remains on shelves for days. It's just dead food.

Perhaps there is a vital life-force in food—some energy that could help heal us. The Chinese believe this, and have developed an entire system of herbal medicine, in which natural food substances are used to promote the healing process.

As Western medicine learns more about what nutrition can accomplish, we may see some major changes in the way we eat. Perhaps Thomas Edison was right when he said, "In the future, man's food will be his medicine, and his medicine will be his food."

Counseling

Pain is not an isolated phenomenon. While that throbbing ache may seem to be located only in your neck or back, it literally affects your entire being, physically, mentally, and socially. The discomfort, regardless of what was initially responsible for it, is thus a multidimensional problem.

However, with appropriate help, the many stresses that are associated with pain can be handled in a positive way. In fact, if they are properly dealt with, they can be used to promote the healing process, rather than hindering it.

Doctors who treat pain may be skilled in managing the physiological aspects of the discomfort. But there are many allied health professionals who are specifically trained to help with the tangential problems. Thus, as an adjunct to pain control therapy, I often refer my patients to these specialized counselors for help.

Sexual Counseling

Malcolm, a forty-four-year-old businessman with excruciating back pain, once told me, "For my wife and me, the two most important things in our relationship have been companionship and sex, not necessarily in that order."

But Malcolm had a serious problem—more serious, he felt, than even the unbearable pain in his back. So devastating was his discomfort that it often interfered with his ability to enjoy sex with his wife. At times, he found it impossible to make love at all. And its absence in their marriage was placing a terrible strain on their relationship.

Malcolm's predicament is not uncommon among pain patients. When you hurt, nearly all aspects of your life are affected, including sex. And when this important and pleasurable part of living disappears, the quality of life often becomes severely diminished.

Pain does not always affect the sexual relationships in a person's life. But when it does, it may represent an extremely important aspect of the illness. I've treated patients with pain who haven't made love in as long as fifteen years. And many of these people are young—in their forties and fifties. In such situations, forced celibacy may be more difficult to live with than the pain itself.

Occasionally, though, the absence of sex is not viewed as a tragedy by the pain patient. In fact, it is sometimes considered to be an indirect benefit or gain of the pain experience. Everyone has heard of the line, "Not tonight, dear, I have a headache." Well, in some cases, chronic pain can become a permanent excuse to avoid undesired intimate relationships.

This commonly occurs among young women whose sexual anxieties are reflected as chronic pelvic pain for which no organic basis can be found. In Chapter 4, I related the tragic story of a young woman with pelvic pain who was subjected to a total hysterectomy. After the operation, her pain still persisted. The surgery was probably unnecessary, and it might have been avoided with the proper analysis of a complete sexual history.

This problem is certainly not restricted to women, however. One of my patients, named Fred, was a lathe operator in the aerospace industry of Southern California. Thirteen years ago, Fred was injured on the job and ever since he had been plagued with chronic and disabling lower back pain. He hadn't made love with his wife in years, and he told me it was unimportant to him:

Fred: Sex doesn't matter to me. The only thing that's important is getting rid of this pain.
Doctor: How does your wife feel about this situation?
Fred: She understands. She's been just wonderful.
Doctor: Are you really attracted to your wife?
Fred: Well, I love her. That's what's important.

Fred refused to confront that last question directly. But later, while reviewing his sexual history, I learned the answer to that and many other questions. Sex disappeared from Fred's marriage fairly early. All he had really wanted out of his marriage was someone to take care of him—a mother substitute—and that was the role that his wife had played. He felt a conflict about enjoying sex with his mother substitute. And so when he was injured on the job, his pain became a convenient excuse for avoiding sex. Over the years, he had forgotten how important and enjoyable sex could be.

When I interviewed Fred's wife, I found her on the verge of leaving him. After a brief affair, she had recognized the importance of sex and how much she had missed it in her relationship with Fred. I referred Fred and his wife to a psychotherapist specializing in sexual counseling, and after a few sessions, they began to rediscover the importance of their sexual needs. Not surprisingly, Fred's back pain and his relationship with his wife both improved dramatically.

Family Counseling

One of the most unique aspects of the program of the UCLA Pain Control Unit is the extent to which we involve not just the patient, but all members of his family as well. (Often, if patients have roommates, we invite them to participate, too.) Clearly, the family environment can significantly contribute to the pain problem, and to its resolution, so we believe it is essential for the family to participate fully in the therapeutic process.

Think for a moment about the many ways in which family members can aggravate an illness. For instance, the family can inadvertently reinforce a pathological behavior pattern, by giving love, affection, and attention to the patient only when he hurts. This conduct tends to reinforce the pain, because the discomfort then becomes the most effective means of ensuring that this positive emotional support will be continued.

Also, various family conflicts, crises, and changes—whether related to the pain or not—can produce profound stress in the entire household, which will certainly tend to exacerbate the pain problem of the patient. The family can also sabotage patient compliance with his prescribed therapy, simply by not offering encouragement for the program. In my opinion, long-term change can be maintained only when the environment supports it. (Try to quit smoking when other family members tease you about it, or themselves continue to smoke.) Without family backing, even the most powerful pain-alleviation programs will probably be ineffective in the long run. Finally, other members of the family can actually profit firsthand from the pain patient's discomfort. By focusing so intently on his illness, they can justifiably divert attention away from other, more critical family issues, like a lack of love, the absence of communication, and excess rivalries.

Although the family can significantly contribute to the pain problem, it may also be the key to overcoming it, with the help of appropriate family therapy. In essence, this counseling is a type of psychotherapy in which the entire family unit is the patient, not just one person. The primary goal is not to change just an individual, but to alter the way the entire family interrelates.

A good family therapist can help the family of a pain patient—and thus the patient himself—in the following ways:

—He can advise the family on how to reinforce a healthy behavior pattern rather than a pathological one. For example, he can encourage family members to give love, affection, and attention to a patient only when he feels good, rather than when he hurts. With this approach, the patient learns that feeling good is the most effective way of attaining this emotional support.

—The therapist can help the family unit deal with its stress as a team effort. Dennis Jaffe, Ph.D., UCLA psychologist and author of *Healing from Within,* encourages and teaches families to meditate together, for he believes that such stress-alleviating techniques are much more potent when performed in this way. According to Jaffe, family meditation is one of the few activities in which the family spends time doing something together silently.

—By encouraging the family to work together as a unit, the therapist can also enhance the likelihood of patient compliance with the recommended therapeutic program. Jaffe believes that family camaraderie can enhance the placebo effect of therapy, by elevating positive expectations and faith in the prescribed treatment.

—Through counseling, the therapist can encourage families to cope more directly with serious problems that have been overshadowed by pain. For instance, if the therapist assists the family in overcoming its communication barriers, pain will no longer be needed as the central focus of family activity.

I have also seen family therapists serve as an educational resource for the family unit, teaching other family members about the role that stress may have played in the patient's illness, and about various aspects of the patient's problems that may have been misunderstood. The therapist can also encourage the family to develop personal health habits that can serve as a model for the patient.

In my opinion, family therapy is always beneficial, if not essential, for successful, long-term improvement in most chronic pain patients. With the help of a sensitive and competent therapist, the family can become an important source of positive support for the patient.

Vocational Counseling

If you have chronic pain, you certainly don't need any extra tension in your life. But such anxiety is often difficult to avoid. For instance, if you don't enjoy your job, that can cause anxiety. If you're disabled or out of work, that can even be worse.

For pain patients whose working world is in this kind of disarray, I often recommend vocational counseling. A job that is interesting and rewarding can offer an individual a strong sense of personal identity. But an unpleasant job, or no job at all, provides little reason for a person even to get out of bed in the morning. Even worse, it fosters feelings of worthlessness and hopelessness, and creates anxiety at a time when it certainly isn't needed.

As is the case with sexual and family problems, vocational problems can also produce situations in which maintaining pain is advantageous. If pain resulting from an on-the-job injury provides complete medical coverage, plus an income without working, some patients prefer to remain at home "disabled" almost indefinitely, particularly when their work situation is a poor one.

Vocational counselors can often help patients to deal more effectively with issues related to their working situation. If a physical disability is involved that limits the type of job a patient can perform, vocational counselors are usually able to recommend other employment possibilities.

I believe that for a person to feel truly fulfilled and happy, both a vocation and an avocation are essential. A vocation is a job that represents your occupation, whether it be a lawyer, salesperson, homemaker, or twenty-four-hour-a-day mother. It should be performed with pride and concern, but you shouldn't identify with it. It's not *you*. An avocation, on the other hand, is your "calling"—a hobby or interest that is just for you. Any income received from it should be incidental, for your avocation is important only because of the pure enjoyment it gives you. In Chapter 9, I'll discuss several avocational possibilities that you may not have even thought about.

Spiritual Counseling

Some patients, in trying to dissect the meaning behind their pain, conclude that they are being chastised for a misdeed or sin. When a person is convinced that his discomfort has such a spiritual basis, it may take more than a physician or a psychologist to help him overcome his problem.

Spiritual counseling can be extremely helpful in such cases. In fact, for some patients, it may be essential to include their clergyman as part of the therapeutic team. Spiritual counseling can help an individual make contact with the meaning and purpose of life, and can provide assistance in resolving the feelings of guilt and self-pity that surround his pain problem.

In Chapter 12, I'll discuss in greater detail the important role that spiritualism plays in the pain experience.

Faith Healing and the Placebo Effect

If you've never seen them in person, you've probably watched them on television. They're called faith healers, and they boast about miracle cures that few physicians would ever claim. A man with crippling arthritis rises from his wheelchair and walks out of an auditorium unassisted. A woman with chronic chest pain feels it disappear for the first time in years, and she sobs with joy. It's a moving experience to watch. But is it fact or fancy?

Although some health care professionals have overcome their initial doubts about unconventional treatments such as acupuncture and biofeedback, they still ridicule the suggestion that faith healing has any true therapeutic validity. I, too, was initially skeptical, and assumed that most of the people who were helped at these faith healing services had "psychosomatic" or functional disorders, rather than "real" medical problems. However, as some documentation now confirms, these services have apparently helped severely afflicted people painlessly to walk, bend, climb stairs, and to leave behind their canes and crutches—an accomplishment their doctors had been unable to achieve. Yes, some faith healers may be nothing more than charlatans, but the results of others—such as Ambrose and Olga Worrall, and Dr. Lawrence LeShan—are truly impressive.

No one really knows exactly how faith healing produces such remarkable changes. My own belief is that faith healing is still another example of how mental attitude can affect bodily processes. Each of us possesses remarkably powerful immune/inflammatory defenses and tissue regeneration systems that are mobilized to promote healing following an injury. Too often, however, fears, anxieties, negative expectations, and beliefs interfere with this self-healing process. But when a person *truly* believes he can be healed by an evangelist (or by a physician or by anyone or anything else), that belief alone may restore the emotional balance necessary to maximize the body's healing powers.

A similar position is taken by Jerome D. Frank, M.D., a psychiatrist at Johns Hopkins University, who has speculated that "miracle cures" are really mislabeled. In a 1975 commencement address at Johns Hopkins, Frank said, "These cures, which although rare are well authenticated, are not really miracles in the sense that the laws of nature are violated, but rather rapid acceleration of normal healing processes . . . It goes without saying that since miracle cures happen in shrines of all religious faiths— and for all we know, in doctors' offices—their occurrence is no evidence for or against any theological position. Two surgeons have published 176 well authenticated cases of cancer which remitted without treatment. Had they occurred at a healing shrine, they would have been regarded as miraculous."

The power of expectant faith is no stranger to the field of medicine. Doctors sometimes give their patients fake pills, or "placebos," to help ease pain, or to treat other psychosomatic disorders. These pills contain inactive substances with no intrinsic therapeutic value, but they are prescribed just as if they contained a potent medication. When an individual takes a placebo and feels better, it's the mind—not the medication—that deserves the credit. This is called the *placebo effect*.

Let's assume, for instance, that I were treating you for duodenal ulcer pain. Which do you think would provide you with the greater pain relief— antacid or placebo? Most likely, you'd assume the antacid would have greater value. But it's possible that both treatments would provide you with the same degree of relief.

Surprised? So were researchers at the Veterans Administration Wadsworth Hospital Center in Los Angeles. They studied the effectiveness of doses of a liquid antacid and a placebo in thirty patients with spontaneous duodenal ulcer pain. No significant differences between the antacid and placebo treatments were found, either in degree or duration of pain relief, or in the time it took for relief to begin.

Oliver Wendell Holmes said of the medications of his time, "If most of the pharmacopoeia was sunk to the bottom of the sea, it would be all the better for mankind and all the worse for the fish." Perhaps his words might apply to some of today's medical procedures as well. In Chapter 4, I described a study by H. K. Beecher, M.D., who, in testing the effectiveness of surgical therapy for angina pain, also discovered just how potent the placebo effect could be. When he performed ligation of the internal mammary artery, it reduced pain by 60 to 90 percent, and according to electrocardiogram readings under exertion, cardiac function had improved, too. Then Beecher told another group of patients that he was going to perform the identical surgery on them, but instead performed only mock operations. The skin was cut but the artery was untouched. The same results—significant pain reduction and improved cardiac function—occurred.

In a separate study by Beecher and Dr. Louis Lasagna, a group of postoperative patients were alternately given morphine and placebos for their pain. The patients who initially were given morphine immediately after surgery showed a 52 percent pain-relief factor; the group who initially received the placebo recorded a 40 percent relief factor. The researchers ascertained that, overall, placebos were 77 percent as effective as morphine, and that placebos became more effective with increasingly severe pain.

In another study, patients with clear, objective evidence of herniated lumbar discs were given a general anesthetic and then injected with a placebo. Seventy percent of them obtained significant long-term pain relief.

Recently, researchers have discovered that placebos may activate the body's own pain-suppression system, releasing endorphins. These substances act on the same nerve receptors that are affected by morphine and thus relieve pain from within. As a result of this finding, an even greater number of health practitioners have begun to recognize the importance of expectant faith in the healing process.

There are literally hundreds of similar studies showing the benefits of placebos. These reports clearly illustrate the powerful influence that positive expectation can have on the healing process. As Dr. Jerome Frank says, "Negative emotions such as depression and anxiety can impede healing, and positive ones such as expectant faith can enhance it. In the patient's eyes we are not only scientifically trained physicians, but ministers of healing. By fostering the faith that heals, we can enhance our therapeutic power, a goal towards which we all continue to strive."

C. Norman Shealy, M.D., in his book *Occult Medicine Can Save Your Life,* comments, "In a very real sense, medicine is now—as it always has been—faith healing. Without the patient's faith in his physician and his treatment, there can be no hope for cure. Surgeons have long known—we have all known—that the will to live, and faith in the healer and the healing, are essential to recovery. They are primary factors without which there is no hope."

Many physicians are beginning to recognize fully the importance of the placebo effect and the ways in which positive expectations and faith can help to promote self-healing. As Herbert Benson, M.D., and Mark D. Epstein editorialized in the *Journal of the American Medical Association,* "The placebo effect demands greater comprehension and must be allowed to survive if medicine is to provide optimal care for patients."

To some extent, *all* systems of therapy (including those reviewed in Chapter 4 and this chapter) owe part of their effectiveness to the faith of the patient, the therapist, or as is usually the case, both. Faith has a critically important influence upon the experience of pain, and in Chapter 6, I will describe how you can make your beliefs and expectations more positive ones.

Integral Medicine

We are living in an exciting era of unprecedented technological advances and explosive increases in scientific knowledge. As a result, most Americans have adopted rising expectations of longer life and better health.

But is this confidence in modern medicine justified? According to its critics, the evidence says no. For although we have witnessed the eradication of many infectious diseases and dramatic decreases in infant mortality, most Americans are not really healthier. Heart disease, stroke, cancer, arthritis, diabetes, and other stress-related illnesses continue to plague us relentlessly, in spite of the therapies that our physicians are able to provide.

Although vast sums of money have been spent on research and treatment, I think the emphasis is often misplaced. For patients with cardiac disease, is it realistic to have devoted so much of our energy to transplanting hearts from the dead to the living, and even from animals to man? Has it been most efficient to systematically poison cancer patients with radiation and drugs, hoping to kill the cancer cells but not the patient?

To stop the angel of death from completing its inevitable journey, almost any type of treatment is accepted. As a result, cadavers are kept alive with artificial respirators, and with heart and kidney machines, long after the human spirit has departed. While so much attention is being paid to the quantity of life, preciously little is given to its quality. And most importantly, only minimal efforts have been made to *prevent* the major diseases of our time by teaching what is known about stress reduction, nutrition, and other relevant issues.

One reason why many patients with chronic pain have not been helped is because of the fragmented, mechanistic way in which their problem is viewed and treated. Typically, patients are partitioned like a jigsaw puzzle, with each broken piece (organ) isolated and sent to the proper specialist for repair. Pain in your knee? See the orthopedist. Pain in your chest? Maybe an internist can help. Pain in your jaw? Check with a dentist. Pain inside your head? You better see a psychiatrist. And so on.

Too often, patients with chronic pain are subjected to frightening, dehumanizing tests and procedures that have little to do with the essence of their pain experience. The results of such tests are usually negative, and they often point out nothing more than the narrow limits of our understanding of the problem. Even when these tests are positive, enabling us to assign the pain problem a name, conventional medicine's track record for curing chronic pain is, unfortunately, a poor one.

Given the complex nature of the chronic pain experience, the conventional approach seems very naive to me. People are not jigsaw puzzles, for their lives involve far more than the mechanical functioning of various organ systems. Their bodies have heads; their minds and hearts have feelings, needs, hopes and dreams. They have families, jobs, and their own unique living conditions and self-concepts. Clearly, doctors must learn to diagnose and treat *people,* not diseases.

This point of view is advocated by a new breed of doctors who practice a more personal, *holistic* type of medicine. Holistic therapists treat the whole individual, rather than his or her individual parts. In addition, they insist that the responsibility for health lies with the patient, not the therapist, and accordingly, they emphasize psychosocial rather than physical aspects of the healing process.

Dr. Kenneth R. Pelletier describes the holistic approach to medicine in *Mind as Healer, Mind as Slayer* thusly:

> Holistic medicine recognizes the inextricable interaction between the person and his psychosocial environment. Mind and body function as an integrated unit, and health exists when they are in harmony, while illness results when stress and conflict disrupt this process. These approaches are essentially humanistic and re-establish an emphasis upon the patient rather than upon medical technology. Modern medicine has tended to view man as a machine with interchangeable parts, and has developed sophisticated procedures for repairing, removing or artificially constructing these parts. These are significant achievements, but in the process the healing professions have lost sight of man as a dynamic, integrated, and complex system with marked capacity for self-healing. Consideration of the whole person emphasizes the healing process, the maintenance of health, and the prevention of illness rather than the treatment of established disorders. The concept of holistic, preventive health care is one of the most important innovations in modern medical research and its clinical applications.

Holistic practitioners rely heavily on the alternative approaches described in this chapter. Although the therapeutic validity of many of these techniques has now been well-established, others have yet to stand the test of time. Nevertheless, it seems clear that at least a few of these alternatives will eventually replace some of the more conventional procedures now in favor. For instance, I predict that most medical schools will include acupuncture training in their curricula within fifteen to twenty years, for in the East, acupuncture ceased to be a fad thousands of years ago. Likewise, many of the surgical treatments now used for pain management will be rejected and forgotten as mental control techniques become even more sophisticated.

This revolutionary process is as old as medicine itself, for many of the highly accepted therapies of past eras have become obsolete by today's standards. Bloodletting, for instance, was a common therapeutic practice until about 1850, used to treat everything from pneumonia to internal bleeding. In 1833 alone, forty-one million bloodsucking leeches were imported into France, and as a result, thousands of people, most of them wealthy, died from this "sophisticated" and expensive procedure.

However, as in every revolution, there is the danger that the oppressed may take on the role of the oppressor. Although its premise implies treating the whole person, holistic medicine is often administered in much the same way as Western medicine—that is, the emphasis becomes technique-oriented. So, instead of prescribing two pain pills to suppress symptoms, the holistic practitioner might recommend two biofeedback sessions. Or four acupuncture treatments. Or three massages. Or ten vitamins.

Without a thorough understanding of the message symptoms convey, there are serious potential dangers inherent in a purely technique-oriented approach. For instance, if I can teach a patient to lower his blood pressure through biofeedback, aren't I also teaching him the means to raise it even higher to satisfy any masochistic, self-destructive tendencies he may have? Or if I can teach a person with cancer to mobilize his immune system to battle those cancer cells, aren't I at the same time teaching him how to weaken his immune system even further? I may not be doing the patient a favor by just teaching him techniques. What really has to be dealt with is the problem in the context of the patient's entire life situation. Before purely symptomatic approaches are used, the responsible therapist must determine the answer to questions like, "To what extent are you feeling self-destructive?" and "Are there reasons why you want to keep your pain?"

I have also found that many holistic practitioners are as ego-oriented as their counterparts in traditional medicine. I have heard proclamations like, "Only X can heal you." Such a statement, in my opinion, can be accurately made only by God.

Despite these problems, the concept of holistic medicine has much to offer. And certainly, conventional medicine has its strengths as well. In my opinion, optimal health care is provided when the therapist is able to combine the best of both the traditional and holistic approaches. This point of view is shared by practitioners of what is now being called *integral medicine.*

Although integral medicine incorporates some aspects of holistic medicine, it does not reject Western medicine as worthless. And while it adopts some of Western medicine's approaches, it is also open to less conventional procedures as well. It combines the old and the new in unique and innovative ways, and thus represents an integration of the two systems.

For some ailments, Western medicine offers the best answers. For others, alternative approaches must be considered. What is most important is to know the person as well as possible, and to choose the best possible treatment with an open mind. To quote Dr. Paul Brenner, assistant clinical professor of obstetrics and gynecology at the University of California at San Diego, "To raise consciousness is to lower malpractice."

The practitioner of integral medicine selects the best that both traditional and holistic medicine have to offer, depending on the individual circumstances of each patient. So, for example, while traditional medicine bases its treatment primarily on drugs and surgery, and holistic medicine focuses upon noninvasive alternative approaches, integral medicine may draw from either or both, choosing the best therapy for the particular needs of each individual. And while traditional medicine holds that disease is caused primarily by physical factors, and holistic medicine emphasizes that mental, emotional, and social factors are primarily to blame, integral medicine views disease as a multicausal process which results from an interaction of all these factors.

Practitioners of integral medicine insist that their patients become equal partners in the therapeutic experience, although each has different responsibilities. In the ideal doctor-patient relationship, the doctor's role is to explore the meaning of each patient's symptoms and to establish a correct diagnosis. He should then discuss the variety of treatments available, and when appropriate, teach the patient self-management techniques. No matter what type of therapy he prescribes, the doctor should thoroughly explain his reasons for recommending it. Finally, he should offer the patient advice, support, and information during the course of the therapeutic program.

The patient must assume specific responsibilities of his own. First, he should consult a variety of doctors who will have differing biases and perspectives concerning the problem. Some of my patients have seen just one doctor, and have blindly placed all of their hopes for healing in just one type of treatment. If you were having your house remodeled, you'd probably seek bids from half a dozen contractors. Doesn't your body deserve to be cared for just as well?

The patient must also provide his doctor with honest information to make an accurate diagnosis possible. When a specific treatment is prescribed, the patient should discuss it thoroughly with his doctor to ensure that he completely understands and agrees to it. He should then follow the treatment program diligently, giving it a thorough trial. Simultaneously, he should provide his doctor with feedback about his progress so that later patients can benefit from his experiences. Also, whenever possible, the patient should utilize appropriate self-management techniques to maximize his own self-healing potential.

Unfortunately, integral medicine is not yet widely available. However, you can help by encouraging your own physician to find out more about it. Franz Kafka once said, "To write prescriptions is easy, but to come to an understanding with people is hard." In a therapeutic partnership with a caring physician familiar with the principles of integral medicine, many patients with chronic pain have found help for the first time.

The unconventional therapies described in this chapter shouldn't be considered only as a last resort. Many meet the criteria of the "ideal analgesic" better than some of the most widely accepted traditional approaches. And thus, you and your doctor should evaluate their possible benefits early in your search for pain relief.

So it's up to you. Are you willing to share some of the responsibility to get rid of your pain? I truly believe that the means for pain relief are available to you. Are you going to use them?

SAMPLE

EXERCISE FOURTEEN: What About Alternative Therapies?

DATE: March 14

TIME: 6 p.m.

	Have Tried Before	Wish to Try Now	Refuse to Try Now	Condition Worsened	No Relief	Temporary Relief	Substantial Relief	Complete Relief	Will Definitely Help	Probably Will Help	Probably Won't Help	Will Definitely Not Help	Don't Know
	EXPERIENCE			**OVERALL RESULTS**					**CURRENT EXPECTATIONS**				
Heat	X					X				X			
Cold	X				X								
Orgone (Reichian) therapy			X										X
Rolfing			X										X
Feldenkrais			X										X
Alexander			X										X
Movement and exercise	X					X				X			
Therapeutic touch		X								X			
Acupuncture		X											X
Acupressure		X											X
Hypnosis		X								X			
Self-hypnosis		X								X			
Relaxation training	X						X		X				
Meditation training	X						X		X				
Guided imagery		X											X
Biofeedback training		X								X			
Nutritional counseling		X								X			
Sexual counseling			X								X		
Family counseling		X											X
Vocational counseling		X											X
Spiritual counseling	X				X							X	
Faith healing		X										X	

EXERCISE FOURTEEN: What About Alternative Therapies?

DATE: _____

TIME: _____

	EXPERIENCE			OVERALL RESULTS					CURRENT EXPECTATIONS				
	Have Tried Before	Wish to Try Now	Refuse to Try Now	Condition Worsened	No Relief	Temporary Relief	Substantial Relief	Complete Relief	Will Definitely Help	Probably Will Help	Probably Won't Help	Will Definitely Not Help	Don't Know
Heat													
Cold													
Orgone (Reichian) therapy													
Rolfing													
Feldenkrais													
Alexander													
Movement and exercise													
Therapeutic touch													
Acupuncture													
Acupressure													
Hypnosis													
Self-hypnosis													
Relaxation training													
Meditation training													
Guided imagery													
Biofeedback training													
Nutritional counseling													
Sexual counseling													
Family counseling													
Vocational counseling													
Spiritual counseling													
Faith healing													

Exercise Fourteen: What About Alternative Therapies?

Exercise Fourteen is designed to summarize some of the different types of alternative therapies available for treatment of chronic pain. As in Exercise Thirteen, please indicate (1) Your experience with each of the therapeutic approaches listed; (2) How successful they have been; and (3) Your expectations as to whether or not each therapy might be of help.

6 *What Can You Do to Help?*

Remember, we're all in this alone.

—Lily Tomlin

If you're like many other people with chronic pain, you've probably visited so many doctors that your personal address book resembles a local medical association directory. After being treated by dozens of doctors— enough to last most people several lifetimes—you have probably acquired so much knowledge about your ailment that you speak about it in technical language usually reserved only for the medical fraternity. About all you haven't learned is the important missing link—how to bring your pain to an end.

You've probably asked every doctor the same questions: "Can anything be done about my pain?" and "Why doesn't it go away?" After perhaps thousands of dollars' worth of treatment, you may be dejected and desperate, and no nearer to a solution to your problem than you ever were.

Some patients blame their physicians for failing to help, for after all, aren't doctors paid to heal people? One angry patient told me, "Doctors are no damn good. They don't know anything, and worse yet, they don't even care about you. The last doctor I saw just gave me more pills which didn't do any good at all."

However, she was speechless when I replied, "Has your own self-treatment fared any better? What have *you* been doing to make yourself well? Don't blame your doctors. They're not the only ones responsible for getting you better. Perhaps they can help, but it's *your* life that's on the line. Are you doing everything you can to regain your health?"

A moment later, I added, "You say your doctors don't know anything.

What do *you* know about yourself? You say your doctors don't care. How much do *you* care about yourself? Take your fair share of the responsibility and let's see what you can do."

I have long believed that within each of us is the power to turn off our own pain. After all, if the nervous system has the ability to generate the experience of pain, it should certainly be able to stop it as well, *if* it is in our best interest to do so. When it doesn't turn pain off, perhaps it's trying to tell you that something is wrong not just in your body, but in your life as well.

Although you may believe that your pain problem is related only to some physical injury or disease, the anguish and suffering you experience may primarily reflect, on a larger scale, some other aspect of your life situation. Pain motivates you to find out what's wrong and to take appropriate action to correct it. When you're finally able to remedy the problem—whether it is physical, mental, emotional, and/or social—the body will at last be free to mobilize its own ability to turn off the pain.

As this book will frequently emphasize, I believe that the natural state of the organism is to be pain-free. Even in the case of severe physical injuries, the body has a remarkable ability to suppress discomfort. I have witnessed several major surgical procedures performed without any chemical anesthetic, using only hypnosis to protect the patients from pain. Well, if a surgeon can cut an undrugged person open with a scalpel and not inflict any discomfort, the body clearly has an astounding ability to arrest even the most severe physical pain.

Several years ago I was driving along a heavily traveled mountain road north of UCLA when I spotted a cat lying by the side of the road. Being somewhat fanatical about injured animals, I stopped my car to see if there was anything I could do to help it. When I reached the cat, I realized it was close to death. It had apparently been struck by a car, and had sustained very severe injuries from the chest down, where few, if any, of its bones remained unbroken.

I thought I'd try to soothe the cat in whatever way possible, so I began to stroke its face gently and scratch it behind the ears. To my surprise, this cat—in spite of its horrible physical injuries—began purring. I was stunned. I had thought the animal must be in excruciating pain. But apparently it was free of discomfort, for its nervous system had mercifully turned its pain off.

That same power exists in us as well. Do you recall the story in Chapter 2 of the severely injured African tribesman? During an initiation ritual, his arm had been torn off by a lion, but he felt no pain. Somehow, his nervous system had suppressed pain that would have been severe enough to drive most people into shock.

Exactly how the nervous system suppresses pain is still unknown, and scientists continue to search for a better understanding of this process.

Why some people—such as yogis or highly hypnotizable individuals—are more adept at controlling pain than others also remains a mystery. But one thing is becoming clear: mounting evidence now strongly suggests that you may be able to regulate your nervous system much more than you ever thought possible. Although all prior attempts at therapy may have been unsuccessful, perhaps the missing ingredient has been *you*.

Throughout the remainder of this book, you will be introduced to many specific techniques designed to provide pain relief. But the most important factors that determine whether they will succeed or fail are your desire to get better and your willingness to give them a fair try. As you'll read in the next few pages, your own ability to alleviate pain may be far more powerful than anything a doctor can offer.

Endorphins: Inner Pain Relievers

One of the most exciting discoveries in the biomedical sciences during the last twenty-five years has suggested that the brain produces its own natural, pain-relieving molecules. These substances—called endorphins—may help explain how the body is able to turn off pain sensations when it's appropriate for it to do so.

Endorphins were first identified in 1975 by researchers interested in discovering how morphine works. While morphine had long been known to be one of medicine's most potent painkillers, no one understood precisely why it was so effective, although earlier research had uncovered a few clues. There was evidence, for instance, that narcotic analgesics like morphine produce electrical changes in a part of the brain called the periaqueductal gray matter (PAGM). In tests on rats with electrodes placed in the PAGM, stimulation generated a significant degree of analgesia in one-half or one quadrant of the body, while the remainder was unaffected. Interestingly, even in the pain-free areas, the body still responded to nonpainful stimuli, like a gentle touch.

How was this possible? No one knew for certain what mechanisms were at work. Early studies indicated that analgesia was produced when nerve impulses traveled down the spinal cord, blocking painful input at the spinal cord level, long before it could reach the brain. But later research revealed even more, namely, that morphine may actually activate this descending system. Scientists discovered that the body had specific morphine receptors—that is, specific sites on cell membranes chemically designed to receive only morphine. These receptors are highly concentrated in areas of the brain, like the PAGM, that suppress pain when electrically stimulated.

Well, why did God (in all Her wisdom) give us receptors for morphine, an extract of the poppy plant? It seems unlikely that we would also have receptors for all other plants (like cabbage, petunias, broccoli, and cauliflower)—so why morphine? It was a real mystery until someone hypothesized that perhaps the body manufactures its *own* painkiller with a chemical structure identical to morphine.

Further research has confirmed that this is, in fact, the case. The human pituitary gland secretes an opiatelike substance that stimulates specific receptors in the same part of the brain which turns pain off. Scientists have actually isolated at least seven different natural pain-killing substances, including enkephalins and complex lipoproteins. Collectively, they make up the endorphins.

There is also growing evidence that some of the alternative modalities I discussed in Chapter 5 may work—not because of their own direct action—but by causing the nervous system to release its own natural painkiller. Endorphins, for instance, may hold the secret to how acupuncture works. Research by Dr. Bruce Pomeranz and his associates at the University of Toronto seems to indicate that acupuncture stimulates the nervous system to secrete endorphins, which in turn suppress pain. In addition, endorphins may be responsible for the pain relief which occurs following the administration of placebos (inactive substances). Soon we may have a more thorough understanding of the dramatic effects that are associated with positive expectant faith.

Interestingly, we have found at UCLA that alternative pain-alleviation techniques are often less effective for patients who chronically use opiate-based analgesics. If you're taking Demerol or Darvon, procedures like acupuncture or guided imagery may not provide much relief. Why? Well, particularly with acupuncture, I think the problem may be that the endorphin receptors become desensitized due to the long-term use of large doses of narcotics. So even though acupuncture may cause the nervous system to release its own natural pain reliever, it can soon become ineffective when the critical receptor sites no longer respond to endorphin release.

For patients who have been taking large amounts of narcotic analgesics, I almost always recommend that they gradually reduce their drug intake in order to reactivate their endorphin receptors once again. After complete withdrawal is achieved, I find that patients typically respond much better to acupuncture, guided imagery, biofeedback, and other minimally invasive procedures.

More is being learned about endorphins every day, and for those of us specializing in pain therapy, this is a very exciting time. Already, endorphins seem to offer an explanation for many of the pain-related phenomena that have gone without explanation for many years. For instance, during World War II, soldiers with extremely severe wounds were operated on with no pain-relieving drugs, enduring the excruciating pain very "bravely." Writes Richard Restak in *Saturday Review:* "Until now, the soldiers' responses have been laid to 'euphoria'—to their relief at still being alive. Now there is an alternative explanation: under conditions of extreme and totally disorganizing pain, the brain can release its own narcotic. Could this mean that the 'strong, brave' individuals who can take torture without breaking down are simply gifted with a large supply of endorphins? And that the 'coward' who 'can't take it' is merely a victim of endorphin deprivation?"

If the body can naturally secrete its own pain reliever—which it apparently can—then the primary task of every person who hurts is to maximize that ability. When there are reasons why the body isn't cooperating in its pain-alleviating role, it's absolutely essential to find out why, and then to set out on the road to better health.

Understanding Pain's Message

One of Western medicine's greatest strengths lies in its ability to treat symptoms using "readjustment" techniques. For example, if you have high blood pressure, your physician can prescribe drugs to adjust your blood pressure down. Or if you have diabetes, he can prescribe insulin to help adjust your insulin level up.

In my opinion, however, this symptomatic approach to health care can be misused. Such is the case when sleeping pills are prescribed for a patient without first finding out *why* he is suffering from insomnia. Equally imprudent is prescribing tranquilizers to an anxious patient without first finding out why he's apprehensive.

To my way of thinking, the best type of therapy involves *change,* not adjustment. And for change to occur, you first need a thorough understanding of the message that symptoms are providing. In Exercise Six on page 70, I asked you to try to decipher the message behind your pain as a way of determining what sort of things need to be changed. What possible messages did you uncover? Were you able to pinpoint any problems in your life that may have contributed to your discomfort?

In my experience, most patients try to think very externally when trying to decipher the subtle inner meaning of their pain. When I recently asked one middle-aged man what he thought was wrong, he replied:

"It's my spouse. I knew my marriage was bad almost from the start. And it seems to be getting worse. I should have gotten a divorce a long time ago. I'm sure I'd start feeling better if I got myself out of this relationship."

Another patient had a different perspective on her pain.

"My job is terrible. I don't like my boss, and I don't like the people I work with. I'm just not happy there. Maybe if I get a new job, my pain will go away."

Still another patient blamed the city she lived in:

"I'm going absolutely crazy living in Los Angeles. I hate fighting the freeway traffic every day. And the smog is the worst. There's also just too many crazy people here. Charlie Manson lived here. If I moved to Arizona, I'd probably feel much better."

All these people had an external vision of the message behind their pain. A divorce, a job change, a move to Arizona—they would all bring about immediate relief. These people also felt a need to do something new. Perhaps they were right. But in many cases, the major problem is not an external one, but an internal one. For instance, perhaps you're worrying too much. Or you're mistrusting your own intuitions. Or maybe your pain is trying to tell you:

"Stop being so self-critical. See your good side, too"; or

"Stop being so perfectionistic. Accept your weaknesses along with your strengths"; or

"Stop feeling so sorry for yourself. The world can be a beautiful place in which to live, if you'll let yourself live. Have fun and the pain will stop."

Although your physician might be able to treat your symptoms, only you can discover and deal with the message behind your discomfort. And until you do, true change can't occur.

Unfortunately, the prospect of major change frightens many people. For some, the fear of change can overwhelm or even paralyze them. Don't let that happen to you. Yes, you hurt, and yes, some personal restructuring may be necessary. But periods of change and transition are as much a part of life as breathing. And when you treat them as natural, necessary occurrences, they won't seem nearly as awesome. Have faith in your ability to cope with change. Take a deep breath, relax, and enjoy life as best you can. Open your mind a bit, take a look at the hard realities, and give the process of change a fair chance.

Galen, the ancient Greek physician, said, "He cures most in whom most are confident." Well, why not show some confidence in your ability to change yourself? As you will see in the ensuing chapters, you really may be able to overcome your pain if you have faith that you can.

Expectations and Belief Systems

There's an old saying in medicine, "The conviction of illness leads to illness, and the conviction of cure leads to cure." From this point of view, the most important first step toward good health is for you to assume the belief that you can and will get better. Yet, so many patients are resigned to believing that little, if anything, can ever ease or erase their pain.

Consider the attitudes of the following two individuals. Which of them do you think has the better chance of getting well?

Patient A: "I'm a helpless victim of incurable pain, and I just have to learn to live with it."

Patient B: "I'll keep looking until I find something that will be able to help me."

Without doubt, Patient B has a greater likelihood for obtaining good health. Why? Because his belief system incorporates the possibility that he may get better. Patient A has stopped even trying.

Although it is important for your expectations to be positive, they must also be realistic. For example, if you have severe arthritis and expect to be entirely cured by the end of the month, that's probably an inappropriate belief. But if you believe that you can gradually learn to overcome the associated discomfort, you may well be able to do so.

To a large extent, how you see your pain problem determines how you experience it. If you see your pain as "an angry lion gnawing on the spine, tearing deeper into the nerves with every bite," that is what you experience. But if you see the same problem as "a cool wind that blows deeply into your back," you may begin to experience it quite differently.

As I mentioned in Chapter 2, "reality" is quite vague. Depending on a number of factors—ranging from parental guidance to peer influences—two people can experience the same reality in very different ways. For instance, someone who grew up believing that hunting is a manly sport and a demonstration of "the survival of the fittest," would probably view the killing of a game animal as a thrilling challenge. But another person, taught to believe that all life is sacred, would be appalled at killing a defenseless animal. It's the same event, experienced in very different ways because of two dissimilar belief systems.

There is an old anecdote about two Jesuit priests who approached their bishop requesting permission to smoke.

"May I smoke while I pray?" the first priest asked.

"Certainly not!" replied the bishop. "When you pray, all of your concentration must be focused on praying."

The second priest approached the bishop.

"May I pray while I smoke?" he asked.

"Of course you may," replied the bishop. "Prayer is appropriate at any time of the day."

Your own impression of reality depends on how you choose to view it. As John C. Lilly, M.D., once said, "In the realm of the mind, what you believe to be true *is* true, or becomes true, within certain experiential and experimental limits that remain to be transcended." To use the vernacular, what you see is what you get. In short, the way you perceive your pain is the way you will continue to experience it.

Do you know how to dematerialize something? How to make it cease to exist in your personal reality? Probably the simplest way is to stop thinking about it. If you presently view your life as filled with pain-racking misery, that is what you'll experience. But if you can learn to stop thinking about your discomfort, it may well disappear. As the saying goes, "Out of sight, out of mind."

But as I'll discuss in the next section, it is very difficult simply to "stop thinking about pain." A more realistic goal is to learn to think of your discomfort in a radically different way. One of my patients, a twenty-eight-year-old college student named Jack, suffered from causalgia pain after an automobile accident in which his right arm was so severely injured that it almost had to be amputated. For months thereafter, he was constantly plagued by an excruciating, burning pain in his arm. Even the lightest touch on his skin would cause terrible agony; if he banged his arm against a desk or some other object, the intense pain that resulted would force him into bed for the next few days.

When I began to work with Jack, it was clear that one of his main problems concerned his beliefs about his future ability to use his arm. Over the next few months, we worked closely together to develop new belief systems and expectations, using some of the techniques presented later in this book. Eventually, Jack learned to experience his arm in a radically different way. Instead of interpreting his discomfort as "painful," he began viewing the feeling as an "electrical tingling." He was ultimately able to say, "Yes, I know that the pain is there, but it doesn't bother me. I hardly ever think about it."

There are several common belief systems that many pain patients share which negatively affect their ability to deal with their discomfort:

—Many pain patients think that the world is out to harm them. It's a hostile place in which to live, they believe, and thus, they are always watchful for the next "horrible event" to strike. This outlook produces a state of chronic stress, which eventually takes a terrible toll upon these people. However, if they could learn to change their perspective so that they see the world as a benevolent, beautiful place designed explicitly for their own enjoyment and self-actualization, then that's how they might begin to experience it.

—Some pain patients believe that their illness is incurable and that their doctors are not to be trusted. If that's what you believe—if you're convinced that you're a hopeless victim of a terrible disease that your doctors are unable to treat—that may become a self-fulfilling prophecy.

—Finally, some pain patients believe that they are personally powerless to do anything to help themselves. These "externalizers" feel that everything that happens to them is the result of divine fate or external influences over which they have no control. Some of these people are like the dogs in Seligman's study described in Chapter 3, for they have developed "learned helplessness." As Seligman wrote in his book *Helplessness*, "The belief that actions are ineffective leads the organism to make no effort to change its situation, dire though it may be."

—At the opposite extreme are the "internalizers" who believe that everything that happens to them, including illness, is a direct result of their own activities and behaviors. These patients often tend to be perfectionists, and readily accept full blame for any flaws or defects in their lives. In effect, they set themselves up for failure, because nobody's perfect. And when they fail, a sense of guilt is typically created. Their pain, in a sense, is a just reward for their own shortcomings and inadequacies, and deep inside, they believe that they really do deserve it.

I try to help my patients adopt a belief system that lies somewhere between these two extremes. Although you may not be responsible for everything that happens to you, you can have a significant influence over how well you deal with your problems. Until you try, you'll never discover your own power. And the first step is to adopt the belief that you *might* be able to succeed.

There's a final point to consider. Even if you are successful in shifting your belief systems in a more positive direction, you may still have to combat the negative attitude of your own doctor. Some physicians inadvertently encourage feelings of helplessness in their patients by telling them that "nothing more can be done." Many patients are actually discouraged from asking questions about their medications or treatment plan. And when patients attempt to take some responsibility for their own care, doctors often accuse them of meddling with the prescribed therapy.

Consider, for example, a patient with back pain. The treatment modalities used by conventional medicine usually include surgery, nerve blocks, drugs, and bed rest, all of which are passive and require no direct patient action or responsibility. Like Seligman's dogs, even if the opportunity to escape pain arises, such patients are inadvertently taught to become helpless and passive. Thus, they may ignore even the most obvious ways to achieve pain relief.

When one of my patients was recently helped by a series of acupuncture treatments, his personal physician told me, "I accept the fact that Robert's pain has disappeared, but I don't believe acupuncture had anything to do with it. I don't know why he got better, but acupuncture couldn't have been the reason." Doctors have their own belief systems, which are often rigidly created in the medical training process. They have their own ways of viewing patients, illnesses, and treatments—and these belief systems are sometimes difficult to change, no matter how impressive an alternative treatment is. When your physician rejects acupuncture, biofeedback, or any other approach as the treatment of choice for you, he is not trying to mislead you or do you harm. He's doing what he absolutely thinks is the best thing for you, according to his own personal belief systems.

Fortunately, as more and more physicians begin to explore unconventional alternatives, the attitude of the medical profession is beginning to change. Dr. Paul Brenner reports that many of his colleagues were initially skeptical about his use of acupuncture to treat pain. Even as he continued to obtain positive results with this modality, the skepticism of his peers barely wavered.

Later, Dr. Brenner began to explore the important role of belief systems on the part of both patients and therapists. On one occasion, he utilized acupuncture to treat a horse with an injured back. The results were profoundly positive, and Dr. Brenner told his startled colleagues, "Perhaps the pain relief was a direct result of my positive expectations. I imagined the horse getting better in my mind's eye, and sure enough, that's what happened."

"Nonsense," these skeptics replied. "It was the acupuncture that did it."

If a doctor tells you that nothing more can be done, that is what he honestly believes. At least, for the moment. But that's no excuse for you to accept his belief system as gospel. Only a fool would fail to explore every possible avenue of pain relief, as long as it is a safe and affordable one. And if you approach each new treatment with the belief that it could help you, it may become a positive, self-fulfilling prophecy.

Breaking a Bad Habit

In a sense, an inappropriate belief is like a bad habit. It may have been acquired many years ago, perhaps even in childhood, and reinforced continuously by doctors, friends, and family. Frequently, I find that the negative attitudes of pain patients toward their illnesses, and toward their personal power to promote self-healing, are often the product of inappropriate conditioning.

How do you go about breaking a bad habit? The best way I know is to learn a new habit that is incompatible with the old one. Consider a rat who has learned to maneuver his way through a maze, and then turn left in order to receive a piece of cheese. The most effective way to change that behavior immediately is not to take away the food (that is, stop rewarding him), because the rat will continue the same behavior for quite a while, still expecting the food to be there. Nor is it to place a barrier where the rat made his left turn, because if he's persistent, he'll chew through it. The best possible solution is to move the food so that a *right*, not a left, turn is required at the end of the maze. By doing so, you have immediately taught the rat a new habit incompatible with the old one. (After all, he can't turn both left and right at the same time.)

Most pain patients are plagued by a variety of bad habits and inappropriate rituals. For example, think back to the many benefits or "gains" associated with chronic pain. Perhaps you've fallen into the habit of using your pain to attain one or more of these benefits, and are thus reinforcing your pain on a regular basis. Maybe your pain attracts attention and sympathy that you might not otherwise receive. Or perhaps it has become a means of manipulating family and friends, a justifiable excuse for being lazy and unproductive, or a way to avoid sexual encounters.

These are the types of bad habits that need to be changed. And to change them, you must create ways other than hurting to meet the needs that your discomfort is now fulfilling. Fortunately, there are ways to do this. One of my patients, a forty-two-year-old housewife named Roberta, realized that her migraine headaches were allowing her to be very self-indulgent. Raising five children, she rarely had time for herself—until her illness gave her a legitimate excuse for getting the extra rest and relaxation that she had deprived herself of for years.

After some soul-searching, Roberta concluded that there might be an easier, less destructive way for her to devote more time to herself. With the support and encouragement of her family, Roberta arranged to set aside one hour each afternoon and two hours each evening for her and her alone. If that meant putting off the laundry for another day, or letting the dirty dishes pile up in the sink, so be it. Her health and well-being came first. Almost predictably, after this new family plan went into effect, Roberta's headaches decreased in frequency and severity.

Roberta's story is not an unusual one, for most pain patients have unwittingly developed many bad habits and ritualistic behaviors. As I said earlier, real change—rather than adjustment—is necessary in such situations. If you want to maximize your nervous system's ability to conquer your pain, you can create alternative habits that may promote rather than hinder the healing experience.

Exercise Fifteen: Breaking Bad Habits

In this exercise, I'd like you to get in touch with your bad habits and to create alternative ways to overcome them. Review your responses to Exercises Six through Eleven. Focus on three of the most damaging bad habits you can identify, and complete the following information in the chart below:

1. What are the bad habits? Obviously, before you can deal with them, you have to identify them clearly.

2. What do you hope to achieve by changing them? For example, will change give you the freedom to engage in enjoyable activities that you've ignored for many months or years? This part of the exercise will serve as

SAMPLE

EXERCISE FIFTEEN: Breaking Bad Habits DATE: <u>March 20</u>

TIME: <u>9 a.m.</u>

	HABIT #1	HABIT #2	HABIT #3
The bad habit	I take too many pain pills.	I feel sorry for myself all the time because I hurt so much.	I use my pain as an excuse for avoiding an active social life.
Your motivation for change	I'm afraid of becoming addicted to pills.	It's a terrible waste of energy to be so preoccupied with my misery. I desperately want to be productive.	I feel very isolated. I want to make new friends (but I'm afraid to).
The new habit	I'm going to do a relaxation exercise whenever I hurt, instead of taking pills.	I'm going to do volunteer work at the local senior citizens home. That won't leave me very much time to feel sorry for myself!	I'm going to join a Parents Without Partners group, and go to meetings at least twice a month.
Rewarding the new habit	I'm going to use the money I used to spend on pain pills to buy season tickets to the local theater.	Everytime somebody at the senior citizens home says, 'Thank you,' that will be a reward, and make me feel I'm using my time well.	I know that once I start meeting new people, I'm going to love it and want to keep active. I've just got to get started.

EXERCISE FIFTEEN: Breaking Bad Habits   **DATE:** _____

     TIME: _____

	HABIT #1	HABIT #2	HABIT #3
The bad habit			
Your motivation for change			
The new habit			
Rewarding the new habit			

an important source of motivation for carrying out your plan of action.

3. What new habits are you going to implement that are incompatible with the old ones?

4. How can you maintain these new habits and reward them so effectively that you won't be tempted to return to your old behaviors?

For instance, if your discomfort has become a convenient excuse for avoiding sex, perhaps you should talk to your partner about why you find sexual relationships so unpleasant. If you can work out this problem in an agreeable way, the need for pain may no longer exist; and the renewed enjoyment of sex may be all the reward you need. Or, as with Roberta, if your discomfort allows you to be alone and self-indulgent, work out a "contract" with your family members that will permit you time to yourself each day. Your happiness over this new life pattern will serve as a powerful reward.

Dealing with Negative Feelings

One of my patients recently told me, "If you can't do anything to help me get rid of this pain, I don't know whether it's worth living anymore. I can't work. I can't enjoy life. I'm a burden on my family. If I can't be helped—if nothing can be done about it—then why shouldn't I just end it all?"

For this individual, and thousands of other patients with pain, moments of optimism occur about as frequently as eclipses of the moon. They are slowly drowning in feelings of depression, helplessness, anxiety, fear, hostility, frustration, shame, embarrassment, and guilt. In effect, negativity now characterizes their entire way of life. Their thinking is defeatist and pessimistic. As Galsworthy said, they are "always building dungeons in the air" around them.

If you're fortunate enough to have avoided this situation, imagine what it must be like living in such a negative environment. Put yourself in the position of awakening each day with little or nothing to look forward to except agonizing pain, a deteriorating relationship with the people around you, phone calls from bill collectors, and despondency and worry that the future might even be bleaker.

It may be hard for you to believe that some people live this way—day after day, month after month, year after year. But I have treated hundreds of them, and there are probably hundreds of thousands of others just like them. I have not yet met even one pain-afflicted person who did not experience severely negative feelings, thoughts, or sensations.

Some patients are embarrassed by the way pain limits their lives. Others experience guilt over the way their illness has impaired the lives of their family members. Still others feel anger, particularly toward acquaintances who show little or no compassion for their plight ("If only that person could feel the discomfort that I do"). But most common are the profound feelings of depression and helplessness that devastate the majority of patients with chronic pain.

Occasionally, suicide is an unfortunate consequence of chronic pain. Faced with continuing discomfort and no hope for relief, some patients decide that life itself is simply no longer worth living. In my opinion, this decision is often made prematurely, for until a person has tried literally every possible pain-alleviation technique, it is foolhardy to say that all hope has been exhausted or that "nothing more can be done."

As a pain therapist, much of my time is spent helping my patients deal more effectively with their negative feelings. If you have chronic pain, you must learn to become less preoccupied with the negative stimuli in your life. Recognize that they exist, absorb their informational value, but don't identify with them. Don't *become* your negative emotions. Observe them as if they were happening to a third party.

For instance, see if you can detect the very real difference between reacting to an emotion in the following ways:

1. "I am depressed."
2. "There are feelings of depression passing through me."

In the first example, the emotion has actually become part of you and you, in turn, have become totally identified with it. In the second, you perceive the emotion, but do not treat it as being intimately tied to your own life.

Here's another instance in which an emotion can be handled in two very different ways:

1. "I am very angry right now."
2. "Hmm, I detect some angry feelings inside of me. How interesting."

Of course, it's not always easy to react in a detached, aloof manner to the turmoil that may be within you. But through practice, you *can* teach yourself to do it. By concentrating, you can "catch" yourself becoming overly involved with a thought or sensation, and can consciously choose to separate yourself from its full impact.

Let's assume, for instance, that you are awaiting a call from your doctor, and as hour after hour passes without the telephone ringing, you become increasingly anxious and upset. By day's end, with the phone call still not having arrived, you very likely might react thusly:

"Damn it. I am furious that that inconsiderate doctor hasn't called!"

But now, let's say about midday, you start noticing these feelings of anxiety beginning to take shape within you. Instead of allowing them to intensify, building upon themselves, you can choose to react in the following way:

"Hmm, there is irritation and anger developing within me. I am aware

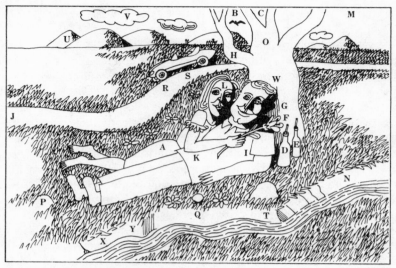

BEGINNER'S EXERCISE IN NEGATIVE THINKING

Without referring to the list below, how many potential hazards can you identify in this scene?

Partial List Of Hazards: (A) Intense sunlight could fade your clothing, grass could permanently stain it; (B) passing bird could soil your head; (C) passing airliner could erroneously jettison its septic tank on your car or person; (D) bottles could tip over and spill on clothes; (E) soft drinks could rot your teeth; (F) pollen could inflame your nasal membranes; (G) nearsighted bee, attracted by flower, could accidentally fly into your ear, become trapped and hysterical; (H) weakened tree limb could fall and fracture your skull; (I) sultry weather could cause embarrassment; (J) great distance from nearest restroom could cause extreme anguish; (K) continuous weight of arm could irritate appendix; (L) companion could suddenly realize how boring you are; (M) freelance photographer could snap embarrassing pictures from helicopter; (N) vice-squad officer submerged in stream could be observing you through periscope; (O) thin bear could be lurking behind tree; (P) you could stub your toe on boulder or get tetanus from stepping on rusty nail; (Q) you could break your teeth on smooth white rock you mistook for hardboiled egg; (R) passing Greyhound bus could careen out of control and demolish your car; (S) mischievous passerby could release handbrake, or paint obscenities in permanent enamel; (T) ground tremor could loosen bank; (U) sudden lava flow could engulf you; (V) stray lightning bolt from cloud could strike tree and electrocute you; (W) plant lice from bark could lodge in scalp; (X) flash flood could carry you away; (Y) rabid herring could leap out of stream and attack your toes.

Fig. 13 *Negative thinkers often carry their worries to extremes, as Dan Greenburg satirically points out in his book,* How to Make Yourself Miserable.

of this, but I'll allow these sensations to pass through me for now. I have more important things to think about, and if I don't hear from him by four thirty, I'll give him a call."

Each time you are aware of experiencing a negative emotion, you have a choice to make. You can allow yourself to be enveloped by anger, depression, or anxiety, letting it capture your entire being. Or you can recognize that such feelings are present, but by firmly deciding that you're not going to identify with them, they will simply pass through you. In this way, the intensity of the negative experience will be significantly reduced.

Humorist Dan Greenburg has proclaimed that lawyers are proficient in the art of negative thinking: they can tell you everything that has gone wrong or could go wrong. However, some pain patients are so negatively oriented that they could put lawyers to shame.

People who hurt often become stuck in a cycle of negativity, and it sours every aspect of their life. For example, have you ever said to yourself, "Maybe I shouldn't go to that party tomorrow night because while I'm there my pain might flare up"? The more you think about that possibility, the greater the chance it will happen. Negative thoughts can be just as powerful as positive ones, and overpowering thought may soon become fact. However, if you realize, "Oh, I'm starting to worry about tomorrow night," you can make a conscious choice not to continue doing so by thinking about something else incompatible with the fear of future pain. In this way, you may actually be able to reduce the chance that your pain will flare up.

In my opinion, emotions are like reality itself—ambiguous and vague. For the way you experience various emotions depends primarily upon your own belief systems and frames of reference. Under one set of circumstances, that same feeling may be experienced as anxiety. Energetically, identical bodily processes occur during both excitement and anxiety—muscles become tense, the heartbeat accelerates, sweat glands are activated—and your mind becomes immediately aware of this increased arousal.

If you choose to identify with the negative end of the spectrum, you'll interpret the feeling as one of anxiety. But if you identify with the positive end of essentially the same emotion, it can just as easily be experienced as excitement. It's up to you.

I also sometimes advise my patients to resist expressing or "acting out" the negative emotions they sense within themselves. Very often, your behavior and actions determine how you feel. So if you act in a negative manner, you may well start to feel that way. Likewise, positive actions can produce positive emotions. Think about it for a moment. Isn't it almost impossible to dislike someone whom you treat really well?

The next time you're feeling depressed, walk over to a mirror, look intently at your own image—and smile. That's all, just smile. Most people find that their grin soon turns into laughter. Once they start laughing, their feelings change as well.

I also encourage my patients to avoid "time warping" as much as possible. Essentially, time warping involves focusing on everything but what is happening to you right now. For patients with pain, it usually entails either regretting the past or worrying about the future—neither of which is relevant to the present moment. The past doesn't exist anymore; it's only there in your imagination. The future hasn't happened yet; it isn't real. The only reality, as vague as it is, reflects what is going on right here, right now. If you focus your thoughts only on the present, you'll find that it is incompatible with regretting the past and worrying about the future. In short, one of the best ways of dealing with your negative thoughts and emotions is to "Be Here Now."

I recall one period of my life when I was experiencing a profound transition. A major romance was breaking up, and at the same time, I was trying to study for some of the most rigorous exams of my student years. I found myself time warping constantly—regretting the past and fearing the future. These thoughts so hurt and haunted me that I finally sought professional help.

By chance, I found my way into a Gestalt therapy group. Although I doubt that this is the type of therapy I'd find useful nowadays, it was the best experience I could have had at that time. The therapist's entire philosophy was based on one idea—"Be Here Now." That's all he would talk about. And he'd ram it into you. It seemed crazy at first, but it really worked. Whenever I'd start to time-warp, I would hear his voice telling me, "Be Here Now." It was just what I needed. And if you're a time warper, that's probably all you need, too.

If you don't think about the past or the future, they essentially won't exist in your personal reality. If you have difficulty avoiding time warping, try to think about positive experiences and expectations rather than negative ones. Recall the good things of the past; contemplate the good possibilities for the future. By doing so, you'll help make negativity incompatible with your inner experience.

Many times I think that the way we should treat ourselves is the way we relate to our best friend. Would you ever tell a friend, "Only think about the worst possible things in your life. Think of how horrible the past was and how miserable your future might be. Dwell upon the negative!"

You'd never say such things to a good friend. So why do you say them to yourself? Wouldn't you give a close friend as much positive support as possible? Then why do you feed yourself so much negativity?

If you want to deal more effectively with your negative feelings, start by beginning to love yourself. Appreciate the good things about yourself, and give yourself some of that positive input that you reserve more often for others. Develop greater faith in yourself and in your ability to create your own destiny. Give yourself more self-love; it may change your entire life.

The Keys to Success

Many patients with chronic pain remind me of ships without captains. They float around on an ocean of negativity, drifting from doctor to doctor, hoping to run aground on a magical island with its own fountain of pain relief. Most of these patients will drift forever, for they have failed to take their share of the responsibility for their own well-being. They have given up actively searching for help. Their situation, they are convinced, is futile. They have stopped trying.

Fortunately, others assume a more assertive, positive role, actively seeking the help and support of many different types of health care practitioners. These patients believe that they can overcome their discomfort, and are willing to explore all possible remedies known to be safe. In short, they become the captains of their ships, and in my opinion, their chances for success are good, no matter how difficult the problem.

No impossibilities exist in their ocean. There are many reports of chronic pain patients who learn to turn their pain off completely, osteoarthritis patients who significantly reduce the swelling in their joints, and cancer victims who "spontaneously remit" from their terrible, degenerative illness.

As a result of my experiences in working with thousands of pain patients, I believe that the major key to success lies in their extraordinary motivation to get better. If you haven't done so already, look deeply within to see how determined *you* are to resume a healthy life-style. If you're currently pessimistic about ever receiving help, an immediate change in attitude is essential. Remember, the best way to change a belief system is by adopting a new one that's incompatible with the old. If you've been thinking, Nothing else can be done to help me, make a conscious effort to accept the possibility that help *is* possible, and you *will* get better.

No, you need not think that every technique and treatment you encounter is the ultimate cure-all. But I believe it is critical for you to assume that the *chance* for success is always there. At the very least, you should be saying, "I don't know whether this will work or not, but I'm going to try it and find out. Only then will I decide if it is worthwhile for me."

Once you have adopted a more positive attitude and belief system, you'll find that there are many new avenues of potential healing available to you. For example, you can personally take the steps necessary to ensure that your body and mind are well-nourished. In Chapter 7, I'll teach you how to relax and meditate, as well as improve your sleep habits. In Chapter 8, I'll discuss the foods and vitamins that can help not only your physical pain, but your depression as well. In Chapter 9, you'll also learn how to enhance your environmental and emotional nourishment, and how to increase the fun in your life. And in Chapters 10 and 11, through techniques like guided imagery, I'll teach you how to retrain your nervous system to learn new habits that are incompatible with your current, pain-producing ones.

As you explore the various recommendations presented in this book, be open-minded and give them an honest try. If your pain eases up as a result of, say, guided imagery, then continue to see how much further it can help in the healing process. Or if no progress is noted after giving sensory awareness a fair chance, then move on to something else.

I also urge you to create your own approaches to pain alleviation. Sometimes we forget how exciting the creative process can be, and we neglect to use it to solve our own problems. Experiment. Try new things. You can determine how successful your own approaches are by evaluating to what extent your nervous system is raising or lowering your discomfort in response.

Few patients have been more creative than Norman Cousins. As you recall from Chapter 4, he had been suffering from a severe illness called ankylosing spondylitis, with only 1 chance in 500 for recovery. But Cousins decided to take control of his fight for survival. With his doctor's consent, he removed himself from the hospital "to find a place somewhat more conducive to a positive outlook on life." Continuing his account in the *New England Journal of Medicine*, Cousins said:

> One of the incidental advantages of the hotel room, I was delighted to find, was that it cost only about one-third as much as the hospital. The other benefits were incalculable. I would not be awakened for a bed bath or for meals or for medication or for a change in the bed sheets or for tests or for examinations by hospital interns. The sense of serenity was delicious and would, I felt certain, contribute to a general improvement.

Self-healing will require hard work on your part. And even if you succeed, you may find yourself occasionally slipping back into your old pain habits. Prepare yourself now to deal with such setbacks. As soon as you sense that your pain is returning, or become aware that your negative feelings are resurfacing, conscientiously implement the therapeutic techniques you'll learn in this book.

Remember. You do have the power of self-healing. I urge you to make the most of it.

Oasis

Time for a rest. From here on, you will be asked to participate in a variety of experiences designed to help you understand and deal more effectively with your discomfort. If you have not yet completed the first fifteen exercises, now is a good time to do so.

When you're ready to return, I'll discuss how you can start getting needed nourishment.

III

Getting Needed Nourishment

7 *The Pause That Refreshes*

Take rest, a field that has rested gives a bountiful crop.

—Ovid

One of my colleagues tells the story of a man brought into an emergency room with severe third-degree burns on both ears. After immediate treatment was administered, a doctor asked the patient how he had sustained such a peculiar injury.

"Well," the man replied, "I tend to be a very nervous individual. I just can't relax. Just about everything that happens is stressful to me. Even the most trivial things make me completely fall apart. I can barely function in the modern world.

"I was home ironing this morning," he continued, "and the telephone rang. I got so nervous, flustered, and confused that instead of lifting up the telephone receiver, I lifted up the iron, and burned my ear."

The doctor was startled by the unusual story. "You certainly do sound like a stressed individual," he said. "But tell me—how did you damage the *other* ear?"

Without hesitation, the patient responded, "I had to call the ambulance, didn't I?"

Humor aside, the stress of modern-day living has become a ferocious enemy of man. Health statistics in the United States scream out that we deal with stress very poorly. Lewis Thomas, president of the Memorial

Sloan-Kettering Cancer Center, believes that relative to the universe, "we are the delicate part, transient and vulnerable as cilia." Too often, we are simply unable to cope, and as a result, stress-related illness has become the major health problem in the modern world.

Life Stress and Illness

For decades, researchers have suspected that there was an important link between stress and physical illness. Now, the relationship has been well-documented by hundreds of studies and thousands of individual medical histories.

In a case you'll probably recall, Dr. Samuel Silverman, a Harvard psychiatrist, predicted the serious illness suffered by Richard Nixon after he resigned from the Presidency in 1974. Silverman told *Time* magazine that post-Watergate pressure was a threat to Nixon's life, and would probably manifest itself in Nixon's legs (because of previous phlebitis problems) and his lungs (because of earlier pneumonia attacks). Several days later, clots in Nixon's legs caused such severe physical problems that the former President nearly died—primarily, according to Silverman, because of psychological stress related to the events surrounding his resignation.

Even the most serious physical ailments may have some relationship to stress. Consider the three sets of twins studied by Dr. William A. Greene, University of Rochester psychiatrist, during the 1960s. One twin from each set was a victim of leukemia. According to Greene, each of the leukemia patients had experienced a major psychological upheaval in her life immediately before the ailment manifested itself. Perhaps, then, concluded Greene, stress might be a precipitating factor in cancer that is even more important than heredity.

His hypothesis has been substantiated by other researchers. Lawrence LeShan, former chief of the psychology department at the Institute of Applied Biology in New York City, has studied hundreds of cancer patients over a period of a dozen years. Interestingly, the majority of these individuals had endured a severe emotional trauma early in life, such as the death of a parent.

In a study of 218 lung cancer patients by David M. Kissen, a British psychologist, many of them had experienced the death or absence of a parent during childhood. There was also a high incidence of work-related problems and particularly long-term marital difficulties in adult life. These patients, said Kissen, also had "poor outlets for emotional discharge," and thus tended to manifest their pent-up emotions in a physical way.

Eugene Pendergrass, former president of the American Cancer Society, has publicly conceded that there may be a relationship between psychological stress and cancer. According to Pendergrass, "Psychological factors sometimes have a marked influence on the behavior and rate of growth of cancer once it has occurred in the human body. It is not unreasonable to postulate that this could result from the interaction of psychological factors and hormonal levels. I want to make it clear that I am not suggesting the psychologic factors act as an initial causative agent in the occurrence of cancer. I am only suggesting that they sometimes have an influence on pre-existing cancer and may have an influence on susceptibility to cancer."

There is also evidence linking high blood pressure, ulcers, and various types of chronic pain to stress. Some experts estimate that 90 percent of all headaches are related to prolonged muscular contraction because of stress. And this muscular tension is not restricted only to the head. If stress has caused your back, your shoulders, or your neck to be tight for a long period of time, pain will very likely be the result. Perhaps you have read the Civil War diary of Ulysses S. Grant, who wrote that on the night before Appomattox when Robert E. Lee had refused to surrender, he went to bed with an excruciating headache. However, as soon as word arrived that Lee had changed his mind, Grant's headache vanished.

A link between stress and coronary artery disease is also quite clear. Dr. Flanders Dunbar at the Columbia Presbyterian Medical Center in New York City noted more than three decades ago that many heart-attack victims were self-made professionals who led very trying lives. According to Dunbar, they were victims of "compulsive striving," and "would rather die than fail."

A 1975 study conducted by a team of researchers at the University of California at Berkeley compared the cultural life-styles and the heart-disease rates of American and Japanese men. Their ten-year study analyzed various factors typically associated with heart disease—including life-style, diet, cholesterol levels, and smoking habits. The researchers concluded that competitive and aggressive American living contributed significantly to the incidence of heart disease. Even Japanese men who ate very high-fat diets still had significantly fewer coronaries than Americans.

Drs. Meyer Friedman and Ray H. Rosenmann, in their book *Type A Behavior and Your Heart*, conclude that people with "striving personalities" are prime candidates for heart disease, hypertension, and other physical ailments. These "Type A" individuals live their lives according to the calendar and the clock. They do everything rapidly—working, walking, eating. They can't do only one thing at a time, and feel guilty about "doing nothing." They are "one-man shows" who tend to do everything themselves, and they go through life with clenched fists and tightened bodies. According to Friedman and Rosenmann, over 90 percent of the males under age sixty who have heart attacks display "Type A" behavior.

Stress is related not only to illness, but also appears to accelerate the aging process. According to pioneer stress researcher Hans Selye, "What we call aging is nothing more than the sum total of all the scars left by the stress of life."

One of the most powerful stressors known is a sudden change in one's life situation. Thomas Holmes, M.D., professor of psychiatry at the University of Washington, has devised a "Schedule of Recent Experience"—a compilation of the forty-four most stressful life events that appear to influence health and illness. He assigned each "life event" a numerical rating or "scale value," ranging from 11 to 100, based upon its impact on the organism.

The death of a spouse ranks highest on the scale, with a score of 100. Modern man faces no more stressful event. Also ranking very high are divorce, a jail term, and personal injury or illness. Ten of the fifteen top crises are related to the family in some way. Interestingly, positive changes in one's life are also stressful—like marriage or an outstanding personal achievement. Although a vacation is usually a desirable, pleasant activity, it represents a change from the norm and it, too, typically involves some stress.

Before reading on, stop for a minute to complete Exercise Sixteen: Your Life Change Score.

Exercise Sixteen: Your Life Change Score

To determine your current life change score, we will use the Schedule of Recent Experience developed by Dr. Holmes. Proceed through the chart on pages 247 and 249. Under Number of Occurrences, indicate how many times in the past twelve months each event has taken place in your life. Multiply that number by the Scale Value of the event, and place the answer in the column titled Your Score. Finally, add the figures in the Your Score column to arrive at your total life change score for the past year.

According to Holmes, if your total life change score is over 300 points for one year, you have almost an 80 percent chance of becoming sick in the near future. If your score falls into the 200- to 299-point range, you have about a fifty-fifty probability of becoming ill. A score in the 150- to 199-point range yields a 37 percent chance of sickness.

This scale can alert you that physical problems might be on the way. And the higher your score, the more serious those ailments may be—that is, if you have a total of over 300 life-change units, you have a greater probability of developing cancer or a heart condition than if you accumulated only 150 points.

By examining the chart closely, you can see how just one stress-producing life event can provoke many others. Let's assume, for instance, that you receive a job transfer that will force you and your family to move across the country. First of all, you will be faced with a business adjustment (39 points) and a change in residence (20). These may be accompanied by a change in your financial status (38), a change in living conditions (25), a new and/or higher mortgage (31), a change in church (19) and social activities (18), and a change in the number of family gatherings (15).

That already totals 205 points. But there may be even more. What if your spouse opposes the cross-country move for some of the reasons mentioned above (change in social activities, etc.). That may cause a variation in the number of marital arguments (35), trouble with the in-laws (29), sexual difficulties (39), and even divorce (73). Suddenly you've accumulated a staggering 381 life-change units—and you're a prime target for illness.

Research by Holmes and his associate, Richard H. Rahe, M.D., indicates that the scale is applicable regardless of race, culture, and age. In study after study, its validity has been substantiated. When Rahe evaluated the stress of twenty-five hundred Navy men on shipboard duty, those who had recently undergone marital or family changes went on sick call 36 percent more often than those without such experiences. Holmes studied the life changes of a hundred college football players just before the start of the season, and based on the scores they received on the Social Readjustment Rating Scale, he classified them as either high, medium, or low risk for injuries. When the season had ended three months later, 9 percent in the low-risk group had been hurt, 25 percent in the medium-risk group, and 50 percent in the high-risk.

Dr. Sidney Cobb has found that the stress of job loss and unemployment has a staggering impact upon automobile workers in Detroit. Cobb, now a professor of community health and psychiatry at Brown University, studied a hundred men who had been laid off from their jobs on the auto assembly lines. He began monitoring their health six weeks *before* the layoffs, and continued doing so for a full two years. The results were startling.

According to Cobb, the unemployed workers committed suicide at a rate thirty times above the norm. Among the hundred men studied, eight cases of arthritis developed, six of severe depression, five of hypertension (which necessitated hospitalization), three of hair falling out, two of high blood pressure, and one of gout. Even the families of these unemployed workers felt the impact. For example, three wives developed peptic ulcers (a rare ailment for women) that required hospitalization.

Clearly, the most significant stressor is usually the loss of a spouse. A British study in the early 1960s researched the lives of forty-five hundred widowers over the age of fifty-four. As might be expected, these men

SAMPLE

EXERCISE SIXTEEN: Your Life Change Score   DATE: _March 29_

TIME: _6 p.m._

LIFE EVENT	NUMBER OF OCCURRENCES	SCALE VALUE	YOUR SCORE
Death of spouse		100	
Divorce		73	
Marital separation from mate		65	
Detention in jail or other institution		63	
Death of a close family member		63	
Major personal injury or illness	1	53	53
Marriage		50	
Being fired at work		47	
Marital reconciliation with mate		45	
Retirement from work		45	
Major change in the health or behavior of a family member		44	
Pregnancy		40	
Sexual difficulties	1	39	39
Gaining a new family member (e.g., through birth, adoption, oldster moving in, etc.)		39	
Major business readjustment (e.g., merger, reorganization, bankruptcy, etc.)		39	
Major change in financial state (e.g., a lot worse off or a lot better off than usual)		38	
Death of a close friend	1	37	37
Changing to a different line of work		36	
Major change in the number of arguments with spouse (e.g., either a lot more or a lot less than usual regarding child-rearing, personal habits, etc.)	2	35	70
Taking on a mortgage greater than $10,000 (e.g., purchasing a house, business, etc.)		31	
Foreclosure on a mortgage or loan		30	
Major change in responsibilities at work (e.g., promotion, demotion, lateral transfer)		29	
Son or daughter leaving home (e.g., marriage, attending college, etc.)	1	29	29
In-law troubles	1	29	29
Subtotal:			

EXERCISE SIXTEEN: Your Life Change Score   DATE: _____

TIME: _____

LIFE EVENT	NUMBER OF OCCURRENCES	SCALE VALUE	YOUR SCORE
Death of spouse		100	
Divorce		73	
Marital separation from mate		65	
Detention in jail or other institution		63	
Death of a close family member		63	
Major personal injury or illness		53	
Marriage		50	
Being fired at work		47	
Marital reconciliation with mate		45	
Retirement from work		45	
Major change in the health or behavior of a family member		44	
Pregnancy		40	
Sexual difficulties		39	
Gaining a new family member (e.g., through birth, adoption, oldster moving in, etc.)		39	
Major business readjustment (e.g., merger, reorganization, bankruptcy, etc.)		39	
Major change in financial state (e.g., a lot worse off or a lot better off than usual)		38	
Death of a close friend		37	
Changing to a different line of work		36	
Major change in the number of arguments with spouse (e.g., either a lot more or a lot less than usual regarding child-rearing, personal habits, etc.)		35	
Taking on a mortgage greater than $10,000 (e.g., purchasing a house, business, etc.)		31	
Foreclosure on a mortgage or loan		30	
Major change in responsibilities at work (e.g., promotion, demotion, lateral transfer)		29	
Son or daughter leaving home (e.g., marriage, attending college, etc.)		29	
In-law troubles		29	
Subtotal:			

SAMPLE

EXERCISE SIXTEEN:—*Continued*

LIFE EVENT	NUMBER OF OCCURRENCES	SCALE VALUE	YOUR SCORE
Total from previous page:			
Outstanding personal achievement		28	
Wife beginning or ceasing work outside the home		26	
Beginning or ceasing formal schooling		26	
Major change in living conditions (e.g., building a new house, remodeling, deterioration of house or neighborhood)		25	
Revision of personal habits (dress, manners, associations, etc.)	1	24	24
Troubles with boss		23	
Major change in working hours or conditions		20	
Change in residence		20	
Changing to a new school		20	
Major change in usual type and/or amount of recreation	2	19	38
Major change in church activities (e.g., a lot more or a lot less than usual)		19	
Major change in social activities (e.g., clubs, dancing, movies, visiting, etc.)	2	18	36
Taking on a mortgage or loan less than $10,000 (e.g., purchasing a car, TV, freezer, etc.)		17	
Major change in sleeping habits (a lot more or a lot less sleep, or change in part of day when asleep)	2	16	32
Major change in number of family get-togethers (e.g., a lot more or a lot less than usual)	2	15	30
Major change in eating habits (a lot more or a lot less food intake, or very different meal hours or surroundings)		15	
Vacation	1	13	13
Christmas	1	12	12
Minor violations of the law (e.g., traffic tickets, jaywalking, disturbing the peace, etc.)	2	11	22
This is your total life change score for the past year			464

SOURCE: *The Schedule of Recent Experience (SRE),* © 1976 by Thomas H. Holmes, M.D.

EXERCISE SIXTEEN:—*Continued*

LIFE EVENT	NUMBER OF OCCURRENCES	SCALE VALUE	YOUR SCORE
Total from previous page:			
Outstanding personal achievement		28	
Wife beginning or ceasing work outside the home		26	
Beginning or ceasing formal schooling		26	
Major change in living conditions (e.g., building a new house, remodeling, deterioration of house or neighborhood)		25	
Revision of personal habits (dress, manners, associations, etc.)		24	
Troubles with boss		23	
Major change in working hours or conditions		20	
Change in residence		20	
Changing to a new school		20	
Major change in usual type and/or amount of recreation		19	
Major change in church activities (e.g., a lot more or a lot less than usual)		19	
Major change in social activities (e.g., clubs, dancing, movies, visiting, etc.)		18	
Taking on a mortgage or loan less than $10,000 (e.g., purchasing a car, TV, freezer, etc.)		17	
Major change in sleeping habits (a lot more or a lot less sleep, or change in part of day when asleep)		16	
Major change in number of family get-togethers (e.g., a lot more or a lot less than usual)		15	
Major change in eating habits (a lot more or a lot less food intake, or very different meal hours or surroundings)		15	
Vacation		13	
Christmas		12	
Minor violations of the law (e.g., traffic tickets, jaywalking, disturbing the peace, etc.)		11	
This is your total life change score for the past year			

SOURCE: *The Schedule of Recent Experience (SRE)*, © 1976 by Thomas H. Holmes, M.D.

experienced significant increases in depression and illness immediately after the death of their wives. But particularly startling was this fact: in the first six months after their spouse's death, the mortality rate of these men was 40 percent higher than the average death rate for men of their age.

Your Unseen Enemy

Chronic psychosocial stress is an unfortunate companion of twentieth-century living. True, stress has been a part of man's existence since prehistoric times, but the caveman was perfectly designed to deal with the acute or short-term stresses he faced. When he sensed the presence of, say, a wild animal nearby, he reacted with "fight or flight." That is, he either fought off the life-threatening enemy or he fled from it.

Physiologically, the sympathetic division of his autonomic nervous system would shift into emergency gear during moments of acute stress. His bloodstream would be inundated with adrenaline and other stress hormones. His pulse and respiration rates would quicken, and his blood pressure would rise rapidly. There would be dramatic changes in his body's electrical activity, and perspiration would dampen his hands and brow. His pupils would dilate, his throat would tighten, and his neck and upper back would become tense. His nostrils would flare out to aid respiration. His pelvis would become rigid, with numb genitals and tight anus. These changes permitted him to react immediately to the crisis situation, and through either fight or flight, it was usually resolved within minutes. His body would then enter a regenerative phase to prepare for future emergencies.

However, modern man is faced with a far different situation. The bodies you and I live in were beautifully designed for survival on this planet ten thousand years ago, but in many ways, they're obsolete for today's world. The major stressors we encounter are not usually resolved by the fight-or-flight response. For example, consider the fear of increasing crime rates and the concern over smog-infested skies. After all, where can most of us run in order to escape crime or increasingly polluted skies? Whom can we fight?

Most people depend for their livelihood on jobs that are incredibly tension-packed—whether you're a policeman whose life is constantly threatened, or an air traffic controller who must flawlessly talk, think, plan, and issue instructions to keep airplanes from tangling with one another. How can you run when faced with family responsibilities? Again, whom can you fight?

Dr. Michael Volen offers another example of the inappropriateness of the fight-or-flight response for modern living. Imagine, he says, driving the crowded freeways of Los Angeles, sitting alone in your automobile during rush hour. Traffic is so heavy that you have completely stopped moving. Your car can't go forward, backward, or to either side. You just sit there, inhaling the nauseating exhaust fumes that pour in from the cars around you. You soon find yourself gripping the steering wheel tightly and gnashing your teeth together, as you feel adrenaline surge through your body. And you want to do one of two things—either you just want to leap out of your car and run away, or you want to walk over and hit somebody. Well, it's inappropriate to take either of these actions on the freeway. You can't fight or run. So you just helplessly sit there—and fume.

How much stress do you think you're experiencing right now. Let's find out. Before you continue reading further, I'd like you to get yourself as comfortable as possible in the chair you're sitting in. Go ahead. . . . Make yourself as comfortable as you can. . . . Right now. . . .

Are you comfortable now? What did you have to do to put yourself at ease? Did you reposition yourself in the chair? Did you stretch the muscles in your arms or legs? If so, why did you have to move at all? Why weren't you naturally comfortable already?

You probably weren't even aware that your body was in a state of tension. But it was, and possibly still is. Millions of other people suffer a similar fate. There are so many pressures inherent in contemporary living that very few people avoid stress-related diseases. Even worse than their number is the fact that many modern-day stressors never seem to end. Our bodies are constantly activated to fight a host of invisible enemies, like inflation or the threat of nuclear holocaust. As adrenaline and other stress hormones race through us, our pulse rate, respiration rate, and blood pressure remain high. Our flexor and extensor muscles are constantly tensed, and the effect is similar to what happens to your car when you step on the accelerator and brake at the same time.

Over time, we slowly burn ourselves out, since our bodies rarely get a chance to relax and restore themselves. As our overloaded systems become exhausted, we develop the characteristic afflictions of civilization: high blood pressure, heart disease, lung disease, ulcers, asthma, arthritis, cancer, depression, and a host of other psychophysiological problems, including, of course, chronic pain.

In short, evolution hasn't kept up with technology. We're stuck in an obsolete body that, while equipped to cope with acute stress, can't adapt to the chronic anxieties of modern life. As I discussed earlier, when feelings of helplessness develop, depression and illness are not far behind. These, in turn, produce even more stress. It's a vicious, destructive cycle.

The relationship between stress and depression cannot be over-emphasized. At a recent conference on stress, Meyer Friedman, M.D., the pioneering investigator in the field of heart disease and stress, told me of some unpublished studies that compared the physiological status of chronically depressed patients with that of the parents of children with leukemia. These parents were subjected to one of the most severe stressors imaginable, for in a final desperate attempt to save their children's lives, the youngsters had been admitted to the hospital for a series of chemotherapy treatments. Yet Friedman found that the physiological indicators of stress were several times higher in the depressed patients than in the parents of these leukemic children! Although the depressed patients didn't appear to be stressed, chronic stress, chronic depression, and chronic illness usually run hand in hand.

The destructive impact of the stress/depression/illness cycle has not yet been fully appreciated by patients or by medical authorities. Tragically, the cycle often stops only when the individual commits suicide, or develops a severe, even fatal, stress-related physical disease. By creating an integrated, therapeutic program that provides comprehensive treatment for stress, depression, and illness, we can deal with this situation in a much more positive, constructive way. In this chapter, you'll learn a simple technique that will help you to overcome chronic stress, your unseen enemy.

What Can You Do About It?

As a practitioner of integral medicine, I think it's important to point out that each person experiences stress in his or her own unique way. Accordingly, there are as many stress-reduction plans as there are people, and each of us must find out for ourselves what works best. Many different techniques have been recommended—including both active and passive types of relaxation. The active approaches range from jogging to swimming to yoga to dancing. They all involve muscular activity, followed by profound muscle relaxation and a sense of well-being. Active relaxing can also occur on a psychological level, in the form of a pastime like reading. Suggestions on how to incorporate active relaxation into your life will be offered in Chapter 9.

Passive stress reduction techniques include massage and manipulation, which directly relax the muscles, and in the process, relax the mind as well. The mind and the body can also be rested by using psychological techniques such as Conditioned Relaxation (presented later in this chapter), meditation, autogenic training, biofeedback, and other approaches like those reviewed in Chapter 5.

It seems obvious to me that stress management techniques can significantly reduce the afflictions of civilization, for they provide an easy and effective way to end the long-term fight-or-flight response which now works against us. Many stress researchers believe that appropriate stress management can help cut cholesterol levels and the incidence of high blood pressure and heart attacks. Relaxation techniques also provide a positive alternative to smoking (which is a major health hazard), and to excessive drinking, drug taking, and overeating (alcohol, other drugs, and obesity contribute significantly to many health problems).

Because prolonged psychosocial stress can increase general muscle tension, people with musculoskeletal pain usually experience an immediate reduction in their discomfort by learning passive relaxation techniques. Several studies also indicate that various methods of relaxation training can reduce the frequency and severity of migraine and chronic tension headaches as well.

As I mentioned earlier in this book, I believe that stress management techniques should be taught to our children at the first-grade level to ensure good physical and mental health. In my opinion, this might be the most profound way to prevent the unnecessary suffering of many patients with stress-related disorders, as well as reduce the staggering costs of modern medical care.

Although most people find active and passive relaxation techniques to be helpful, I must emphasize again that everyone is different. What may work well for one patient may not be appropriate for another. Hans Selye once stated that there are two kinds of people—racehorses and turtles. Although it can be stressful when the turtle must run like a racehorse, the converse is equally true. Many doctors tell patients who have had heart attacks to retire from work and "take it easy." However, having the hard-driving, Type A person slow down, stop working, and do nothing may be more stressful than continuing his present life-style.

How, then, can you determine what works best for you? By trying different techniques and then seeing the results. Try massage, meditation, Conditioned Relaxation, autogenic training, or biofeedback and see what happens. Exercise Seventeen can be very helpful in this regard. By periodically assessing your Stress Index, you can keep track of how well you are doing. Take a moment to find out how you score now. Later, after you have begun practicing the Conditioned Relaxation exercise, or any other stress-reduction technique that you feel will be beneficial, calculate your Stress Index again to see how well you are doing.

Exercise Seventeen: Your Stress Index

The Stress Index will help you to chart the changes in the amount of stress you experience as you work with various stress-reduction techniques. I recommend that you calculate and graph your score once each week. To obtain your score, proceed through each of the twenty-two

SAMPLE

EXERCISE SEVENTEEN: Your Stress Index *CODE:* 3 = *often*
2 = *once or twice this week*
1 = *rarely*
0 = *not at all*

STATEMENT	DATES	4/2	4/9	4/16	4/23	4/30	5/7	5/14	5/21	5/28	
I feel tense or anxious		2	1	2	3	2	2	2	1	1	
I feel angry or irritable		2	2	1	1	1	1	1	2	1	
I feel depressed or helpless		3	3	2	3	3	2	1	0	1	
I find it difficult to relax		2	1	1	2	1	1	1	0	1	
I find it hard to concentrate on one thing		0	0	0	0	0	0	0	0	0	
I find it hard to meet deadlines or quotas		0	1	2	1	0	0	0	0	0	
People at work make me feel tense		2	2	2	1	2	1	1	0	1	
People at home make me feel tense		3	1	2	3	2	2	1	0	0	
I have indigestion		0	0	0	0	0	0	0	0	0	
I have headaches		3	3	3	3	3	3	2	2	2	
I have high blood pressure		0	0	0	0	0	0	0	0	0	
I have rashes or other skin problems		0	0	0	0	0	0	0	0	0	
I have tension-related neck or shoulder pain		1	0	0	1	0	0	1	0	1	
My hands tend to be cool or perspiring		1	1	1	1	0	1	0	0	0	
I have difficulty falling asleep		3	3	3	2	2	2	1	1	1	
I wake up very early in the morning		3	3	3	3	3	3	2	2	1	
I eat when I feel tense		2	2	2	2	1	1	1	0	1	
I smoke when I feel tense		0	0	0	0	0	0	0	0	0	
I drink alcoholic beverages when I feel tense		2	2	1	2	1	2	1	1	1	
I take drugs when I feel tense		0	0	0	0	0	0	0	0	0	
I chew my nails when I feel tense		3	3	3	3	3	3	3	3	3	
I worry about the future		3	3	3	3	3	3	3	3	3	
Stress Index Score		35	31	31	34	27	27	21	15	18	

SOURCE: *The Stress Index*, © 1978 by David E. Bresler, Ph.D.

EXERCISE SEVENTEEN: Your Stress Index

CODE: 3 = *often*
2 = *once or twice this week*
1 = *rarely*
0 = *not at all*

STATEMENT	DATES								
I feel tense or anxious									
I feel angry or irritable									
I feel depressed or helpless									
I find it difficult to relax									
I find it hard to concentrate on one thing									
I find it hard to meet deadlines or quotas									
People at work make me feel tense									
People at home make me feel tense									
I have indigestion									
I have headaches									
I have high blood pressure									
I have rashes or other skin problems									
I have tension-related neck or shoulder pain									
My hands tend to be cool or perspiring									
I have difficulty falling asleep									
I wake up very early in the morning									
I eat when I feel tense									
I smoke when I feel tense									
I drink alcoholic beverages when I feel tense									
I take drugs when I feel tense									
I chew my nails when I feel tense									
I worry about the future									
Stress Index Score									

SOURCE: *The Stress Index,* © 1978 by David E. Bresler, Ph.D.

statements and enter a score of 3 if the statement applies to you often, 2 if it applies once or twice a week, 1 if it applies rarely, or 0 if it does not apply at all. There is no specific significance to any particular range of scores; rather, it is the *changes* in the scores over time that are important.

The Importance of Sleep

Perhaps one of the most natural ways we deal with stress is by getting a good night's sleep. There are several theories about the purpose of sleep, but probably the most popular one is that various recuperative or restorative processes occur during this time. According to this hypothesis, our bodies are fatigued, stressed, and exhausted by day's end, and without sleep, they would never have a chance to recover.

Sleep is particularly important during times of illness. While we are asleep, most of our metabolic energy can be directed toward the healing process, as antibodies are built up, bacteria are disposed of, and new cells are produced to replace damaged ones.

I believe that REM (rapid eye movement) sleep—the stage of sleep during which most dreaming occurs—is often a time of intense stress release. When we have more stress than can normally be discharged during a normal sleep period, sleep itself is disturbed, for we dream so violently that we wake ourselves up. No wonder so many highly stressed chronic pain patients have difficulty sleeping.

When people are deprived of REM sleep in laboratory studies, their need for REM sleep becomes even more intense. On subsequent nights, when allowed to sleep normally, these test subjects experience an increased amount of REM, as if the body was trying to make up for the earlier deprivation.

Ironically, when people sleep poorly, they often resort to the use of sleeping pills, which typically only compound their problems. Most hypnotic drugs significantly suppress REM sleep, causing fewer and shorter REM periods. Consequently, there is a reduced opportunity for stress release. (Even drugs like flurazepam [Dalmane] that do not suppress REM sleep reduce stages III and IV of sleep, which are the deepest stages of sleep.)

Rather than relying on sleeping pills, my patients are encouraged to practice a relaxation technique at bedtime. Instead of a prescription for sleeping pills, they are given a prerecorded cassette tape containing the Conditioned Relaxation exercise that you are about to learn. This type of exercise does not interfere with sleep cycles; rather, it strongly promotes natural sleep. Not surprisingly, many people who once called themselves insomniacs can regularly fall asleep within minutes of beginning this relaxation exercise. If you have trouble falling asleep, it will almost certainly be of great benefit to you as well.

Why Conditioned Relaxation?

There is no shortage of effective relaxation techniques. Probably the best known of these is Transcendental Meditation, introduced to the Western world by the Maharishi Mahesh Yogi. Studies reviewed in Chapter 5 indicate that TM significantly reduces many of the body's metabolic and nervous system activities.

However, despite the enormous publicity surrounding TM, it is not necessarily any more effective than many other relaxation exercises. Approaches ranging from autogenic training to Edmund Jacobson's "progressive relaxation" to Herbert Benson's "relaxation response" have all produced impressive benefits.

My own relaxation system—called Conditioned Relaxation—has emerged from my experiences at UCLA as a method particularly effective for pain patients. Unlike TM, it does not require a mantra. And once it is mastered through diligent practice, a state of relaxation can be achieved almost instantaneously by taking a single "signal breath."

Most people are familiar with the work of Pavlov, the Russian psychophysiologist, whose experiments with dogs demonstrated the conditioning process. He would ring a bell, show a hungry dog some meat, and, of course, the animal would salivate. After repeating this procedure many times, Pavlov eliminated the middle step—that is, he rang the bell but did not show the meat to the dog. Because of the repeated pairing of the bell and the meat, the dog had become conditioned to salivate whenever he heard the bell.

Conditioning is the most fundamental form of learning on the planet. Most sophisticated life-forms—from worms to guinea pigs to cats to dogs—learn this way. (When your cat—or even your goldfish—sees you approaching at feeding time, he will usually become highly excited even before seeing the food.) Our primitive nervous system learns this way as well. In Conditioned Relaxation, these same principles of classical conditioning are applied to allow you to relax on command—even when you're unable to go through an entire relaxation exercise. Just as the bell became an automatic signal for Pavlov's dog to salivate, a "signal breath" can be used to help your body relax instantaneously.

There are enormous benefits in learning to relax on command. For example, if you feel a sudden surge of pain or stress while driving on the freeway, you would obviously be unable to perform an entire relaxation technique. But it would certainly be possible for you to take a quick signal breath that would immediately induce relaxation.

Everyone can learn Conditioned Relaxation and benefit from it. No unusual mental capabilities are necessary, and no particular educational experiences are required. It makes no difference whether your pain is in your shoulder, neck, back, head, chest, or anywhere else. If you are persistent, and give your mind and body time to learn the technique, it will almost certainly help you. If you *allow* the exercise to work, rather than *pursuing* relaxation, you may be pleasantly surprised by what you can accomplish.

Relaxation cannot be forced. Although you can voluntarily tighten or tense many of your muscles, you can't voluntarily relax them. You can only *allow* them to relax by not contracting them. To me, it's like trying to force yourself to urinate, to remember a name, or to go to sleep. You can't make it happen. In the same way, you can't make yourself relax; you can only allow it to occur.

Ideally, when performing this exercise, I'd like you to achieve the state of relaxation described by the English poet William Wordsworth, when he wrote:

> A sense sublime
> Of something far more deeply interfused,
> Whose dwelling is the light of setting suns,
> And the round ocean and the living air,
> And the blue sky, and in the mind of man . . .

But whatever the experience is for you, keep in mind that my patients at UCLA almost universally achieve some degree of pain relief by learning to relax. Like many of them, you may reap the benefits of Conditioned Relaxation the first time or two you try it. But if you're like others and don't achieve results immediately, *don't give up.* You'll only be cheating yourself if you do. Just as with hitting a tennis ball, you have to practice patiently and allow your muscles to learn to perform as you want them to. Once they've developed the necessary skills, you don't need to work nearly as hard to keep them performing at an optimum level.

Make a pledge that you will conscientiously practice this technique *at least* twice a day (preferably more), *every day*, for several weeks. Begin now by starting to work on the way that you breathe, for breathing is the key to relaxation.

The Breath of Life

Breathing is literally the way of life. As I emphasized in Chapter 3, the air around us is a vital source of nourishment. Each time we breathe, we draw oxygen into the body's cells and tissues, where it is used in the burning of the body's fuel and the production of energy.

According to the philosophy of yoga, breathing controls the flow of prana—the cosmic life force—into the body. The nose, it is believed, is the proper instrument for breathing, not the mouth. Animals breathe through their nostrils, and they are certainly masters of relaxation.

If you pay close attention to your breathing, you'll notice that it varies according to your moods. You breathe differently, for example, when you're happy as opposed to sad, bored as opposed to excited, or calm as opposed to angry.

Proper breathing can actually help to control negative emotions, including anger, hatred, jealousy, grief, and frustration. Simply by slowing down the rhythm of breathing, which in turn reduces the heart rate, you can often eliminate tension, nervousness, and pain altogether.

Compare your own breathing to that of a baby. Most likely, your breathing is centered in your upper chest, and only the thorax is involved in taking short, shallow breaths. Infants, however, instinctively know how to breathe properly. They push their diaphragm down with each inhalation, then relax it as they exhale. Try it and you'll find that this type of deep, abdominal breathing is highly relaxing.

Let's take a few moments now to begin working with your breathing. Sit upright in a comfortable chair, and begin breathing slowly and deeply from the abdomen. Let your breathing become very rhythmic, as each inhalation equals each exhalation in length. You may find it helpful to count as you breathe, so as you inhale, count "one thousand, two thousand, three thousand . . . Exhale, one thousand, two thousand, three thousand . . ." Allow each breath to be natural, flowing deep into your abdomen and flowing out on its own. Adjust your rate of breathing until your body finds its own smooth, regular, and easy rhythm.

In my opinion, this type of breathing is an important prerequisite for any type of relaxation exercise, as well as many of the other pain-alleviation techniques presented later in this book. So before you proceed further, spend some time working on your breathing until you feel that you have mastered the ability to breathe slowly, deeply, and easily from the abdomen.

How to Learn Conditioned Relaxation

Each time you practice Conditioned Relaxation, find a quiet spot in which to do it. Don't allow yourself to be interrupted before you've completed the exercise. Take the phone off the hook and ask the children to play in another part of the house. I often park my car at the beach on my way to UCLA, and perform the relaxation technique there. It's about the only place I've found where I am virtually guaranteed that I won't be distracted for several minutes.

Get yourself as comfortable as you can before beginning the exercise. Loosen any tight clothing or shoes, and remove any jewelry you may be wearing.

I recommend that you perform this exercise in a seated position, unless your discomfort is such that it is very uncomfortable for you to do so. If you lie down, you'll find that you may fall asleep before the exercise is completed. Later on, you can use this exercise to induce sleep, and at that time, the reclining position is obviously preferable. However, you can't learn the full technique if you fall asleep, so while practicing, a comfortable seated position is recommended.

Whereas Transcendental Meditation uses a mantra to quiet the mind, Conditioned Relaxation uses your own breathing. At the onset of the exercise, you will concentrate on your breathing, as a means of keeping your mind from wandering to any stressful thoughts. At various other times throughout the exercise, you will refocus on the simple and natural act of inhaling and exhaling.

Keep in mind that there are two ways to breathe—from your chest and from your abdomen. For this exercise, try to breathe only from your abdomen, meaning that your stomach will move in and out with each breath you take. Allow your breathing to become slow and rhythmic.

The text of the relaxation exercise is printed below. If you like, you can read it through several times, and then try it. However, I would suggest that you have someone read it to you as you perform it. Or, because most people find it difficult to arrange for another person to read the exercise to them two or three times a day, I strongly recommend that you read the text into a cassette tape recorder, and then perform the exercise while the tape is being played back. Information about obtaining a professionally recorded version of the Conditioned Relaxation exercise can be found in the Appendix.

It's advisable to work initially with a friend or a tape recorder for two reasons: first of all, it is difficult to remember the entire exercise, and second, it's often hard to pace yourself properly. If you learn the exercise the wrong way, you'll only be hurting yourself. A friend or the tape recorder can serve as an important guide to keep you on the proper track.

If you (or your friend) are a fast reader, now is the time to slow down. As you read the following text into the microphone of your tape recorder, do it slowly and deliberately. Let each thought penetrate deep into your mind before you begin the next one. As a general rule, speak slowly, pause about three seconds each time there is an ellipsis (. . .), and about six seconds between paragraphs.

Now, let's get started.

Conditioned Relaxation

This tape contains a Conditioned Relaxation exercise which you can use any time you wish to reach a deep state of gentle relaxation . . .

Before beginning, take a moment to get comfortable and relax . . . Sit upright in a comfortable chair and loosen any tight clothing or jewelry or shoes that might distract you. Make sure you won't be interrupted for a few minutes . . . Take the telephone off the hook if necessary . . . Now take a few slow, deep abdominal breaths . . . Inhale . . . Exhale . . . Inhale . . . Exhale . . .

Focus your attention on your breathing throughout this exercise, and recognize how easily slow, deep breathing alone can help to produce relaxation. Let your body breathe itself, according to its own natural rhythm . . . Slowly and deeply . . .

Now let's begin the exercise with what we call a "signal breath," a special message that tells the body we are ready to enter a state of deep relaxation. The signal breath is taken as follows . . . Exhale . . . Take a deep breath in through your nose . . . Then blow it out through your mouth.

You may notice a kind of "tingling" sensation when you take the signal breath. Whatever you feel is a signal or message to your body that will become associated with relaxation, so that as you practice this exercise over and over again, simply taking the signal breath alone will produce the same degree of relaxation that you'll be able to get by completing the entire exercise.

Breathe slowly and deeply . . . As you concentrate your attention on your breathing, focus your eyes on an imaginary spot in the center of your forehead . . . Look at the spot as if you are trying to see it from the inside of your head . . . Raise your eyes way up so as to stare at that spot from the inside of your head. Concentrate your attention on it . . . The more you are able to concentrate on the spot, the better your relaxation response will be . . .

As you continue to focus your attention on the spot, you might notice that your eyelids have become quite tense . . . That's fine, for what we want to do is to teach your body the difference between tension and relaxation. Your eyelids are controlled by some of the smallest muscles in your body, and they become easily tired and fatigued as they become more and more tense. When I count to three, we'll demonstrate the difference between tension and relaxation by allowing your eyelids to close gently, allowing the feelings of tension to melt away quickly.

One . . . Two . . . Three . . . Close your eyelids firmly but not too tightly, and as they close, sense a soothing feeling of relaxation radiate all around your eyes . . . the top of your eyes . . . the bottom . . . the sides . . . the front and back . . .

Breathe slowly and deeply . . . Feel the relaxation in your eyes, and how nice it feels . . . Let these feelings of gentle relaxation radiate all around your eyes and out to your forehead . . . to your scalp . . . all around the back of your head . . . to your ears and temples . . . to your cheeks and nose . . . to your mouth and chin . . . and around to your jaw . . . As you feel all the tension flow out of your face and the area around your mouth, relax your jaw muscles . . . As you do so, let your jaw gently open slightly so that all the tension can smoothly flow away . . .

Remember your breathing, slowly and deeply . . . Relax the muscles in your neck, and as you relax the back of your neck, let your head tip gently forward until your chin just about touches your chest . . . As you do so, feel all the tension flow away from the muscles in the back of your neck . . . Let this nice, gentle feeling of relaxation now radiate down into your shoulders . . . Feel the heaviness of your shoulders on your trunk as the shoulder muscles gently relax . . . This is one of the most important areas of the body to relax since we all tend to store a lot of tension in our necks and shoulders . . . Feel all the tension flow away, and sense the nice, gentle feeling of deep relaxation . . .

Remember your breathing, slowly and deeply . . . Let this feeling of relaxation now radiate down your arms . . . to your elbows . . . forearms . . . wrists . . . and hands . . . Spend a moment to relax each of your fingers . . . your thumb, index finger, middle finger, ring finger, little finger . . . As your hands and arms completely and gently relax, you may notice feelings of warmth and heaviness . . . Some people report pulsations or tingly sensations . . . Some can even sense their heartbeat in their fingertips . . . Others report even magnetic or pulling sensations . . . Whatever you experience is your own body's way of expressing relaxation . . . Remember, you cannot *force* yourself to relax, you can only *allow* yourself to relax . . . Trust your body . . . It knows what to do . . .

Remember your breathing, slowly and deeply . . . Relax your chest . . . and abdomen . . . and let this feeling of relaxation radiate around your sides and ribs, as waves of relaxation cross your shoulder blades to meet at your upper back . . . middle back . . . and lower back . . . Feel all the muscles on either side of your spine softly relax . . . Let your spine carry the weight of your trunk as your back muscles relax more and more deeply . . . Let this feeling of gentle relaxation now radiate down into your pelvic area . . . to your buttocks . . . sphincter muscle . . . genitals . . . Feel your whole pelvic area open up and gently relax . . . Relax your thighs . . . knees . . . calves . . . ankles . . . and feet . . . Spend a moment to relax each toe . . . your big toe, second toe, third toe, fourth toe, and little toe . . . Breathe slowly and deeply . . . Relax and enjoy it . . .

Now that your body is gently relaxed and quiet, take a moment, starting from the top of your head working down, to check lightly to see how much relaxation you have obtained . . .

If there is any part of your body that is not yet fully relaxed and comfortable, simply inhale a deep breath and send it into that area, bringing soothing, relaxing, nourishing, healing oxygen into every cell of that area, comforting and relaxing it . . . As you exhale, imagine blowing out, right through your skin, any tension, tightness, pain, or discomfort in that area. Again, as you inhale, bring relaxing, healing oxygen into every cell of that area, and as you exhale, blow away, right through the skin, any tension or discomfort.

In this way you can send your breath to relax any part of your body which is not yet as fully relaxed and comfortable as it can be . . . Breathe slowly and deeply, and with each breath, allow yourself to become twice as relaxed as you were before . . . Inhale . . . Exhale . . . Twice as relaxed . . . Inhale . . . Exhale . . . Twice as relaxed . . .

When you find yourself quiet and fully relaxed, take a moment to enjoy it . . . Sense the gentle warmth and feeling of well-being all through your body . . . If any extraneous thoughts try to interfere, simply allow them to pass through and out of you . . . Ignore them and go back to your breathing, slowly and deeply . . . Slowly and deeply . . . Enjoy this nice state of gentle relaxation . . .

Now, as you concentrate on your breathing, paint a picture in your head of how you want to be . . . See yourself or any part of your body as you want *it* to be . . . Freely use your imagination . . . See the possibilities of being exactly as you want to be . . . See more clearly the vision in the center of your mind's eye . . .

Breathe slowly and deeply . . . Remember your wish, what you want for your life . . . Strengthen it . . . Tell yourself that "every day, in every way, I will feel better and better" . . . "Every day, in every way, I will feel better and better" . . . "Every day in every way, my wish will grow stronger and stronger" . . . "Every day, in every way, my wish will grow stronger and stronger" . . . Add any other suggestions you want to make to yourself . . .

Remember your breathing, slowly and deeply . . . When you end this exercise, you may be surprised to notice that you feel not only relaxed and comfortable, but energized with such a powerful sense of well-being that you will easily be able to meet any demands that arise . . . To end the exercise, tell yourself that you can reach this nice gentle state of Conditioned Relaxation any time you wish by simply taking the signal breath . . . Reinforce that signal breath by concluding the exercise with it . . . Exhale . . . Inhale deeply through your nose . . . Blow out through the mouth . . . And be well . . .

Now that you've experienced Conditioned Relaxation for the first time, how do you feel? Are you more relaxed, tranquil, and calm? Many people are after just one experience with this exercise. How about the intensity of your pain? Did the relaxation affect it in any way?

As you continue to practice this technique, you'll probably find yourself increasingly able to reduce your level of discomfort. Not only is this a wonderful sensation in itself, but it is also an undeniable indication of the control you can have over your pain. As many of my patients begin to experience the benefits of Conditioned Relaxation, they also begin to overcome the feelings of helplessness and hopelessness that have tormented them for years. No longer do they feel like victims who are at the mercy of internal and external stressors. No longer do they feel incurable, praying for a miracle pill that some doctor will give them. Now, they know there is something that *they* can do that really helps when they hurt. With diligent practice, Conditioned Relaxation may very well help you, too.

The Art of Diligent Practicing

If your initial experiences with Conditioned Relaxation are positive, you may be convinced that nothing will ever keep you from practicing it at least two times a day. Well, I hope you're right. But despite the best of intentions, be prepared for those difficult times when setting aside ten minutes for the exercise will seem like the most impossible task you've ever faced.

Here's a typical scenario that you should be prepared for: You oversleep one morning, you race in and out of the shower, dress quickly, fix yourself a fast breakfast, separate the kids who are already fighting, curse the paperboy for throwing the *Times* on the roof again, call the repairman about a malfunction in the hot water heater, and grab your shovel to dig your car out of the three-foot snowstorm that struck the previous night. Now—honestly—on a day like that, are you going to find ten minutes to practice Conditioned Relaxation?

Probably not. And that's very unfortunate, since the stress of such a morning makes the relaxation exercise all the more necessary and beneficial. I urge you to force yourself to practice the relaxation exercise twice a day, even if only in an abbreviated fashion. Although it may seem inconvenient, you will never regret doing it. The exercise should never be thought of as a chore, but rather as precious time devoted to improving your life. Nothing is more important than your health and well-being, so why not give yourself this valuable gift twice each day?

I'm reminded of the young man who once asked James Fadiman if he meditates, to which Fadiman replied, "Yes, for three minutes every day." The man laughed, expressing his doubts that any positive benefit could be obtained from only three minutes of meditation. But Fadiman responded, "I find it much better to relax for three minutes than to *not* relax for half an hour."

Some of my patients have told me they practice the Conditioned Relaxation exercise only when their discomfort flares up. But under such circumstances, it's not unlike the leaking roof syndrome—when it's raining outside, it can't be repaired, yet when it's not raining, there's no need to fix it. When the relaxation exercise is practiced only randomly, it may be ineffective when it's really needed.

So practice, practice, practice. When you feel comfortable—practice. And when you hurt—practice. You *can* teach your body to ease your own pain, but you must be willing to extend the effort to do it.

Some people are so skeptical that they won't give the exercise a chance to work. This is understandable, for when a patient's orientation for years and years has centered around pills and injections, he or she is conditioned to reject such a simple, uncomplicated procedure. As the reasoning goes, "If strong medication doesn't help me, how can a few deep breaths and a relaxed limb or two do any good?"

All I ask is that you try this relaxation technique. Allow yourself to really experience it fully, and then, *you* be the judge as to whether or not it is right for you. Make the relaxation exercise as much a part of your daily routine as eating and brushing your teeth. If you relax at the same times each day, it will become a positive habit rather than an intrusion on your other activities.

If you car-pool to and from work, find yourself a quiet corner in the back seat each morning and evening, plug in your cassette recorder earphone, and relax! If you're a homemaker, do the exercise in the morning after the kids have left for school, and at night after they are all tucked into bed. If you're a student, find an empty classroom during the last few minutes of your lunch hour, start your cassette recorder rolling, and make the most of the quiet time you have available; repeat the process at night before beginning your homework.

After diligent practicing, you may notice something wonderful happening. Each time you proceed through the exercise, your pain may significantly diminish. It may even disappear completely. And as you continue practicing from one day to the next, you may soon find that simply taking the initial signal breath will instantly relieve your discomfort. The rest of the exercise won't even be necessary. You will have controlled your own pain with just a single, deep breath.

One of my patients, an elderly woman with terrible facial pain, recently told me, "Whenever I eat and my jaw moves up and down, I get this horrible pain on the left side of my face. But all I have to do is take the signal breath, and within twenty seconds, the pain is gone, and I can continue eating. It's just amazing!"

After several weeks of practicing the Conditioned Relaxation technique, you may want to shorten it or change it to suit your needs better. Feel free to do so. Introduce other types of relaxation experiences that you think will be helpful. An excellent source book of relaxation techniques is *Relax*, edited by John White and James Fadiman.

Problem-Solving

Although Conditioned Relaxation can be learned by almost anyone motivated enough to practice it, some people do meet problems along their road to pain relief. Let me mention some of the difficulties you might encounter in learning relaxation, and how best to cope with them:

1. Probably the most common problem for pain patients is that they hurt so much that they find it extremely difficult to concentrate solely on the exercise itself. In such cases, the key is to stick with it. If you practice and keep practicing the exercise, you'll find it progressively easier to turn your attention away from your pain and toward the technique itself. Begin just by working with your breathing, and as you become more comfortable, continue by working through the entire exercise.

2. The mind is like a child. It has grown accustomed to receiving all of your attention, and it may throw it's own kind of temper tantrum when you try to quiet it for a few moments. Even when you make every effort to concentrate on your breathing, your mind may wander without warning, distracting you in any way possible in order to reclaim your attention. For instance, in the middle of the exercise, your mind may interrupt you with thoughts like these:

> I forgot to unplug the toaster downstairs in the kitchen. And right now the toaster plug is waving in the breeze that's blowing through the window. . . . Oh, no, the plug is frayed, and sparks are shooting out. They've set the cord on fire . . . The fire is spreading to the drapes . . . The drapes are burning now. . . . The fire has now spread to the kitchen cabinets. . . . If I get up right now and run downstairs, I can probably throw enough water on the fire to put it out. But if I keep doing this nonsensical exercise. . . . Oh, no, the fire has now spread to the walls. . . .

This entire monologue all occurs in a flash. And it's an example of what your mind will do to try to bring you out of the exercise. Although you don't consciously or deliberately make thoughts enter your mind, you may suddenly become aware that your mind has successfully kidnapped your attention and that you are lost in thought.

The best way to deal with this situation is just to let your thoughts pass through you, as if you are invisible. Don't identify with them. Experience them as butterflies, flittering around, then see them fly away, leaving you quietly behind. Don't get angry, frustrated, guilty, or worried. Don't resist them, fight them, or try to stop them. Any response you make will take you out of the relaxation experience. So instead, just go back to your breathing, without interacting with your thoughts.

Also, don't worry about forgetting something important that comes to mind while doing the exercise. Simply tell yourself that this isn't the time to think about it, and return to your breathing. You'll remember it when you finish the exercise. It will not be lost forever, no matter how hard your mind may try to convince you of that.

After you have been doing the relaxation exercise for quite some time, your mind may change its tactics. In my case, my mind has learned that the best way to distract me is with its sense of humor. On one occasion, I was flowing through the exercise very smoothly when suddenly my mind flashed: "I forgot to get the air in my car tires changed!" It was such an outlandish thought that I could not keep from laughing, which took me right out of the relaxation experience. But I regained my composure almost immediately, returned my concentration to my breathing, and let the thoughts pass. Just like a child who gradually learns rules of behavior, so the mind will learn to be still. As you continue to practice in the upcoming weeks, such distractions will become significantly less frequent.

3. Some people simply don't know what it feels like to relax. They may never have really relaxed in their lives. As a friend once said, telling a tense, nervous person to relax is like telling him to stop breathing. He can't do it.

For people like this, I often recommend a few sessions of biofeedback. It helps provide them with instantaneous information as to when their various muscles are relaxing, and what it feels like when they do. Biofeedback can open up the doors of perception, allowing you to taste what relaxation really is. Once it's learned, then Conditioned Relaxation can be used to its fullest potential.

4. People who don't use a tape recorder as a guide often race through the exercise, and thus reap little if any benefit from it. If you don't have a tape recorder, you can buy an inexpensive cassette recorder for about $20 at many discount electronics stores. (You probably spend almost that much on pain pills every month.) Make your own tape or purchase a prerecorded copy as I suggested earlier.

Eventually, as you become more familiar with the exercise, practice once a day with the tape and once without it to become accustomed gradually to performing the exercise on your own.

What Can You Gain?

In follow-up reports from individuals who have practiced Conditioned Relaxation for at least several weeks, the results have often been astounding. Pain relief has been the general rule rather than the exception. Many patients have learned to reduce or even stop spasticity in their muscles. Others have used the exercise to help them sleep at night. Still others report an enormous sense of well-being and rekindled feelings of self-confidence.

Conditioned Relaxation can also help you to achieve a state of nonidentification as described in Chapter 6; that is, the ability to let thoughts and feelings pass through your mind without identifying with them and acting upon them. Just as importantly, learning to relax is essential for mastery of other pain-alleviation techniques to be presented in subsequent chapters.

Most pain problems are clearly stress-related. Often, the degree of stress determines the degree of discomfort. My patients typically report that their pain becomes worse when they are under increased stress.

In my opinion, excessive psychological stress can often be identified as the *primary* cause of pain. Your discomfort is a natural reaction to this stress, and a powerful way in which your body is trying to tell you to relax and rest for a while.

Here is one way in which stress leads to body fatigue and pain: Stress causes your muscles to become tense, which in turn produces capillary constriction and an impairment of local blood circulation. Meanwhile, because the tensed muscles require metabolic energy, their cells use up vital nutrients and excrete a large number of toxic wastes. Since blood circulation has decreased, these toxins accumulate over time. Finally, as vital nutrients become more scarce, the body becomes fatigued and pain develops, carrying the message, "Stop! Relax! You need to rest!"

If you heed the message and relax your muscles, local circulation will be increased, and the muscle cells will be better able to excrete accumulated waste products. Since relaxed muscles require less metabolic energy, more vital nutrients are available to nourish the cells and promote healing. Thus, it is not hard to see how relaxation can significantly help alleviate musculoskeletal pain.

Pain may also be a message that your mind is fatigued, for the mind, too, requires regular periods of rest in order to function properly. Symptoms of mental fatigue include headaches, a lack of concentration, chronic worrying, daydreaming, and general irritability. Likewise, emotional fatigue can develop following extended periods of anger, anxiety, grief, or emotional conflict.

Pain's message, then, is often a simple one: Rest. When your back pain or headache flares up, or when you become irritable or depressed, your body may be trying to force you to do what you were unwilling to do—namely, stop everything and relax. If you don't, your discomfort will, in all likelihood, flare up even more.

To determine if this relationship applies to your own pain, try a simple experiment. At the instant you become aware of any increased discomfort, immediately stop what you are doing, take the signal breath, and give yourself a few minutes to rest and relax while you concentrate on your breathing. If your symptoms disappear, or are reduced, you are on the right track. In such cases, it's clearly to your advantage to work as hard as you can to learn to relax. However, if the symptoms remain unchanged, then the message underlying your discomfort may have little to do with a need to relax. This experiment will help you make that determination.

Most of my patients are surprised to find out how remarkably effective relaxation can be in helping them deal with their pain problems. "I was doubtful at first," reported a woman in her sixties plagued with lower back pain. "But I hurt so much I was willing to try anything. Now I can just relax the pain away in no time. I just can't find the words to explain how wonderful I feel."

Another woman, whose pain in her neck and back bothered her for over ten years, told me, "Now that I've mastered the relaxation exercise, I haven't had to use a pain pill in the last four months. It's a wonderful feeling knowing that I can finally control it."

Don't be foolish. In my opinion, *everyone* can benefit by learning how to relax. Even you.

Exercise Eighteen: Charting Your Progress

The Conditioned Relaxation exercise (or some suitable alternative) should be practiced *at least* twice daily. Before each practice session, rate your subjective levels of tension or relaxation using a −10 to +10 scale. Thus, if you feel slightly tense, rate it −1. If you're as tense as you have ever been, rate it −10. Anything in between should be so rated. In the same way, use a +1 to +10 scale for relaxation. So if you feel slightly relaxed, rate it +1, and if you are totally and completely relaxed, rate it +10. Again, rate anything in between accordingly.

In addition, rate your subjective levels of pain or pleasure on a −10 to +10 scale as described in Exercise One, with −10 representing extreme discomfort and +10 representing extreme feelings of pleasure. Post these ratings on the Weekly Rating Chart, and note any recent stressful events in your day.

SAMPLE

EXERCISE EIGHTEEN: Charting Your Progress

WEEKLY RATING CHART

Rating Code

Tension −10	0	Relaxation +10
Pain −10	0	Pleasure +10

Day	Date	Time		Tension/Relaxation Level		Pain/Pleasure Level		Recent Stressful Events	Notes & Comments
				Before	After	Before	After		
1	4/3	7:30	A.M.	−5	−5	−6	−5	responsibilities at work	
		8	P.M.	−8	−6	−7	−7	argument at dinner table	
2	4/4	7:30	A.M.	−4	−2	−4	−1		
		8	P.M.	−7	0	−4	+2	doctor bill in mail	
3	4/5	7:30	A.M.	−1	+3	−2	+4		
		8	P.M.	−7	−2	−7	−2	argument with spouse	
4	4/6	7:30	A.M.	0	+5	+2	+3		
		8	P.M.	−3	+5	0	+4		
5	4/7	8	A.M.	0	+6	0	+6		
		6:30	P.M.	+1	+4	+2	+5		
6	4/8	8	A.M.	0	+1	+1	+4		
		6:30	P.M.	+2	+3	+2	+3		
7	4/9	7:30	A.M.	0	+4	−2	+1	car broke down	
		8	P.M.	−3	+6	−4	+5		
Total weekly ratings				−35	+22	−29	+22		
No. of practice sessions				14	14	14	14		
Average weekly ratings				−2.5	+1.6	−2.1	+1.6		

Week of _____ April 3–9 _____

EXERCISE EIGHTEEN: Charting Your Progress

WEEKLY RATING CHART

Rating Code

Tension	Relaxation
—10	0 +10

Pain	Pleasure
—10	0 +10

Day	Date	Time	Tension/Relaxation Level		Pain/Pleasure Level		Recent Stressful Events	Notes & Comments
			Before	After	Before	After		
1		A.M.						
		P.M.						
2		A.M.						
		P.M.						
3		A.M.						
		P.M.						
4		A.M.						
		P.M.						
5		A.M.						
		P.M.						
6		A.M.						
		P.M.						
7		A.M.						
		P.M.						
Total weekly ratings								
No. of practice sessions								
Average weekly ratings								

Week of _____

SAMPLE

EXERCISE EIGHTEEN:
Charting Your Progress Graph

Code for entering average
weekly rating scores:

x – – – x *Tension/Relaxation Level Before*
x ——— x *Tension/Relaxation Level After*
o – – – o *Pain/Pleasure Level Before*
o ——— o *Pain/Pleasure Level After*

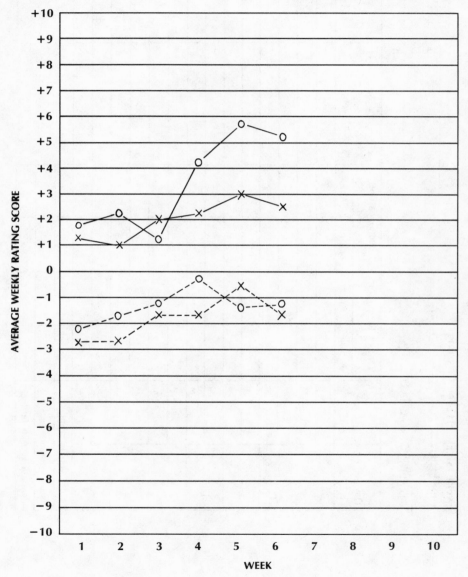

EXERCISE EIGHTEEN:
Charting Your Progress Graph

Code for entering average
weekly rating scores:

x – – – x Tension/Relaxation Level Before
x ——— x Tension/Relaxation Level After
o – – – o Pain/Pleasure Level Before
o ——— o Pain/Pleasure Level After

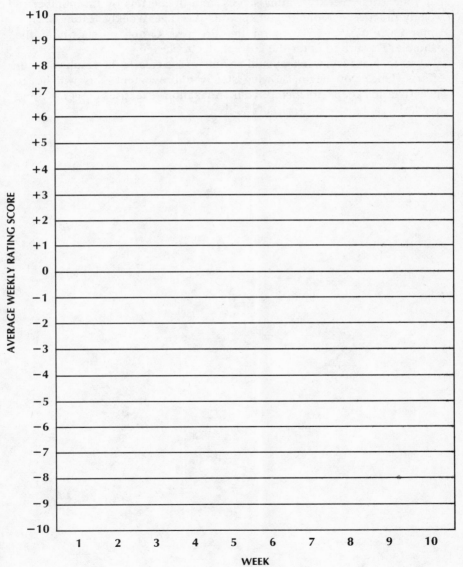

After completing the relaxation exercise, rate your subjective levels of tension/relaxation and pain/pleasure again, and note any changes, experiences, or feelings of importance. This will be helpful in interpreting sudden fluctuations in your overall progress.

At the end of each week, calculate the algebraic sum of each column to get your Total Weekly Rating scores, and divide this by the number of weekly practice sessions to obtain your Average Weekly Rating scores. Enter each of these scores on the Progress Graph as shown in the example. Be sure to enter the correct algebraic sign.

Over the next few weeks, you'll be able to see clearly the results of your efforts. Once you begin showing steady improvement, this will be an incentive to keep practicing your relaxation exercise diligently and regularly.

8 *You Are What You Eat*

"Modern medicine has become a major threat to health, and its potential for social, even physical, disruption is rivalled only by the perils inherent in the industrialized production of food."

I think these words by Ivan Illich crystallize a glaring tragedy of twentieth-century life. Contemporary medicine, relying far too heavily on drugs and surgery, still hasn't solved some of the most critical medical mysteries of our times. Despite medicine's apparent sophistication, serious health problems ranging from cancer to chronic pain are still shrouded in unanswered questions.

But perhaps, as Illich suggests, the industrialized production of food may be partly responsible for our ills—although few health professionals have yet recognized this possibility. In my opinion, nutrition is the most neglected factor in health and illness. I firmly believe that you are what you eat. If you consume nutritious, unadulterated food, your body will look and feel good. If you eat poorly, your body and your emotional well-being will reflect that, too. It's sad to realize that so many Americans have forgotten, or have never known, the wonderful feeling of a body overflowing with the energy of positive good health that comes from being genuinely well-nourished.

What's your diet like? Are you eating sufficient quantities of the foods that can help you to feel better? Frankly, I often shudder when patients with pain describe their diets to me. "Junk foods" with very little if any nutritional value frequently dominate, at the expense of foods that could promote the healing process. But as one patient told me, "Eating is one of the only pleasures I have left in my life. So I eat the things I like, even though I know some of them aren't the healthiest."

That kind of reasoning is enough to make you sick. Literally. The U.S. Department of Agriculture has estimated that one-half of the calories consumed in the average American daily diet are "naked" or "hollow," meaning they have minimal nutritional value. When a similar diet was fed to young rats, they matured less than half as fast as rats on a more nutritious diet.

A 1977 study conducted by the Senate Select Committee on Nutrition indicated that six of the ten leading causes of death in the United States are linked to what we eat. Another federal government report described this country as a "malnourished nation with the resources to buy sufficient food, but lacking the knowledge to choose the foods that are best for us."

In every cell of our bodies, complex biochemical processes are constantly at work which require a steady supply of a variety of essential nutrients. If they are absent or exist at inadequate levels, symptoms of serious diseases are almost inevitable.

Interestingly, all living creatures have basic nutritional instincts that communicate when and what to eat. With man, these instincts are present from birth. They tell us when we're hungry or thirsty, and when these basic needs have been fulfilled. Just as importantly, the body is perfectly designed to tell us when we may be eating the wrong things. (If you eat too much sugar or salt, for instance, your body will probably react with either nausea or vomiting.)

Some of my patients have doubted that the body has such sophisticated, innate wisdom. However, they often change their minds once I ask them to observe the eating habits of infants. During the first year of life, babies will consistently be more receptive to eating, say, fresh fruit and raw vegetables than highly processed white bread and candy.

However, as they grow older, these natural instincts are violently distorted by an onslaught of adulterated foods. Over a period of years, they gradually acquire a taste for refined foods, and usually by school age, their innate food preferences have disappeared. Ask the typical five-year-old whether he'd rather have a piece of chocolate fudge or an apple, and sadly, he'll probably choose the candy. Into adulthood, he'll continue to reach for the foods low in nutrition, eating them with zeal.

Unfortunately, we live in a society that encourages us at every turn to develop an appetite for these substandard foods. TV advertising bombards us with slick promotions for one type of adulterated food or another. And across the nutritional wasteland, we follow this advice like sheep.

Think for a minute about how you reward your children for doing something right (getting good grades, going to bed on time) or on special occasions (in Easter baskets and Christmas stockings). If you're like most parents, you probably give them candy. Throughout their childhood, candy is associated with love, approval, and reward, and this conditioning carries over into adulthood. Whenever we feel the need for love and support, we reach for a candy bar. Yes, that candy may make you feel better momentarily. But over a period of years, it can contribute to everything from tooth decay to obesity to diabetes.

Even if junk foods have become a way of life for you, there is still a glimmer of hope amid the Hershey's chocolates and the Big Macs. For although the body's natural instincts have been suppressed by your unhealthy eating habits, they have not been destroyed. Time after time, when I have placed my patients on nutritious diets, their bodies have "unlearned" the bad eating habits developed over many years. In fact, after just a few weeks, those junk foods once as addicting as narcotics have totally lost their appeal and have faded into the past for good.

Caution: Supermarkets May Be Hazardous to Your Health

Through the magic of modern technology, the food we eat has been so transformed from its natural state that it often is incapable of adequately nourishing us. In the past, food was produced by individual families or on nearby farms, and was eaten fresh and close to its natural state. Over the last few decades, however, enormous changes in the production of food, and consequently in our diets, have occurred. The frightening state of contemporary foods can turn even the strongest stomach. With each bite of the typical American diet, we may be contributing significantly to the decline and fall of our own good health.

At last count, there were more than three thousand additives used by U.S. food manufacturers. These include laboratory-produced substances like preservatives, flavoring agents, buffers, stabilizers, surfactants, thickeners, extenders, deodorants, noxious sprays, maturing agents, sweeteners, neutralizers, moisteners, drying agents, chelating agents, emulsifiers, antioxidants, dyes, fungicides, defoliants, and fortifiers.

The food industry, the largest retail enterprise in the United States, interestingly refuses to use words like "additives" or "chemicals" to describe these substances. Instead, they revert to less-alarming terms such as "food ingredients." But no matter how they are labeled, we are swallowing them with abandon. According to the Department of Agriculture, the typical American consumes three pounds of these substances a year—about 0.25 percent of his total food intake.

Frederick W. Richmond, a New York Congressman, concisely described the way Americans eat, at a conference sponsored by the Community Nutrition Institute in 1977: "Start the day with an orange-flavored drink containing as many components as the spacecraft that—for some reason—carried it to the moon . . . Eggs over and crisp bacon: cholesterol and sodium nitrate . . . Toast made from a mix containing fifty percent water and wood cellulose . . . Water itself that is possibly contaminated with PCBs . . . Saccharin . . . Sugar . . . More fat . . . Additives . . . Preservatives . . . All held together with an alphabet soup of emulsifiers and stabilizers."

What purpose do these synthetic substances serve? Well, none of them makes our food more nutritious. None of them causes us to feel any healthier. Their major purpose is to make your food look and taste better, so that more of it can be sold. It's as simple and sad as that.

By the time most food reaches the supermarket shelves, it has been heated and frozen, beaten and bruised, manipulated and mutilated, and wrapped in a glamorous package that may cost more than the food itself. True, it may look inviting, smell wonderful, and taste delightful. But in the process, so much of its nutritive value has been destroyed that often the food has had to be artificially "enriched" or "fortified" in order to restore at least some of its nourishment. And as an extra bonus, we consume a vast array of artificial additives whose role in the development of various diseases is becoming increasingly apparent.

The Poisons in Your Food

As my patients have heard me say so often, few health-related phenomena upset me quite as much as what is being done to our food. None of us really knows the impact that the accumulation of these unnatural, laboratory-produced chemicals is having on our bodies, but if what we have learned so far is any indication of future findings, it is almost certainly a negative one. I watch very carefully what I eat and encourage my patients to do the same. As a result, they have reduced or eliminated some of the most common foods from their diets—like gelatins saturated with dyes that have caused birth defects in animals; ham, hot dogs, and bacon that include cancer-causing nitrites; and peanut butter or corn that may be polluted with aflatoxin, another chemical suspected of producing cancer.

Actually, food additives are nothing new. Man has been supplementing his food with foreign ingredients for centuries. Probably the first such additives were spices and herbs designed to make food more tasteful. Man later learned that certain spices helped preserve his food. However, these early additives were natural substances, while today, most are artificially-created and laboratory-produced.

I have talked to many representatives of food manufacturers who defend these additives with gusto. They have told me that antispoilants, for instance, curtail the reproduction of bacteria, allowing certain products to be stored for months. Other types of additives, they say, can increase or decrease the levels of moisture in foods (for example, the moisture-controlling properties of calcium silicate can prevent table salt from caking). Additives are used to either hasten or retard the ripening or growing process of various fruits and vegetables—like maleic hydride, which discourages sprouting in stored potatoes. Still others are utilized to make food look more delicious—for instance, sodium nitrate, which adds a rich, red color to processed meats. There are also nearly two thousand synthetic flavoring agents that are added to foods solely for taste.

While some people may be grateful for these benefits of food technology, I prefer to leave my trust in the hands of Mother Nature. To my way of thinking, the benefits of food additives are far outweighed by the well-documented negative effects of these substances. How, for example, can food manufacturers defend additives that prevent vitamins and enzymes from nourishing the body in the ways they were intended? Without such nourishment, a variety of ailments can develop, from headaches to insomnia to fatigue. When these deficiencies occur for long periods of time, the impact upon the body can be devastating. I agree wholeheartedly with Dr. James L. Goddard, former Food and Drug Administration commissioner, who once said, "In a number of cases the additives have only an economic benefit to the food producers and no benefit at all to the person who eats the final product."

I am surprised to find that many of my patients are unmoved by this information. After all, they reason, doesn't the FDA exist to protect us? Wouldn't the FDA ban any substance that's dangerous to our well-being?

Unfortunately, the matter isn't that simple. Yes, there are food safety laws and the FDA was created to protect us from perils in our food. But, according to Dr. Herbert Ley, Commissioner of Food and Drugs during the Nixon Administration, "The thing that bugs me is that the people think the FDA is protecting them—it isn't. What the FDA is doing and what the public thinks it's doing are as different as night and day."

Additives are allowed into our foods before they are ever subjected to long-term studies. The FDA and food manufacturers contend that it would be impractical to test a substance for several decades before allowing it onto the marketplace. However, there is evidence that malignant tumors may take as long as thirty years to develop following exposure to a carcinogenic agent. The full effects of new additives, then, cannot be known until after decades of use.

In a sense, we are inviting a catastrophe to happen. No test results have ever stated conclusively that a particular chemical is safe when used over an extended period of time. Even the FDA itself, in its Fact Sheet of October 1971, admitted in typical bureaucratic lingo that "there is no way in which absolute safety can be guaranteed. Premarketing clearance . . .

does assure that risk of adverse effects occurring is at an acceptably small level."

The GRAS List

The year 1958 was the best and the worst of times. Congress passed the Food Additive Amendments in that year, intended to provide protection for the public against impure substances in their foods. Under these amendments, food manufacturers must show "proof of a reasonable certainty that no harm will result from the proposed use of an additive." However, within these amendments was a terrible loophole. Many food additives in use before 1958 were placed on a "generally recognized as safe" (GRAS) list. These substances had been in use long enough for the FDA to consider them harmless—even though most of them had never been tested. The hundreds of substances on the GRAS list were exempt from all food additive orders, and were permitted to be used without restrictions, in any amount desired, in foods for which they had been approved. Over the years, new items have regularly been added to that list.

Well, at first glance, the GRAS list doesn't appear particularly threatening. After all, it includes substances like pepper and vinegar, which seem harmless enough. However, as long ago as 1969, the FDA's Bureau of Science admitted that some of the substances on the list were "suspect," while "substantial grounds for concern" existed for others.

Let me tell you about an additive called nordihydroguaiaretic acid or NDGA. For two decades it was used as an antioxidant to prevent deterioration in fatty foods, and it was placed on the GRAS list in 1958. However, a dozen years after the FDA proclaimed that it had "information to show safety," NDGA was removed from the GRAS list when further tests showed it caused inflamed cysts and kidney lesions in laboratory rats.

Other substances on the GRAS list have shared similar fates. For instance, have you ever heard of saforale? It's a flavoring agent used for many years in root beer, until studies revealed that it was responsible for everything from cirrhosis to testicular atrophy to liver cancer in animals.

Other substances, like brominated vegetable oils and oil of calmus (a flavoring agent for candy and beverages), have also been quietly removed from the GRAS list once studies revealed that, alas, they were not safe at all. I'm sure you're also familiar with the most notorious of all additives formerly on the GRAS list—cyclamate and saccharin. Cyclamate, because of its status as a "safe" substance, was the most widely used artificial sweetener in the United States in the late 1960s. Initially, it was intended to be consumed only by people forced to limit their sugar consumption for medical reasons. But it was soon being pumped into a wide range of food products such as Diet Pepsi, Kool-Aid, Metrecal, candy, ice cream, jams, and even children's vitamin tablets. When the additive was eventually banned, primarily because of studies linking it to bladder cancer in rats, fifteen million pounds of it were being swallowed every year in the United States and almost three out of every four families were consuming it.

As if these facts aren't enough to distress you, there's still a nasty coup de grace concerning substances on the GRAS list. You probably think that to find out what a food's ingredients are, all you must do is read the label. Right? Wrong.

The FDA, in a stroke of sheer madness, has agreed that all items on the GRAS list need not be incorporated onto the label. A product can contain dozens of additives on the GRAS list without any obligation to list them. Cyclamate, for instance, was not listed as an ingredient on most of the foods that contained it.

To add to the confusion, the FDA has created another monstrosity it calls "standards of identity." Here's how this system works: The FDA has accumulated a list of several hundred food products so common that the agency has decided their manufacturers do not need to place *any* of their ingredients on their wrappers or containers. That's right—none!

What does this mean? Well, walk through the supermarket and look at products like bread, mayonnaise, spaghetti, milk, cheeses, or frozen desserts. Also examine the labels of canned fruits and vegetables, fruit juices, nonalcoholic beverages, margarine, fruit preserves, or food dressings. These and dozens of other food items do not have to mention even a single ingredient, including additives, on their labels—no matter how many substances they contain or what these ingredients are. If the manufacturer doesn't want to tell you what he's put in his food, you'll never find out, short of writing him a personal letter demanding the information.

One final note I want to emphasize: Although the FDA does not *require* these ingredients to be listed, it does *allow* the manufacturers to list as many or as few as they want to. So when a jar of mayonnaise or a loaf of bread lists its ingredients, it may only be listing *some* of them—perhaps only those that flatter the food as much as possible.

Consider the case of Coca-Cola, the all-American drink. Coke used to list only one ingredient on its label:

"Contents: Caramel colored."

But then as the era of consumerism became a reality and people began reading labels more carefully, the manufacturers of Coca-Cola expanded their ingredient list: "Carbonated water, sugar, caramel color, phosphoric acid, natural flavorings, caffeine."

Well, consumers cheered loudly, for it appeared that the ingredients of Coca-Cola were finally being fully disclosed. But were they?

According to the FDA, soft drinks can and often do include the following substances, without any mandate that they be listed on the label: acetic acid, ammoniated glycyrrhizin, brominated vegetable oils, dimethylpolysiloxane, dioctyl sodium sulfosuccinate, enzyme-modified soy protein, ethyl alcohol, glycerol ester of wood rosin, guar gum, gum ghatti, licorice, malic acid, propylene glycol, quillaia (soap bark), tartaric acid, and yucca.

Those are the facts, the sad facts. As Ralph Nader stated at a recent Congressional hearing, "All chemicals added to food should be on the label of the container. The current enforcement of the law is irrational allowing over two hundred ingredients to be added to food at the will of the manufacturer without labeling, and several hundred more that can only be found by reference to the Federal Register."

The Additives You Eat

Thanks to rulings by the FDA, our food is saturated with substances which we could very well do without, including:

—*Flavor enhancers,* the largest single category of additives, which encompass everything from cloves to inosinate and disodium guanylate. The best-known of these flavoring agents is monosodium glutamate (MSG), which is on the GRAS list even though it was considered dangerous enough to be removed from all baby foods. It is still widely used in large amounts in thousands of other convenience foods—including frozen and canned foods, soups, mayonnaise, and crackers—while evidence mounts that MSG has caused headaches in man and irreversible brain damage in infant laboratory animals.

—*Color additives,* which are used because food manufacturers believe that you and I are interested in buying only attractively colored foods—that is, orange juice that's colored orange rather than green; yellow margarine rather than white; and green frozen peas instead of brown. According to the food companies, consumers demand food that looks appetizing, and these wishes are simply being met. In the process, coloring—most of it synthetic—is injected into most of the foods we eat—from bread to meat to fruit. Even when a product carries the label "U.S. certified artificial color," some impurities are still permitted into the coloring agent.

—*Preservatives and antioxidants,* intended to prevent spoilage and extend the shelf life of food. For instance, sodium propionate is used in many breads to retard molding. Although such substances are much more effective as long-term preservatives than salt or vinegar, there is concern over the negative symptoms caused by some of them. Among the most common antioxidants, and certainly the most controversial ones, are BHA (butylated hydroxyanisole) and BHT (butylated hydroxytoluene), used in foods like breakfast cereals, enriched rice, dehydrated potatoes, and desserts and beverages prepared from dry mixes. Although they are part of the FDA's GRAS list, they have been linked with severe allergic reactions in some people. Also, we don't yet know the long-term effects of these preservatives.

—*Emulsifiers, stabilizers,* and *surfactants,* designed to enhance the texture and consistency of foods. They are used in puddings to improve creaminess, in cereals to retard formation of clumps, and in bread to make it softer. They are also common in meats, ice cream, frozen desserts, cakes, doughnuts, margarines, and salad dressings.

The use of these substances is usually more for cosmetic reasons than anything else. And that outrages me. I firmly believe that we would be far healthier if most additives were eliminated from our diets. Those attractive vegetables and well-preserved meats on your dinner table may seem like a blessing for the moment, but they might be causing serious illnesses that provoke pain and other symptoms.

Additives often cover up changes in foods which we really should know about. For example, when food spoils, and when its color, taste, and odor have deteriorated, additives can mask these symptoms by turning green hot dogs into red ones, or a rancid steak into a pleasant-smelling one. Although this doctored food may appear more appetizing, it's certainly not healthier for you. Your own instincts would immediately tell you not to eat spoiled food if they weren't being fooled by the additives that disguise its real nature. In my opinion, food manufacturers who use cosmetic additives to artificially make food look good, smell good, and taste good are doing the consumer a great disservice.

As I often tell my patients, "If a food contains an additive whose name you can't pronounce, or if the food can never spoil, don't eat it." To me, restricting additives from your nutritional program is a simple, but important form of nutritional insurance.

To snarl this issue further, additives can affect our bodies much like drugs do. "On the surface, additives and drugs may appear as disparate categories," commented Benjamin Feingold, M.D., chief of the Department of Allergy at Kaiser Foundation Hospitals in northern California, at a recent conference. "However, except for terminology, there are no differences between a compound used as a medication and one introduced into our food as an additive—both are low molecular weight compounds. This is important to recognize, since in spite of this identity, not one of the thousands of compounds introduced into our foods as additives has ever been subjected to pharmacological studies such as those required of compounds licensed for use as medications. We actually know nothing of the behavior of these compounds in the body."

Despite our relative lack of knowledge, I shudder to imagine the effects these additives may be having. Consider that the ice cream that you buy often contains an emulsifier called diethyl glycol, used in place of eggs;

this same additive is also used in paint remover and antifreeze. Then there's piperonal, added to ice cream in place of vanilla, but which also is used as a killer of lice. Aldehyde, used as a cherry flavor, is actually an inflammable liquid also found in plastics and rubber. Other ice-cream flavoring agents—including butyraldehyde (nut flavor), amyl acetate (banana), benzyl acetate (strawberry), and ethyl acetate (pineapple)—are also used in rubber cement, cleaning fluids, and oil paint solvents.

Many people are very conscious of environmental pollution, and concede that, say, the smog they breathe may be harming their well-being. But they often overlook the problem of internal pollution, caused by the unhealthy food they consume. If they could see the poisons in their bodies as clearly as the poisons in the sky, they might be motivated to choose their foods more carefully.

Food Allergies

Medical journals are filled with case studies of people afflicted with allergies to certain foods or the substances in them. Often an individual can be ill for years without ever learning that his ailment is being caused by something he is eating. To compound his dilemma, even if he is fortunate enough to learn what food substances he is allergic to, he may still be inadvertently consuming them in inadequately labeled products.

For instance, consider the case of a sixteen-year-old boy who was so allergic to peanuts that his body reacted violently whenever he mistakenly ate them. He carefully read the labels of every food he consumed to ensure that it didn't contain peanuts. However, one day after eating a slice of packaged cake, he felt his throat actually closing up on him. His parents quickly administered an antihistamine, and then two Adrenalin shots, but nothing helped. The boy was hospitalized and placed in an oxygen tent. He was near death for several hours.

After the boy had recovered, his parents were determined to find out what had caused the violent reaction. They eventually learned that although peanuts were not mentioned as an ingredient of the cake, the "vegetable shortening" listed was actually a peanut oil–cottonseed oil mixture.

A list of allergic reactions to food substances could fill an entire volume in itself. If you have pain, you should certainly not ignore allergies as a possible contributing factor to your discomfort. For example, sodium nitrate, used to keep meat and fish looking fresh and appealing, may be responsible for a rheumatic allergic reaction, with terrible pain in the joints. A Connecticut woman suffered severe aches in her arms and legs every time she went to the movies. The cause of her discomfort was eventually linked to the popcorn she ate during each visit to the theater.

Allergic reactions can also cause headaches, abdominal pain, and emotional problems ranging from irritability to depression. A visitor from the Soviet Union recently told me that Russian nutritionists believe that some types of schizophrenia may be related to food allergies—particularly in reaction to foods like red meat and sugar. A strict restructuring of the patient's diet can cause him to lose his schizophrenic symptoms within thirty days, according to this report.

Unfortunately, there are very few ways to test what foods you may be allergic to. The common skin tests involve simply grinding the food into paste, scratching it into the skin, and waiting to see if an allergic reaction develops. But this may tell you only what your skin, not the rest of your body, is allergic to.

Frankly, I'm not very concerned about the surface reactions of your skin to a food substance it has never before been exposed to. I'm more interested in how your whole body reacts to a particular food. If you are allergic to a certain food, your internal defense system will treat it as an enemy and will mobilize against it. Chronic pain may be the way your body is trying to get you to stop eating a food you are allergic to, especially if you experience gastrointestinal discomfort or headaches.

If your pain is due to injury or illness, you require the maximum support of your immune/inflammatory system to optimize your body's ability to heal itself. If your body's defenses are required to wage an additional battle against an allergic food substance, it's like fighting two separate wars at once. So, if you can eliminate food allergies, much more of your body's defenses will be free to deal with overcoming your pain.

William G. Crook, M.D., an allergist and pediatrician, and author of *Your Allergic Child,* believes that the most common food allergies in both adults and children are caused by beef, pork, eggs, corn, wheat, nuts, chocolate, citrus, cola, or milk. Why not try eliminating some or all of these items from your diet for two to three weeks and see what effect it has on you? You may be surprised to find that you begin feeling better. Then reintroduce these items into your diet gradually—say, one eliminated food every two to three days. If your pain worsens after the reintroduction of one of these items, then you may have finally pinpointed a potential cause of your pain. Don't be foolish—find out if foods and food additives may be disrupting your life. If you're like many of my patients, you'll prefer a slightly restricted diet to a life filled with chronic pain.

Eating for Good Health

Food—the right kind of food—is good medicine. Often, it's the *best* medicine. If you eat carefully and healthfully, food may be more effective in the long run than any other healing agent.

Unfortunately, research into the curative potential of good eating habits is still in its infancy. Studies with contradictory conclusions abound, leaving the consumer in nutritional limbo. Even so, there is mounting evidence that nutrition may someday join and even surpass pharmacology as a major tool in medical therapeutics. If and when that day occurs, your doctor may prescribe natural foods rather than chemicals to cure your ills.

Think of it: You eat three meals a day (plus periodic snacks), 365 days a year, for many decades. That gives you tens of thousands of opportunities to nourish your body with some of nature's own "medicine." Why not make the most of those opportunities?

Some of the suggestions I will make in the remainder of this chapter are common-sense ones. Certainly, they carry no guarantees. I'm not proclaiming that with the proper diet you can completely eliminate the pain in your body. However, it may help you to mobilize your body to the fullest extent possible to combat illness and promote well-being.

As a general rule, the closer your food is to its original source, and the less that has been done to it, the better it will be for the body. Kaptain Korny (a very forgettable breakfast cereal) may be made of pure corn, but it has been mutilated beyond nutritional recognition by the time it reaches the supermarket shelves. Likewise, a highly processed corn chip contains far fewer nutrients than a fresh ear of corn. And a store-bought "orange drink" is much less healthful than a glass of freshly squeezed orange juice.

So what should you be eating?

There are certain nutrients as essential to your well-being as oxygen. In order for necessary biochemical processes to occur, a variety of basic nutrients must be present, including fiber, protein, carbohydrates, and fat.

Fiber

It is now known that proper amounts of fiber or bulk can produce better health. Fiber (or "roughage," as it is sometimes called) is found in varying amounts in raw, unprocessed vegetables and fruits, as well as in many whole grains like oats, brown rice, and particularly wheat bran. It is not digested, and as it passes through the intestines, it promotes regular bowel movements and prevents constipation. There is also preliminary evidence indicating that a high-fiber diet may prevent diverticulitis, appendicitis, cancer of the bowel, other diseases of the large bowel, and heart disease. In a study in the Netherlands, 140 grams of high-fiber rolled oats significantly cut cholesterol levels in only three weeks.

Unfortunately, fiber is scarce in the typical American diet. Even though fiber yields no protein, calories, or vitamins, I recommend that you regularly include whole grains, raw fruits, coarse vegetables, and other high-fiber foods in your meals. Bran, for instance, is effective and relatively inexpensive, and can be added very simply to your diet by sprinkling it over cereal, or putting it in casseroles or meat loaves. About three or four tablespoons of bran should be part of your diet each day.

Protein

Protein is the primary substance in the body's muscles, organs, skin, nails, and other tissue. Next to water, it is the most abundant substance in the body. It is necessary for the growth, maintenance, and repair of the body.

Did you know, for instance, that all of the body's disease-fighting antibodies are proteins? So are enzymes, which promote the chemical breakdown of food. Two proteins, actin and myosin, are necessary for muscle contractions to occur. The oxygen-carrying activity of blood cells is due to a protein called hemoglobin.

All proteins are composed of chemical building blocks called amino acids. Many of these amino acids are essential for the body to function properly, and they must be obtained through the food we eat, because the body cannot manufacture them. Although vegetables are a source of amino acids, most are deficient in one or more of them, and thus vegetables must be consumed in variety in order to obtain everything the body needs. The soybean is one of the rare "complete protein" vegetables. By contrast, most animal protein contains all the necessary amino acids.

What are the richest sources of protein? Meats, fish, poultry, eggs, and dairy products—all animal protein—are close to human protein in their structure, and in general they are easily digested by the body. Vegetable protein is most abundant in foods like whole grains, seeds, nuts, dry beans, peas, legumes, and peanut butter.

Carbohydrates

Carbohydrates are the body's major sources of fuel and energy. As well as providing some of the building materials for body tissue, they also assist in food digestion. If you're a typical American, about 50 to 60 percent of your diet is composed of carbohydrates.

Essentially, carbohydrates are supplied in two forms—starch and sugar. Starches are obtained primarily from grains and vegetables, including items like bread, cereals, potatoes, peas, and beans. Starches must be cooked in order to be digested easily.

Sugars occur in their simplest and most natural form in fruits and honey, and are very easily digested in the body. However, Americans have become much more accustomed to a very different form of sugar— refined sugar—that is liberally added to prepared foods. Unfortunately, during commercial preparation, this sugar is robbed of much of its nutritive value. The vitamins and minerals essential to good health have been drained away, leaving behind only "empty calories" that are often detrimental to the body. As far as I'm concerned, this type of sugar is simply another food additive—and a potentially dangerous one.

How does $C_{12}H_{22}O_{11}$—alias table sugar—harm the body? Well, we know that a liberal consumption of sugar contributes to ailments like diabetes, ulcers, and tooth decay. Also, according to Dr. John Yudkin, University of London emeritus professor of nutrition, sugar may be a greater cause of arteriosclerosis and heart attacks than saturated fats. According to Yudkin, East African tribes on a high-fat diet suffer almost no heart disease because their sugar consumption is minimal. By comparison, the citizens of St. Helena Island in the south Atlantic eat very little fat (as well as exercise heavily and smoke very little), but experience a high level of heart disease—possibly related to a high sugar intake.

Yudkin's studies show that coronary death rates in fifteen countries increased steadily with a rise in the nation's average consumption of sugar. He contends that a person eating four ounces of sugar daily, from all sources, has more than five times the chance of developing heart disease than if he consumed only half as much sugar.

Despite such evidence, a friend of mine is convinced that sugar is good for him. He recently told me that after eating food heavy in sugar, he feels tremendously energized, even more so than if he consumes protein.

The sugar industry, of course, couldn't agree more. A recent industry ad announced: "Snack on some candy about an hour before lunch. Sugar's quick energy can be the willpower you need to eat less . . . The sugar in a soft drink or ice cream cone, shortly before mealtime, turns into energy fast. And that energy could be just the energy you need to say 'no' to those extra helpings at mealtime."

The Federal Trade Commission banned that ad as "false, misleading and deceptive." Yes, refined sugar may provide a temporary rise in energy, but it also tends to reinforce the desire for sweets, creating a psychological dependence, and can even lead to a physical addiction. In addition, because the body utilizes sugar very rapidly, the rush of energy is short-lived. It is followed by a quick letdown, during which the body's energy level plummets even lower than it was before the sugar was consumed. In the process, a state of depression frequently occurs.

If you're like most Americans, you probably consume much more sugar than you realize—certainly a lot more than the teaspoonful stirred into your morning cup of coffee. In fact, from the early morning breakfast cereal to the midnight snack, sugar is the dominant substance in the American diet. The typical adult now consumes 2.4 pounds of sugar per week (as compared to 2.1 pounds of beef). Most of this sugar is hidden in commercially produced foods, particularly convenience foods that require little or no preparation. Every time you drink a six-ounce bottle of Coca-Cola, you're swallowing 3½ teaspoons of sugar. A single ice-cream cone also contains 3½ teaspoons of sugar, and ½ cup of sherbet contains 9 teaspoons. There are 4 teaspoons of sugar in a cup of canned, sweet fruit juice, and 25 teaspoons in 6 Fig Newtons. You consume two teaspoons in ½ cup of stewed fruits, and 4½ teaspoons in ½ cup of fruit gelatin.

That's only the beginning. Add several hundred more sugar-saturated items to this list—including various brands of baby foods, canned and frozen fruits and vegetables, bread, peanut butter, breakfast cereals, chili sauce, cottage cheese, ketchup, frozen desserts, and even salt—and you'll understand better why there are so many "sugar junkies" among us. Food manufacturers used over twelve billion pounds of sugar in 1977 just as a food additive. Even if you take your coffee black, and avoid rich desserts like cake and cookies, you still probably consume more sugar every day than any other single food item.

In summary, then, the body does rely on carbohydrates in the diet to supply calories and energy essential for the body to function properly. But an overindulgence in sweet and starchy foods, particularly sugar, will tend to crowd out the nutritious foods high in essential vitamins and minerals that the body needs.

Fats

Like carbohydrates, fats are a primary supplier of energy, as well as a source of fatty acids that promote healthy skin. Fats also serve as carriers for certain vitamins—A, D, E, and K—and by assisting in the absorption of vitamin D, they help provide calcium to bones and teeth. Many Americans obtain as much as one-half of their fuel needs from fats—which is an overreliance on this single energy source.

The fats we consume are either from animal fats (like those in butter, lard, cream) or vegetable fats (like those in soybeans, peanuts, corn, safflower). Most animal fats are "saturated" (filled with hydrogen atoms); most vegetable fats are "unsaturated." Saturated fats increase blood cholesterol levels; unsaturated fats may actually reduce cholesterol levels.

Fats are usually harder to digest than many other foodstuffs, particularly when they are cooked at high temperatures. You should limit your intake of fats to 25 to 30 percent of your calories, and be particularly cautious not to overeat saturated fats.

Vitamins

Vitamins.

It's one of those words that we all grew up with, knowing little of what it meant. Yes, we were told that vitamins were important for the proper functioning of our body. But what is that alphabet soup of substances really all about?

Well, let's start at the beginning. By definition, vitamins are organic compounds that are essential in minute quantities for good health and proper body growth. Their scarcity or total absence can rapidly cause both physical and mental disturbances, including serious diseases like scurvy, beriberi, rickets, and xerophthalmia.

With very few exceptions, the body cannot synthesize vitamins, so they must be provided through one's diet and in dietary supplements. Even though vitamins have no intrinsic caloric or energy value, they are a critical component of enzymes, which in turn are vital to various metabolic reactions in the body.

Contrary to popular belief, the body requires only small quantities of vitamins. Even those doctors who advocate high-potency vitamin regimens recommend a vitamin consumption that is relatively low when compared to the body's much larger intake of carbohydrates, protein, and fats. Still, even though our vitamin requirements are small, the typical American diet cannot be relied upon to supply an optimal amount of these nutrients. Many people don't eat the right kinds of foods, and even when they do, vitamins are often burned away in cooking. Even before that, the commercial processing of food usually reduces vitamin content significantly.

Scientists have identified at least twenty different vitamins. Let's review the most essential ones:

Vitamin A

The major sources of vitamin A are egg yolks and liver, as well as butter, cream, whole milk, and cheese made from cream or whole milk. Dark green, leafy vegetables (like spinach) and yellow vegetables (including carrots) are also rich in this vitamin.

The functions of vitamin A are not completely known, but some aspects of its importance are clear. For instance, vitamin A plays a vital role in growth during childhood. Also, it is essential for normal vision, particularly in dim light. Vitamin A also helps maintain clear and smooth skin, and keeps the mucous membranes of the nose, mouth, and various organs healthy and resistant to infection.

Vitamin A deficiency has been linked to minor health problems like colds and sore throats, as well as to serious ailments like stress-related ulcers. Also, if you're a victim of rheumatoid arthritis, a shortage of vitamin A may be playing a role in your illness. In one study, a vitamin A deficiency was detected in the blood of fifty-two of fifty-eight rheumatoid arthritics.

Some research indicates that severe stress can significantly reduce the supply of vitamin A in the body, and larger than normal dosages of the vitamin may be necessary during particularly stressful times. A growing number of scientists believe that most diseases (and chronic pain) put increased stress on the body, thus necessitating increases in vitamin A intake.

One final point: vitamin A in excess can cause as many problems as a deficiency of the substance. Researchers have concluded that very large doses of vitamin A (more than 40,000–50,000 units daily) can contribute to headaches, irritability, and liver damage. Unlike several other vitamins (like vitamin C and the B vitamins), a surplus of A in the body is not simply excreted; it often remains in the body, possibly causing damage when very large amounts are consumed. Because of its possible dangers, the Food and Drug Administration does not permit the sale of vitamin A tablets and capsules in strengths over 10,000 units (except by prescription).

Vitamin B

Once there was only one vitamin B—or at least that's what nutritionists thought. But now we know that at least twelve different vitamins make up the B family. Although they are closely related, they each have their own unique functions and characteristics.

Vitamin B$_1$ (thiamine), for instance, assists the proper functioning of the nervous system, and it facilitates the digestive processes. One of the richest sources of B$_1$ is pork, but it is also plentiful in other meats, as well as in fish, poultry, eggs, peas, dried beans, and grains.

Vitamin B$_2$ (riboflavin) aids the body's cells in making maximum use of oxygen. It also promotes a healthy skin, eyes, and mouth, and is necessary for the metabolism of protein, carbohydrates, and fats. The richest sources of B$_2$ are meat, dairy products, green leafy vegetables, yeast, wheat germ, and fish.

Niacin, or *vitamin B$_3$,* also aids in the breakdown and utilization of proteins, carbohydrates, and fats. It also improves circulation and promotes a reduction in blood cholesterol levels. It plays an important role in maintaining the health of the skin, tongue, and digestive system. Foods like peanuts, lean meat, poultry, fish, and milk are excellent sources of niacin.

Vitamin B$_6$, or *pyridoxine,* must be present in the formation of red blood cells and various antibodies. Like other B vitamins, it plays a role in protein, carbohydrate, and fat metabolism. It promotes the good health of the skin, nerves, and muscles. Meats and whole grains are important sources of vitamin B$_6$.

Vitamin B$_{12}$ (cyanocobalamin) helps maintain a healthy nervous system. It has been used to treat victims of anemia, by promoting the maturing process of red blood cells. One of the richest sources of vitamin B_{12} is liver, although it is also plentiful in kidneys and other organ meats, fish, eggs, and dairy products.

There are other B complex vitamins, including *orotic acid, biotin, choline, folic acid, inositol, pantothenic acid,* and *para-aminobenzoic acid.* These B vitamins are not understood as well as those discussed above, but they seem just as essential to the well-being of the body. Significantly, all the B vitamins work together, and if even one is deficient, the remainder do not function at peak levels.

When a deficiency in B vitamins exists—which is not uncommon in the typical American diet—an individual can experience depression, irritability, fatigue, and even suicidal tendencies. Insomnia, anemia, and high cholesterol levels are other signs of a shortage of vitamin B. Tragically, the processing of foods often dissolves the B vitamins that they naturally contain. In addition, sugar, so common in most of our diets, is one of the major enemies of the vitamin B family.

All B vitamins are water-soluble. Therefore, they need to be part of the diet each day, since the body does not store them.

Can the B complex vitamins help your present physical and mental ailments? Very possibly. They have been able to improve some heart problems, by enhancing the functioning of the nerves related to the heart. People under unusual stress or who are very nervous usually respond well to supplemental doses of the B vitamins.

Certainly the most astonishing research into vitamin B involves riboflavin. Because this vitamin (B_2) plays an important role in cellular respiration, some researchers believe that its scarcity may influence the growth of cancer. As Nobel Prize Winner Dr. Otto Warburg suggested in 1966, "Though there are hundreds, perhaps thousands of secondary causes that stimulate cancer growth, there is only *one primary cause,* and that is oxygen starvation of a cell or a particular tissue." By encouraging proper oxygen respiration, Warburg suggests that riboflavin may provide a defense against cancer.

Studies with laboratory animals at Florida Southern College revealed that riboflavin reduced the incidence of cancer in animals injected with cancer-producing substances. Lionel A. Poirier of the National Cancer Institute reported in 1976 that riboflavin had repressed the development and growth of liver cancer in test animals exposed to cancer-causing chemicals. As research continues, the role that riboflavin plays in cancer may be more clearly defined.

Vitamin C

Vitamin C, also called ascorbic acid, is available in plentiful amounts in all citrus fruits (oranges, lemons, limes, grapefruit, etc.), as well as in lettuce, tomatoes, strawberries, broccoli, cabbage, and raw potatoes. It is essential in the maintenance of healthy teeth and gums, bones, and blood vessels. It also guards against infection, and is necessary for the building of collagen, which is the primary component of connective tissue in the body.

As is the case with so many other necessary nutrients, vitamin C deficiency is not rare. The body cannot manufacture or store vitamin C, and according to one estimate, more than half of all Americans consume inadequate amounts of C. If you smoke cigarettes, inhaling the smoke burns up the vitamin C in your body very rapidly. Just a single cigarette can consume 25 milligrams of vitamin C. A deficiency in vitamin C also lowers the body's resistance to infection—whether from the common cold or from more serious ailments.

Stress and anxiety take their toll on vitamin C as well. If you're a patient with pain, and anxious about your illness, that stress may be using up large quantities of vitamin C in your body.

Adequate amounts of C may, in fact, help to ease pain. A Houston neurosurgeon, James Greenwood, has found that most of his back pain patients experience a reduction in their discomfort when they consume about 1 gram of vitamin C per day.

You may have heard of the research of biochemist Linus Pauling, winner of two Nobel Prizes, who believes that vitamin C not only prevents colds but also stops them in their early stages. In his book, *Vitamin C and the Common Cold,* Pauling recommends taking 1000 milligrams (1 gram) of vitamin C every hour at the first sign of a cold. As a preventive measure, he suggests the regular consumption of at least 1000 to 2000 milligrams per day.

An important study along these lines was conducted in 1961 by a Swiss investigator, Dr. G. Ritzel. Using 279 skiers as the subjects for his investigation, he had half of them consume 1000 milligrams of vitamin C each day, and the other half take an identical-looking placebo. The skiers in the vitamin C group experienced a 61 percent reduction in the number of days they were ill from upper respiratory infections.

Pauling's confidence in the healing ability of vitamin C goes far beyond the common cold. In 1971, noting that ascorbic acid apparently strengthens the body's immune system, and that it is the building block for collagen, the substance that secures cells together, he suggested that it may prevent cancer or at least curtail its growth.

Since then, other researchers have supported this notion. Biochemist Irwin Stone, in his 1972 book, *The Healing Factor: Vitamin C Against Disease,* discussed studies by German physicians indicating that vitamin C in doses of 1 to 4 grams per day (and sometimes accompanied by increased doses of vitamin A) appear to control cancer in some cases.

Other studies by Dr. Ewan Cameron, chief surgeon of Leven Hospital in Loch Lomonside, Scotland, tested 100 patients with cancer in its late stages. Each patient received 10 grams of vitamin C daily, beginning on the day when their doctors decided they could no longer be helped by conventional treatment. Their subsequent progress was compared with that of 1000 control patients of similar age, sex, and type of cancer, who were cared for in an identical manner except they were not administered vitamin C supplements.

What happened? On the average, the patients receiving vitamin C lived four times longer than patients in the control group. A dozen of the patients treated with vitamin C were still alive when the study ended, and they seemed completely cancer-free. Not a single one of the 1000 control patients remained alive. In Cameron's study, vitamin C was most helpful in treating cancer of the colon. It was also extremely beneficial in cases of breast cancer and cancer of the kidney.

Cameron also reported that vitamin C effectively eases pain. Patients who had been taking large doses of morphine and diamorphine found vitamin C so effective as a pain reliever that they were able to stop taking these potent drugs. There was also evidence suggesting that large doses of vitamin C can build up the body's defenses so as to minimize the chances of getting cancer. Vitamin C's ability to strengthen the body's cells apparently inhibits cancer cell enzymes from successfully attacking them.

Cancer is not the only disease that may be responsive to nutritional therapy. Drs. E. Abrams and J. Sandson, writing in the *Annals of Rheumatic Disease,* reported that arthritis improves with high daily doses of vitamin C. In still another study, by Dr. L. C. Gass, pain associated with arthritis was eased using large daily doses of vitamin C.

Except for man and the primates, most other animals can synthesize their own vitamin C. Pauling has speculated that man probably once had the ability to produce it, but lost it through mutation. He has calculated that for optimum good health, dosages from 1 to 10 grams a day of vitamin C may be needed. Although a great deal more research needs to be conducted, large doses of vitamin C probably do little harm, except in patients who have a tendency to form kidney or gallstones.

Vitamin D

Vitamin D plays an important role in the proper utilization of calcium and phosphorus in the body. Without it, serious diseases ranging from rickets to spasmophilia can occur.

The body needs only a very small amount of vitamin D to maintain good health. Yet many people do not obtain even the tiny dosage necessary. Interestingly, the body manufactures its own vitamin D when exposed to the sun. A substance called ergosterol in the skin is converted to vitamin D by the sun's ultraviolet rays. But in our modern society, where people clothe themselves heavily and spend much of their days indoors, vitamin D deficiency is not uncommon.

When the body does not produce enough vitamin D on its own, it must be obtained from other sources. Plentiful supplies of it are found in milk, egg yolks, fish, liver, and oils.

Incidentally, because vitamin D is stored in the body's liver, I generally advise patients to avoid consuming excessive amounts of it (more than 400 units per day). A surplus, particularly when consumed in pill form or via cod liver oil, can produce symptoms such as nausea, severe headaches, vomiting, and fatigue.

Vitamin E

Much is still being learned about the importance of vitamin E. But as more and more information is uncovered, vitamin E is clearly earning the distinction of being essential to good health. It helps in the regulation of sexual development, and its absence can cause sterility. It is also important in both preventing and curing various heart and blood vessel ailments.

Vitamin E also serves as an antioxidant for certain air pollutants. If you live in a city with high levels of smog, vitamin E may help reduce smog's negative impact upon your body. Daniel B. Menzel, Ph.D., of Duke University Medical Center, has conducted several tests indicating that vitamin E can protect the lungs and blood against air pollutants. His results have shown that when diets are supplemented with even 100 units of vitamin E, resistance to smog damage increases significantly. However, in comments on the typical American's consumption of vitamin E, Menzel says, "The present dietary intake of vitamin E is inadequate to provide maximal protection against ozonides."

The richest sources of vitamin E include whole wheat, brown rice, green leafy vegetables, fresh beef, liver, and eggs.

Vitamins, then, are so necessary to the body that when they are deficient in the diet, vitamin supplements are essential. Although each individual has his own unique nutritional requirements, the Food and Nutrition Board of the National Research Council has issued its recommended dietary allowances (RDAs), which serve as rough guidelines for the amount of vitamins and minerals that should be consumed daily. There is a continuing controversy over the validity of these figures, which many people believe are far too low. (Linus Pauling has stated that the RDA of vitamin C, rather than keeping people in "ordinary good health," actually keeps them in "ordinary poor health.") Keep in mind that the RDAs are only "recommendations," and have never been promoted as flawless yardsticks of the body's needs.

Generally, I recommend a higher intake of certain vitamins than the RDA levels. While the RDAs may be helpful in determining *minimal* vitamin requirements, I am more interested in *optimal* amounts. A deficiency of vitamins can be devastating to the body, and therefore I usually advise a trial of supplementary vitamins for pain patients. Their bodies need all the help they can get to facilitate the healing process.

Everyone's needs for vitamin supplements are different. While a certain amount may be optimal for me, you may need much more or much less. No two people are alike. Also, your own unique requirements for vitamins may change, depending on the demands being made on your body at a given time.

I recall that when I first read Pauling's recommendations of taking high doses of vitamin C, I was very skeptical, but thought I would at least give it a try. I started by taking 1 gram of vitamin C an hour, and almost immediately began excreting it in my urine. However, a month later, when I felt the early symptoms of a cold, I once again started taking 1 gram of vitamin C an hour. But this time, about nine hours passed before I began excreting away excess amounts. My needs during illness had increased significantly.

Since no one really knows the optimal levels of vitamins for people with chronic pain, I encourage my patients to experiment with various levels of vitamin supplements to determine what their individual needs are. As long as they are careful to avoid taking excessive amounts (particularly of vitamins A and D), about the worst thing that can happen is that they will have expensive urine. Frequently, however, my patients report that moderate levels of vitamin supplements help them sleep more soundly at night and feel more energetic during the day.

Minerals

Some people are fanatical about vitamins. They take incredible care to ensure that they are consuming the proper amounts. Each morning, they swallow a handful of vitamin tablets with the enthusiasm of a child eating candy. But interestingly, many of these same people pay much less, if any, attention to minerals, some of which are equally essential to good health.

When was the last time you examined your own diet to determine whether you are consuming adequate amounts of minerals? Have you ever done so? Let's look more closely at some of the more important minerals in your diet.

Calcium

Calcium is the most abundant mineral in the body. It is necessary for growth and reproduction. It aids in the bloodclotting process, and is essential for bone repair and the maintenance of cell membranes. A deficiency of calcium can aggravate certain types of arthritis, and can contribute to nervousness, muscle cramps, and insomnia.

The primary sources of calcium are milk products—like milk, cheese, and ice cream. It is also present in broccoli, turnips, mustard greens, nuts, and egg yolks. For calcium to be properly absorbed and utilized, magnesium, phosphorous, vitamins A and D, and certain proteins must also be present.

Iron

This is an essential mineral often deficient in the American diet. It (along with copper) must be present for the manufacture of hemoglobin. The richest sources of iron include organ meats, liver and kidney, as well as most green leafy vegetables, including spinach and cabbage. Iron deficiency can lead to anemia (low red blood cell count), accompanied by fatigue and weakness. Coffee and tea can also block the proper absorption of iron.

Iodine

The need for iodine can vary considerably from person to person. One of this mineral's primary roles is to regulate the rate at which energy is used by the body. Insufficient amounts of iodine often result in fatigue, constipation, weight gain, and intolerance of cold temperature. Seafoods and kelp are rich sources of iodine. Interestingly, the need for this mineral appears to decrease with age.

Magnesium

This mineral is necessary for many metabolic processes, and a deficiency of it can produce tremors, muscle cramps, weakness, nervousness, heightened sensitivity to noise, and seizures. Recent research studies have shown that magnesium can help combat emotional problems, skin disorders, kidney stones, and senility. Magnesium is found in milk, whole grain, seeds, nuts, and green, leafy vegetables.

Manganese

Manganese plays important roles in the development of bones and nerves, the strength of ligaments, the functions of the pituitary gland, and digestion. A deficiency of manganese can contribute to increased sugar in the bloodstream and increased fats in the body, and can also interfere with the activity of other minerals. Manganese is found in egg yolks, whole grains, and green, leafy vegetables.

Zinc

Zinc is necessary for the proper functioning of several enzymes and proteins. It is also needed to transport vitamin A from the liver (where it is stored) to the rest of the body. Zinc contributes to various healing and digestive functions, and can aid in the treatment of alcoholism, acne, and even sickle-cell anemia. It is present in meat, fish, whole grain, brewer's yeast, and wheat bran.

If you are taking mineral supplements, I recommend that you choose chelated minerals. This simply means that the minerals are combined with proteins (which they normally are in foods) in order to facilitate absorption.

L-Tryptophan: Nature's Pain Reliever

As basic research into the biochemistry of chronic pain continues, I believe that the most effective pharmacologic approaches to pain relief will be ultimately found in naturally occurring substances. Recent research studies indicate that an essential amino acid called L-tryptophan may significantly alleviate not only pain, but some of its companions as well, including depression and insomnia.

You're probably consuming some L-tryptophan every day in your diet, but possibly not in sufficient amounts. Many natural foods are rich sources of tryptophan, including bananas, green leafy vegetables, red meat, milk, eggs, avocados, and pineapples.

Why is L-tryptophan so effective? Think back to my hypothesis in Chapter 2 of the two different types of pleasure. One type of pleasure I described—the relaxed, secure, mellow, morphinelike variety—may be mediated by a brain neurotransmitter called serotonin. Because serotonin is synthesized from tryptophan, the amount of tryptophan that is consumed determines how much serotonin is produced in the brain. When tryptophan intake is deficient, and particularly during periods of stress, serotonin levels can drop, resulting in depression, anxiety, insecurity, agitation, hyperactivity, insomnia—and pain.

One way to cope with this serotonin deficiency is to supplement your diet with L-tryptophan. Large doses of this amino acid, when combined with appropriate vitamin supplements (niacin and B_6) that enhance its conversion to serotonin, may help to alleviate pain and many of the problems that accompany it.

For example, some studies indicate that tryptophan can be as effective as certain antidepressant drugs, while lacking any unpleasant side effects.

Two researchers at the West Suffolk Hospital in Suffolk, England, compared the antidepressant qualities of tryptophan and a drug commonly used for such symptoms, called imipramine (Tofranil, Presamine). The researchers, Bapuji Rao and A. D. Broadhurst, administered a tablet containing less than a quarter of an ounce of tryptophan to nine depressed patients, and imipramine to seven others.

Findings reported in the *British Medical Journal* revealed improvement in both groups after a four-week period. The authors concluded that the naturally occurring amino acid was just as effective as the laboratory-produced drug. These findings are particularly significant since imipramine can often cause serious side effects, including blurring of vision, dryness of mouth, low blood pressure, urinary retention, and occasionally heart palpitation, hepatitis with jaundice, and seizures.

Similar conclusions were reached by a study reported in *Lancet,* which analyzed the effects of tryptophan on depressed patients in hospitals in Sweden, Norway, Finland, and Denmark. After three weeks of administering tryptophan to one group of patients and imipramine to another, the nine doctors conducting the study stated, "The imipramine as well as the tryptophan group showed highly statistically significant improvements . . . Side effects in the tryptophan group were less frequent than in the imipramine group."

In another study, a group of twenty-seven severely depressed patients in England were divided into two groups. For nearly a month, one group was given daily dosages of 3 grams of tryptophan and 1 gram of nicotinamide (a form of niacin). The other group was treated in a more conventional way—with twice-weekly, electroconvulsive shock treatments. By the end of the test period, the tryptophan-nicotinamide group had shown significantly more improvement than those receiving shock therapy.

At the North Nassau (New York) Mental Health Center, two hundred patients with obsessive-compulsive behavior were treated for low serotonin levels with tryptophan by biochemist Hemmige R. Bhagavan, Ph.D. Each patient was given between 3 and 9 grams of tryptophan per day, along with 1000 milligrams of nicotinic acid and 200 milligrams of vitamin B_6. Between 70 and 80 percent of the patients experienced "considerable improvement" after only a month on this therapeutic program.

Tryptophan's ability to combat insomnia is equally impressive. Drs. Althea Wagman and Clinton Brown of the Maryland Psychiatric Research Center in Catonsville gave tryptophan doses ranging from 1 to 3 grams to women who had difficulty falling asleep. Those subjects taking the large doses of the amino acid reduced their usual sleep onset time from thirty to thirty-five minutes to an average of thirteen minutes. They also slept later in the morning by as much as forty-five minutes.

Ernest Hartmann, M.D., of Boston State Hospital, has conducted several studies that have arrived at similar conclusions. He discovered that just 1 gram of tryptophan reduced sleep onset time in ten male subjects by about 50 percent. The men also slept more soundly during the night, with less awakenings. The architecture of their sleep was not as distorted as with prescription sleeping pills—that is, the various sleep stages—like REM (dreaming) sleep and deep sleep—remained intact. This had led Hartmann to label the amino acid a "natural hypnotic."

Because tryptophan is convenient, safe, and free of serious side effects, I recommend that my patients try to ascertain for themselves what impact it may have on their own depression, insomnia, and pain. The most obvious approach would be to increase your intake of foods high in tryptophan, particularly steak, fish, eggs, chicken, soybeans, cottage cheese, milk, mixed nuts, baked beans, and soy protein. However, it isn't that simple, as Richard J. Wurtman, Ph.D., of the Massachusetts Institute of Technology, emphasizes. Tryptophan is one of twenty-two amino acids, and according to Wurtman, most proteins consist of only about 1 percent tryptophan. Foods like steak or fish include so many other amino acids that tryptophan becomes competitively overpowered, and not all of it is transported to the brain.

That's why I recommend that my patients take tryptophan in capsule form, and on an empty stomach. Tryptophan capsules are available without a prescription at many health food stores (although as of this writing, they are extremely expensive food supplements).

For my patients with pain, I recommend 500 milligrams of tryptophan with 50 milligrams of B$_6$ and 100 milligrams of niacin two hours before sleep. After a week on this regimen, if their body tolerates these levels well, I recommend another 500 milligrams just before retiring for the night. If you have chronic pain, depression, and insomnia, why not try it for two weeks to see how effective it is for you? Should you develop any side effects, simply stop taking it or check with your doctor.

A Recommended Nutritional Program

No nutritional program is perfect for everyone. Still, I have found it helpful to prepare a general diet appropriate for the typical patient with pain (if such a person exists). I suggest that you study it, and make changes relative to your own tastes, needs, and bodily reaction to the program. Never underestimate the role your body can play in communicating what is good for it and what is not. When in doubt, trust the wisdom of your body, and watch carefully how it responds to what you do.

You'll notice several foods absent from my recommended program which may presently be part of your own daily regimen. They are as common to most dinner tables as silverware, but I suggest that my patients avoid them as much as possible. They include items like the following:

—Sugar and items that contain sugar, which are the most overconsumed (and one of the unhealthiest) foods in America. These include candy, Cokes, ice cream, sherbet, pies, cakes, and so forth. (Try eating fruit instead.)

—Highly processed and refined foods that are drained of nutrients and saturated with additives of doubtful value.

—Coffee, tea (except herb teas that have no tannic acid), and soft drinks.

—White flour products, including white bread, macaroni, spaghetti, cookies, cake, and pastries. Like sugar, avoid white flour like the plague. Even flour products that carry the word "enriched" on their labels have had more than a dozen vitamins and minerals removed from them.

—Excessive table salt, which the average American consumes at a rate of 14.5 grams per day. It is only needed by the body at a rate of 1 gram per day. Avoid canned vegetables because of their high salt content; use fresh vegetables whenever possible.

—Cheese (except cottage cheese, Jarlsberg, or other low-fat cheese).

—Fats, like butter, cream, bacon, and margarine.

A few other reminders:

First, don't overeat, even if you are underweight. According to an old adage, you shouldn't eat more than 80 percent of your stomach's capacity; eight parts of a full stomach sustain the man; the other two parts sustain the doctor.

That's very good advice. Most people eat more than they can use, hoarding calories as if they were gold. The results keep doctors very busy.

Also, relax before you eat. Take a few deep breaths, or if you'd like to, do the Conditioned Relaxation exercise described in Chapter 7. If you eat when you're anxious and tense, the capillaries in your digestive organs are constricted. But if you relax, which in the process sends more blood to your digestive organs, your body will process your food more efficiently.

I also suggest that you add vitamin and mineral supplements to your diet. Except for tryptophan, dietary supplements should be taken with meals. Since Vitamins A, D and E are fat soluble, be sure to include some low-fat food (for example, low-fat milk instead of water) to be sure that they are properly absorbed by the body. You'll have to experiment to find out what levels of supplements (if any) are best for you, but listed below, as a rough guide, are the amounts I take each day.

THE BRESLER HEALTH MENU

BREAKFAST

Juice (6–8 oz. glass of any unsweetened fruit or vegetable juice on list)

Fruit or berries

Entree

Beverage

Take vitamin supplements (with milk)

LUNCH

Fruit or berries

Vegetables

Entree

Beverage

ONE SNACK (Any fruit or berries with 2 tbsp. nonfat milk or yogurt)

DINNER

Salad (vegetables with tbsp. vinegar and any herbs or peppers to taste)

Vegetables

Starch

Entree

Fruit or berries

Beverage

TWO SNACKS

FOOD SOURCES

FRUITS OR BERRIES

One cup of:
  blackberries (85 calories)
  blueberries (85)
  boysenberries (65)
  cherries (140)
  grapes (110)
  pineapple (75)
  strawberries (56)

Or one slice:
  cantaloupe (½ med.—
    5"—65)
  honeydew (½ small—
    5"—65)
  watermelon (4" x 8"—
    115)

Or 6 oz.:
  grapefruit juice (80)
  orange juice (90)
  pineapple juice (90)
  tomato juice (30)

Or one:
  apple (70)
  apricot (18)
  banana (100)
  grapefruit (½—40)
  nectarine (40)
  orange (70)
  pear (100)
  peach (40)
  plum (25)

VEGETABLES (Steamed or Raw)

One ½ Cup Serving of:
  beans (30 calories)
  bean sprouts (30)
  brussels sprouts (28)
  carrots (33)
  eggplant (25)
  onions (30)
  peas (58)
  tomatoes (1 med.—33)

Or one cup of:
  asparagus (30)
  broccoli (40)
  cabbage (30)
  cauliflower (26)
  celery (18)
  chicory (10)
  cucumber (1 av.—30)
  greens (44)
  lettuce (1 head—30)
  mushrooms (56)
  peppers (1 whole—15)
  radishes (20)
  sauerkraut (40)
  spinach (40)
  squash (60)
  watercress (10)
  zucchini (24)

ENTREE

*One 3–4 oz. (uncooked)
  serving of:*
  beef (250 calories)
  chicken (175)
  fish (175)
  veal (200)
  (Broiled, baked, roasted,
  or boiled, without skin,
  with grease strained off
  and fat cut off)

Or: 2 eggs (80 each)
  (Poached or boiled once
  per day only & not
  more than 6 per week).

Or: 4 oz. cottage cheese
  (120)
Or: 2 oz. Jarlsberg
  cheese (107)

STARCH

One medium-sized
  baked potato (90) with
  1 oz. yogurt (22)

Or: one small piece corn
  bread (2" x 3"–150)

Vitamin Supplements

	Daily Recommendations
Vitamin A	7500–10,000 units
Vitamin D	300–400 units
Vitamin E	200–400 units
Vitamin C	1000–4000 mg.
Vitamin B$_1$	25–75 mg.
Vitamin B$_2$	25–75 mg.
Vitamin B$_6$	50–150 mg.
Vitamin B$_{12}$	50–100 mcg.
Niacinamide	50–100 mg.
Pantothenic acid	15–50 mg.
Biotin	0.1–0.3 mg.
Folic acid	0.2–0.5 mg.
*Choline	100–250 mg.
*Inositol	100–250 mg.
*P-aminobenzoic acid	20–30 mg.
*Rutin	25–200 mg.

*Need in nutrition not established.

Mineral Supplements

	Daily Recommendations
Calcium	250–400 mg.
Magnesium	150–250 mg.
Iron	10–15 mg.
Zinc	0.1–0.5 mg.
Copper	0.5–2 mg.
Iodine	0.10–0.15 mg.
Manganese	2–5 mg.

True, my overall dietary recommendations are somewhat restrictive—some of the foods that you like may have to be sacrificed. However, many of my patients find that they feel remarkably better after trying my program for just a few weeks, and that they quickly develop a taste for healthy foods—particularly sugar-free foods—that they may never have been attracted to before.

Exercise Nineteen will help you to take a careful look at what you've been eating. After reviewing your diet, modify my recommendations in any way that you feel is best. Then try your new eating program for a month and see what happens.

I often tell my patients that after a month on their new nutritional program, they can then reintroduce, one by one, some of the foods they had eliminated from their meals. If they maintain their feeling of improved well-being, then they can continue eating these favorite foods. But if they start feeling ill again, they should permanently remove that particular food from their daily menu.

If your new eating program helps to reduce your discomfort—great! Stay with it. If not, continue to modify it until you feel you've honestly given this approach a fair try. If your discomfort remains unchanged, then your body is telling you to look elsewhere for the message behind your pain.

Exercise Nineteen: A Nutritional Evaluation

This exercise will help you to take a closer look at exactly what you've been putting into your body. The first step is to record every item of food you eat over a seven-day period. Be sure to include all snacks. Then analyze what you've been eating. Have you been eating as healthily as you possibly could? Do you consume an excess of sugar, coffee, fats, and the other food substances that can be harmful? What additional foods may be beneficial?

Finally, make a schedule of a new nutritional program that you're willing to try for a month, beginning immediately. Base it on my recommended Health Menu if you wish, but feel free to modify it in any way that you think is best.

SAMPLE

EXERCISE NINETEEN: A Nutritional
Evaluation

DATE: _April 11_

TIME: _9 a.m._

Part One: Seven-Day Food Intake

	BREAKFAST	SNACKS	LUNCH	SNACKS	DINNER	SNACKS
Day 1	orange juice, cereal, toast, coffee		no lunch		TV dinner, coffee	
Day 2	orange juice, cereal, toast, coffee		fruit salad, coke		turkey, canned vegetable, coffee	ice cream
Day 3	orange juice, cereal, toast, coffee		turkey sandwich, coke		turkey, canned vegetable, coffee	cookies
Day 4	orange juice, donut, coffee	donut	ham sandwich, potato salad, coke	donut	TV dinner, coffee	cookies
Day 5	orange juice, cold cereal, coffee		turkey sandwich, coke	cookies	TV dinner, potatoes, coffee	ice cream
Day 6	orange juice, cereal, toast, coffee		green, leafy salad, coke	cookies	cheese sandwich, salad, coffee	ice cream
Day 7	orange juice, donut, coffee	donut	toast, coke		TV dinner, potato, coffee	cookies

Part Two: Dietary Analysis

What foods should I stop eating?		
donuts	coffee	ice cream
bacon	coke	TV dinners
cold cereal	cookies	canned vegetables

What foods should I start eating?		
fresh fruit	fish	eggs
fresh vegetables	veal	vitamin supplements
	beef	cottage cheese

EXERCISE NINETEEN: A Nutritional Evaluation

DATE: _____

TIME: _____

Part One: Seven-Day Food Intake

	BREAKFAST	SNACKS	LUNCH	SNACKS	DINNER	SNACKS
Day 1						
Day 2						
Day 3						
Day 4						
Day 5						
Day 6						
Day 7						

Part Two: Dietary Analysis

What foods should I stop eating?

What foods should I start eating?

SAMPLE

EXERCISE NINETEEN—*Continued*
Part Three: Your New Nutritional Program

Breakfast choices

orange juice
fruit
eggs

Lunch choices

fresh fruit   cottage cheese
fresh vegetables
milk
beef / veal / fish / chicken

Dinner choices

salad   fruits
fresh vegetables   beef / veal / fish / chicken
baked potato
corn bread

Snacks

cantaloupe

watermelon

SAMPLE

EXERCISE NINETEEN—*Continued*
Part Three: Your New Nutritional Program

Breakfast choices

orange juice
fruit
eggs

Lunch choices

fresh fruit   cottage cheese
fresh vegetables
milk
beef / veal / fish / chicken

Dinner choices

salad   fruits
fresh vegetables   beef / veal / fish / chicken
baked potato
corn bread

Snacks

cantaloupe

watermelon

9 *It Never Hurts When You Laugh*

We must laugh and we must sing,
We are blest by everything,
Everything we look upon is blest.
—William Butler Yeats

One of my colleagues recently proclaimed, "He who laughs, lasts."

This aphorism may be more profound than even he realizes. For while laughter may not be the best medicine, it certainly can be a more powerful healing agent than most of us ever imagined. As reported in *Science Digest*, "Laughter is good for both body and mind. It eliminates nervous tensions which upset body functions and it clears the mind of annoyances and resentments. . . . Laughter leaves a feeling of well-being, of personal satisfaction, and of contentment."

As you're learning throughout this book, pain relief can be achieved in many ways that you may never have known existed until now. It is hoped you've already used some of them and have made real progress toward conquering your discomfort. You may even be convinced by now that you have the power to transform, alter, and change how you feel through techniques you had never tried before.

However, even a recuperating pain patient can still be overwhelmed by the negativity that besets him. The adversities around him become obsessions, at the expense of the pleasure he could be experiencing. In a sense, he inadvertently commits emotional suicide—ravaging himself with worry and depression.

If this sounds like a description of you, why aren't you allowing more positive energy into your life? Where are the pleasant and joyous moments to counterbalance the negativity? Despite your pain, why are you allowing the joys that life still holds for you to be consumed by anxieties and fears?

People with chronic pain have often lost their ability to laugh. I have found, however, that if they can recover their sense of humor, it can improve their physical as well as psychological health. Hearty laughter can clear the respiratory system, exercise vital organs (for example, the lungs), reduce tension, and provide a positive emotional release.

One of the most amazing stories about laughter's benefits is told by Norman Cousins, again in his account of his illness published in the *New England Journal of Medicine*:

> [My doctor and I developed a] program calling for the full exercise of the affirmative emotions as a factor in enhancing body chemistry. It was easy enough to hope and love and have faith, but what about laughter? Nothing is less funny than being flat on your back with all the bones in your spine and joints hurting. A systematic program was indicated. A good place to begin, I thought, was with amusing movies. Allen Funt, producer of the spoofing television program "Candid Camera," sent films of some of his CC classics, along with a motion-picture projector. The nurse was instructed in its use.
>
> It worked. I made the joyous discovery that ten minutes of genuine belly laughter had an anesthetic effect and would give me at least two hours of pain-free sleep. When the pain-killing effect of the laughter wore off, we would switch on the motion-picture projector again, and, not infrequently, it would lead to another pain-free sleep interval. Sometimes, the nurse read to me out of a trove of humor books. Especially useful were E. B. and Katherine White's *Subtreasury of American Humor* and Max Eastman's *The Enjoyment of Laughter*.
>
> How scientific was it to believe that laughter—as well as the positive emotions in general—was affecting my body chemistry for the better? If laughter did in fact have a salutary effect on the body's chemistry, it seemed at least theoretically likely that it would enhance the system's ability to fight the inflammation. So we took sedimentation-rate readings just before as well as several hours after the laughter episodes. Each time, there was a drop of at least five points. The drop by itself was not substantial, but it held and was cumulative.
>
> I was greatly elated by the discovery that there is a physiologic basis for the ancient theory that laughter is good medicine.

Emotional nourishment, then, is a critical element of your health program. Add some laughter to your life, and see what an important difference it can make in how you feel.

Overcoming Depression, Fear, and Anger

Depression. Fear. Anger.

They all can be terribly destructive emotions, paralyzing people into a life-style that is profoundly more miserable than the one they could be enjoying.

Depression is the most serious mental health problem in the United States. There are at least twenty million men and women who are severely depressed, only 40 percent of whom are being treated for their problem.

Not surprisingly, the major causes of depression are all related to either physical or emotional pain. The common triggers of depression include sexual identity threats (that is, a man becoming impotent, a woman learning she cannot bear children); the end of a close relationship; moving from one home to another; confronting a painful situation that had once been repressed; mild or serious physical illness; and an inability to perform one's job well.

Very often, physical pain is an important symptom of depression. Depressed people frequently report cramps or a tightening of the chest or stomach. They may also complain of fatigue, insomnia, and a variety of other physical maladies.

Like depression, unresolved fear and anger also make it difficult for you to enjoy the world around you. Wouldn't it be nice to become an infinite sponge, soaking up the love, laughter, friendship, music, and poetry that are here for the taking? But fear and anger are phenomena that feed upon themselves, diminishing the quality of life. Fear, for instance, generates only more fear, until eventually you're drowning in an infinite sea of phobias. How far-reaching can these phobias become? Marvin Kitman, author of *The Coward's Almanac*, has outlined some of the more common, contemporary fears in his tongue-in-cheek personality test titled, "What Are You—a Coward?" Do any of these sound familiar?

1. Sometimes I feel sad for no reason.
2. My favorite color is yellow.
3. If I cover my head with blankets, nothing can harm me (I hope).
4. Large, fierce police dogs have it in for me.
5. I would throw all this up and go seek my future in Brazil if I didn't have sinus trouble.
6. Revolving doors have it in for me.
7. Better safe than sorry.
8. ABC means always be careful.
9. I am seriously worried that the birds are plotting something.
10. Sanitation men have it in for me.
11. Somewhere, right now, a big computer is looking for my card.

12. The CIA has decided I am the only American qualified to carry out a suicide mission.

13. In reality, pop-top beer cans are not as safe as they make them out to be.

14. I have a routine blood test; my doctor will discover that I have tertiary syphilis.

15. A big bad wolf is to be feared.

16. They have it in for me.

Let's face it. Even the most negative emotions are not totally bad. They all have some positive aspects. As Maslow said, "All growth is associated with pain. If you're not hurting, you're not growing." Emotional pain and negativity can help you to learn more about yourself at the deepest level of personal understanding. When you're severely depressed, for example, your soul-searching is intensely honest and real. And that can certainly be worthwhile. However, it must not go on forever. After a reasonable period of mourning, anger, or fear, it's time to move on. Release those emotions, and start to develop a more positive outlook on life.

Unfortunately, many people do not know *how* to swim away from the ocean of negativity in which they are drowning. Breaking out of the stale molds they've lived in for so many years isn't easy. With anger, for instance, screaming at the individuals with whom you're irritated may not be the most appropriate behavior, for it can create more problems than it cures. I suggest that my patients share their feelings with the person or persons involved, but in a way that is sensitive to the feelings of the other individual(s). If anger must be released in a physical way, I encourage my patients to hit *things*, not people. Some achieve the release they need by jogging or playing an aggressive game of tennis or racket ball.

However you choose to express negativity, do it in a way that will permit you quickly to separate yourself from it as soon as it's been released. Then make a conscious effort to direct your body and mind toward positive, enjoyable experiences. As I've written previously in this book, the best way to break a bad habit is to create a new one incompatible with the bad one.

Exercise Twenty: Changing Feelings Through Actions

Emotions are often manifested through certain types of behavior. For example, anger can cause shouts of frustration. And fear can provoke uncontrollable trembling.

But just as clearly, the opposite is also true—that is, feelings can follow actions. Thus, by acting depressed, angry, or fearful, you'll often begin to feel that way as well. Sometimes, it's necessary to begin to act according to the way you *want* to feel—to replace your negativity with a behavior that's incompatible with negative actions. In the process, you'll often find that your feelings change, too.

In this exercise, you will see how effective this technique can be. In the next few days, select three separate times when you're feeling (a) frightened, (b) angry, (c) depressed.

As soon as you recognize each of these emotions, write a paragraph describing exactly how you feel. Then simply walk over to a mirror and smile at yourself. That's right—force a smile. Do it for at least twenty seconds. Then write another paragraph describing your feelings after the twenty seconds of smiling. How did they change?

Serum Fun Levels

To help measure the joys you're experiencing in life, Richard J. Kroening, M.D., and his wife, Beverly, created the concept of "serum fun levels." According to the Kroenings, serum fun levels are a logical extension of conventional medical measurements like serum cholesterol levels—an important indicator of your well-being. Serum fun levels, though, concentrate on the amount of pleasure in a person's life. They focus on the positive input that can rebalance the system and nourish it with invigorating and strengthening energy.

Do you, for instance, have a hobby that you participate in—not because you have to, but simply because it's fun? Do you go places and meet people for no other reason than the enjoyment it brings? One patient told me she started going out to coffee shops at night—a very simple activity she had once enjoyed, but which she had forsaken since pain had invaded her life. "I never realized how much I like going to the coffee shop," she said. "The waitresses are so kind to me, and the coffee shop has a soothing atmosphere. I feel very content there."

Unfortunately, many people with pain become accustomed to their own self-imposed limitations, and soon begin believing that it's impossible to incorporate pleasure into their days and nights. For instance:

"How can I ever go bike riding with this terrible headache?" or:

"I can't sit and play cards for hours with this pain in my side," or:

"I'm sure the stress of my job makes my pain worse, but I have to work, don't I?"

However, no matter how severe your pain and how gloomy your life appears to be, there's always room for joy. And when there's pleasure and happiness in your life, problems that may befall you will be minimized.

Let me relate the story of Tom, a forty-six-year-old truck driver, who fell and injured his back on the job ten years ago. Tom was the company's best driver, a reliable and conscientious employee. Despite his severe

SAMPLE

**EXERCISE TWENTY: Changing Feelings
Through Actions**

Fear	Date: April 12	Time: 8:30 a.m.
Before	**After**	**Change**
I am very afraid of the possibility of having surgery again. It would be my second operation, and the thought terrifies me.	I feel calmer now. I made it through the first operation; if I need another one, I'll make it through again.	My fear really diminished in just a few seconds. I feel more confident now.

Anger	Date: April 14	Time: 7 p.m.
Before	**After**	**Change**
I'm so mad at Bill. He doesn't seem sensitive enough to what I'm going through. Can't he be more understanding?	I'm still angry, but this crisis is no worse than any other we've had, and we've weathered them all before. I think it'll be O.K.	I feel I have a better perspective now. My anger is warranted, I think, but I can't let it bother me so much.

Depression	Date: April 17	Time: 6 p.m.
Before	**After**	**Change**
I'm really dejected about my job. The responsibilities are getting bigger, and I feel overwhelmed by them.	Why am I letting this bother me so much? My boss said he'd hire an assistant if my work load got too heavy. If I'm still upset tomorrow, I'll tell him I need extra help.	I'm still somewhat tense, but I have a plan of action now. The few moments in front of the mirror got me out of the bad depression.

EXERCISE TWENTY: Changing Feelings
Through Actions

Fear	Date:	Time:
Before	After	Change

Anger	Date:	Time:
Before	After	Change

Depression	Date:	Time:
Before	After	Change

back pain, the company doctor concluded that his injury wasn't a serious one and directed him to return to work. Tom followed this instruction, but his severe discomfort persisted during the ensuing months.

Nine months after the original injury occurred, while tightening the load on his truck, he felt his back go out again. But this time the pain was immobilizing. Tom told the company doctor and his insurance carrier that the new injury was related to the previous one. They refused to believe him, claiming he was able to work nine months after the first accident without any serious symptoms. They even denied that the new injury was serious, even though the driver's own personal physician concluded it was so severe that surgery might be necessary. The insurance firm refused to pay any medical benefits, and Tom was forced to sue the insurer to try to get the money to which he felt entitled.

The case remained in litigation for nearly nine years before the court finally ruled in Tom's favor. He had won the battle, but in the process, he lost the most precious parts of his life—his wife had left him, his job was gone, and he was forced to abandon his life-style of fancy cars and hand-tailored suits.

Tom now has his medical bills paid for life, and after an inexcusable delay, he is receiving the best possible care for his back pain. The insurance company is paying $160 a day for a room for him, but it is in a psychiatric hospital, which he describes as "a living hell." His room is the size of a small bathroom, furnished with nothing but a bed and a coat rack. He has no TV, no books, no visitors. He spends his days convincing himself that the insurance company has ruined his life. And he has more bitterness in him than anyone I've ever met.

What Tom needs, more than anything else, is to raise his "serum fun levels"—to begin having fun again for the first time in years. He must learn to regain his love for life and to get away from the lonely desolation of his gloomy room. Tom needs to experience the world once again, and long walks with a friend, an evening at the movies, or a picnic at the park would all be highly therapeutic. In my opinion, if Tom can begin to enjoy himself again, his pain will become significantly diminished, if not eradicated altogether.

Get the point? You are what you eat, and you don't only nourish yourself with food. Everything you do in life can nurture you—either positively or negatively. What kind of nourishment are you giving yourself?

If It Feels Good, It Can't Be Bad

Most of us have grown up in a culture in which self-indulgence has been discouraged. We have been taught to feel guilty about almost anything that gives us pleasure.

No wonder, then, that people with chronic pain so often refuse to engage in any action or activity that would bring them physical or emotional pleasure. Even though such behavior might help to relieve their terrible discomfort, their cultural upbringing often sabotages any thoughts of self-gratification.

As I discussed in Chapter 5, physical therapy is one of the simplest yet most effective treatments for people in pain. Yet I am often surprised at how reluctant pain patients are to enter such a program, particularly if it involves their active participation.

I strongly encourage my patients to become somewhat self-indulgent and to nourish themselves with positive energy whenever possible. A technique as simple as applying heat or cold to their bodies can often provide immediate pain relief. To me, they're foolish if they pass up such a safe and effective opportunity to help themselves.

Here are my suggestions for the two types of pain described in Chapter 2:

If you're feeling helpless, hopeless, lethargic, and overcome by despair and depression, apply cold to your body. Take a cold shower, or swim a few laps in a cool swimming pool. As uncomfortable as that cold water may be at first, you'll notice a significant improvement in how you feel afterward—refreshed with a profound sense of invigoration. In addition to the application of cold, I also recommend a brief session of hearty exercise—walking, running, climbing stairs, or even hitting something. Any of these may greatly improve the way you feel.

For the opposite kind of pain—manifested as anxiety, agitation, tension, insomnia, and hyperreactivity—the application of heat is one of the best approaches. Take a warm bath, a sauna, or whirlpool, or place a warm heating pad on your body. The Conditioned Relaxation exercise can also help you to overcome these kinds of feelings.

Other physical experiences are important for the pain patient, too. Sexual activity, for example, can be one of the most important and beneficial sources of physical and emotional nourishment. Yet so many of my patients simply don't maintain an active sex life. Not only are the cultural taboos against self-indulgence at work here, but in addition, people who hurt have often convinced themselves that sexual pleasures are incompatible with their aches and pains. They couldn't be more wrong.

I recall one of my patients, victimized by severe shoulder pain, who had not made love with his wife for more than six months. He was convinced that it would be impossible to enjoy sex while his shoulder ached with discomfort, and he was demoralized, since he knew his wife had missed it. He was even afraid to discuss the subject with her.

I did more than suggest that he revive his sex life. At his request, I wrote out a prescription for it. When I next saw him a week later, he reported that he and his wife both wanted to thank me. Not only was he still able to enjoy making love, but he felt wonderfully invigorated by it.

If your own sex life has been in neutral for a while, I urge you to shift it back into gear. If you're interested in raising your "serum fun levels," sex can be one of the ultimate joys. It is probably the best and safest activity done purely for enjoyment (can you think of anything more pleasurable?).

When engaging in sex, do whatever makes you feel good. Let your desires and instincts be your guide. Make up your own rules. Be uninhibited, and enjoy it!

Try giving sexual pleasure openly, and you'll find your own pleasure will increase as well. Masters and Johnson call this "give to get"—giving enjoyment so as to get get it in return. Communicate with your partner through words, gestures, and sounds. Let each other know what makes each of you feel good, and do it.

Also, totally immerse yourself in the lovemaking experience. Ignore your pain, and don't be surprised if the discomfort disappears. The more intense your sexual experience, the less intense your pain will be. An active and happy sex life is good for your pain and good for your life.

If you want to read more on this subject, I recommend *The Joy of Sex* and *More Joy of Sex*, both authored by Alex Comfort.

Exercise Twenty-One: Nourishing Yourself

Based on what you've learned in this chapter thus far, make a list of five ways in which you might be able to alleviate your physical or psychological discomfort by becoming more self-indulgent. Then during the next week, actualize each one of these goals, and record how effective each of them was in relieving your pain.

The Power of Touch

Our skin is the largest organ of our bodies. It requires constant nourishment, in the form of touches, caresses, and cuddles. Yet in our society, this basic need is rarely met. In most American families, there usually is only minimal touching. Older children, in particular, often make little, if any, physical contact with their parents. Some authorities believe that when people are deprived of physical touch that is given in either a loving or friendly manner, they may become motivated to touch in anger; this may be contributing to the epidemic of physical violence now so evident in our culture.

Most of us have at some time experienced the pleasant sensations and undeniable benefits of touching and being touched. If, for example, your spouse is feeling tension and tightness in the neck and shoulders, your gentle stroking of that area can soon dissolve away that tension, replacing it with a deeply soothing feeling of relaxation.

In an experiment supervised by Dolores Krieger, professor of nursing education at New York University Medical Center, sixty-four patients were divided into two groups, one of which received "therapeutic touch" from nurses twice a day. The other group received only routine nursing care. After just one day, the patients who had been touched showed significant increases in the hemoglobin levels of their blood (hemoglobin, located in the red blood cells, transports oxygen from the lungs to the body tissues). No such changes were found in the other group.

How often are you touched by friends or family members? When, for instance, was the last time you were massaged? Massage, with a history as old as man, has become a highly fashionable healing art in recent years. There have been a dozen or more books written on the subject, some packaged and sold with their own bottles of rubbing oil. Schools across the country are teaching the art of massage to thousands of interested people.

When massage is tenderly shared with a friend or a loved one, it can be enriching and soothing to both the spirit and the physical being. It's a wonderful experience, and it's delightfully habit-forming.

Although a number of massage manuals can provide you with detailed explanations of massage techniques, feel free simply to do what comes naturally. The pleasant sensation of another person's hands is so delightful that special skills are usually not required. Just allow things to happen naturally—and your "serum fun levels" will soar.

The best way to receive a massage is in the nude. If you're self-conscious and thus feel the need to be partially clothed, then do so. But the full benefits of a massage can be best enjoyed when the entire body is involved, unrestrained by clothing.

During the massage, keep your eyes closed, focus your mind on your breathing, and then get in tune with each part of your body as it is being touched. Concentrate only on the present moment—and enjoy what you feel.

Incidentally, some of my patients complain that they do not have a spouse or a friend to massage them. Must they therefore be deprived of the massage experience? Not at all. Self-massage can also be extremely enjoyable. You can rub, knead, and squeeze your own body reasonably

SAMPLE

EXERCISE TWENTY-ONE:
Nourishing Yourself

DATE: _April 18_

TIME: _6 p.m._

	This week I plan to:
1	Read some of my old Max Shulman humor novels that I love.
2	Make a real effort to make my lovemaking with my spouse more enjoyable.
3	Take a whirlpool bath at Jan's house.
4	Surprise my spouse with breakfast in bed on Sunday.
5	Walk along the beach by myself Saturday morning.

	When I:	It affected my pain in the following way:
1	Read my humorous novels	I laughed a lot, and took my mind off my pain for awhile.
2	Made love	The pain disappeared, not only while we enjoyed each other, but hours after!
3	Took a whirlpool bath	I still felt pain, but I think the hot bath lessened it. I slept better that night.
4	Served breakfast in bed	I felt great! It made my spouse so happy that I forgot my pain all morning.
5	Walked along the beach	The pain remained about the same, but at least I enjoyed the scenery.

EXERCISE TWENTY-ONE:
Nourishing Yourself

DATE: _____

TIME: _____

This week I plan to:
1
2
3
4
5

When I:	It affected my pain in the following way:
1	
2	
3	
4	
5	

well, although there are certain parts of the body that are difficult to reach.

Exercise Twenty-two: Healing Through Touch

In this exercise, I want you to examine your body, searching for areas of tension, pain, or discomfort. You can do this by either lightly touching yourself or by keeping your hand an inch or two away from your skin as you scan its surface.

When an area of tension is located, you may feel a tingling sensation in your fingers. Some people describe the feeling as "focused heat"; others describe it as "sharp cold." Indicate on the charts below areas of pain and tension you have located. In addition, assign each of the areas a subjective pain intensity rating from -1 to -10, with -10 being the most severe discomfort you've ever experienced.

Now try to dissolve away the tension by moving your hands in circular motions, either directly on the skin or an inch or two above it. This technique has been called "the laying on of hands." Many patients report that after touching the area lightly, or gently stimulating the space around it, localized feelings of tension and discomfort disappear.

Try it for yourself. Gently pass your hands over each stressed area of your body for a few minutes, and as you do, sense all the pain or tension melt away beneath your fingers.

Then complete the second set of drawings, again indicating the areas of distress and a rating of their pain intensity. How much change occurred?

Four Hugs a Day

The importance of close physical contact cannot be overemphasized. Its positive impact both upon our bodies and psyches still sometimes amazes me, even though I have seen it work wonderfully well with hundreds of patients.

We can all benefit by learning to express and meet our physical needs in a loving, caressing way. Thus, I give many of my patients a homework assignment: During the upcoming weeks, they are to get and give four hugs a day. I even write out a formal prescription that says simply, "Four hugs a day—without fail." Don't ever underestimate how powerful this "therapy" can be, and the role it can play in the healing process. And it's a safe prescription, too. To my knowledge, no one has ever died of an overdose of hugging. However, as one of my patients told me, "It is addicting. Once you start hugging, it's a hard habit to break!"

Not long ago, I received a call from the husband of one of my patients. To put it mildly, he was quite irate. "What kind of crazy doctor are you?" he said. "Four hugs a day! What are you people out at UCLA doing anyway? I thought this was a respectable medical school. Who ever heard of telling someone they need four hugs a day to get better!

"The only reason I'm not pulling my wife out of your Pain Control Unit is that she really believes this nonsense will help her. I'm going along with it just because she wants me to. But I want you to know that I don't approve one bit of any of this crazy stuff!"

Five days later, I received a call from the same man. But this time, his demeanor was very different: "Hey, Doctor, this is really hard for me, but I just wanted to say I'm really sorry about the way I talked to you the other day. My wife has become a totally different person. She feels so much better. And she's fun to be around. The last few days have been wonderful. I thought this four-hugs-a-day routine was stupid. But maybe it's not. I think it works."

I sometimes tell my patients that during the upcoming week, I'd like them to hug four people they've never hugged before. And *they* have to initiate the action. I recall what happened to Marie, a wonderful sixty-six-year-old patient of mine, who had developed severe arthritis in her hands. She was very self-conscious about her physical condition, and had become quite introverted. But when I gave her an excuse to break out of her shell, she didn't hesitate for a moment.

She would approach total strangers, and say, "Hi, my name is Marie, and I know this sounds a little strange, but my doctor tells me that it may help my pain problem if I can get hugged four times a day. Here's my written prescription. Could you help me out? I need a hug."

She was never turned down.

I recommend that when you're feeling angry, rather than lashing out physically in a state of rage, try holding on to that negative emotion for a few minutes or hours until you can physically express yourself in a loving, caressing way. In some Far Eastern cultures, the "reprimand hug" is widely used, in which anger is gently expressed while tightly holding the target of your displeasure. Medical writer Helen Colton writes:

> What a charming, humanistic idea! Some time when you're upset with your spouse or lover, try the "reprimand hug." Hold off discussing your anger until you're in bed tenderly stroking each other. A woman might then be able to say calmly: "I felt hurt and threatened when you paid so much attention to Cathy at the party."
>
> Or a man might say gently, caressing his wife's face: "I had a tough day with cranky customers. I was looking forward so much to walking in the door, seeing the table set for a good dinner, just being with you. So I was boiling with disappointment and rage when you weren't even home."

SAMPLE

EXERCISE TWENTY-TWO: Healing Through Touch

DATE: _May 1_

TIME: _10 a.m._

BEFORE

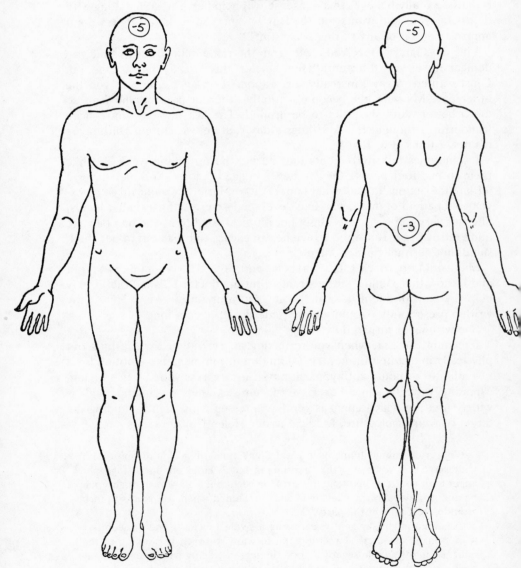

**EXERCISE TWENTY-TWO: Healing
Through Touch**

DATE: _____

TIME: _____

BEFORE

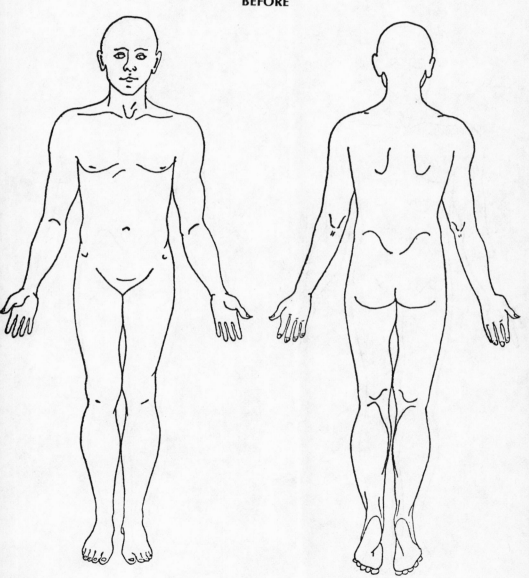

SAMPLE

EXERCISE TWENTY-TWO—*Continued*

DATE: <u>May 1</u>

TIME: <u>10 a.m.</u>

AFTER

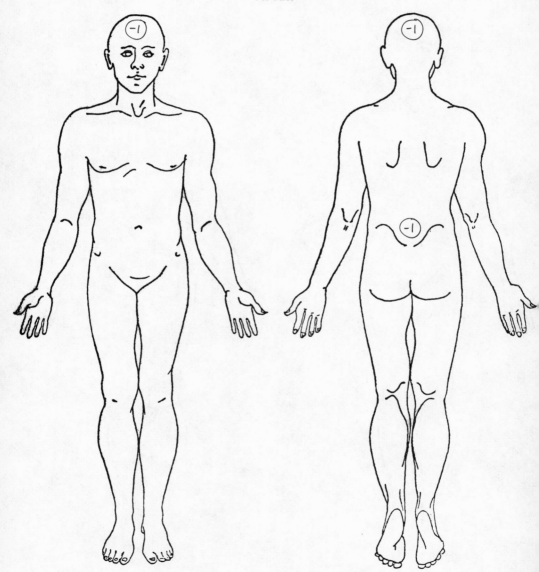

EXERCISE TWENTY-TWO—*Continued*

DATE: _____

TIME: _____

AFTER

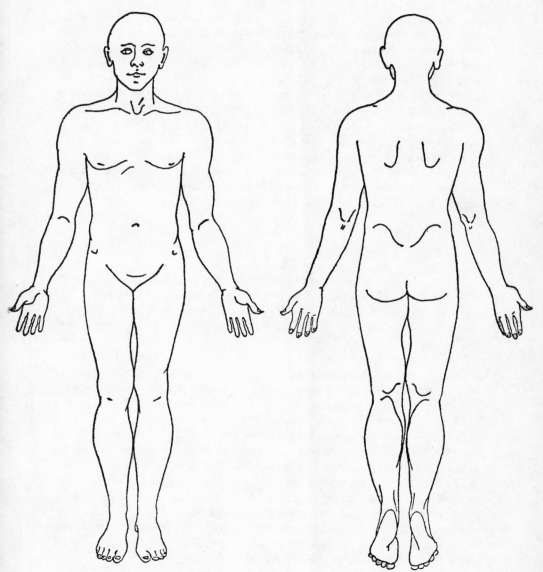

Just how important is touch? For a child, the most effective pain reliever of all is not a physician's injection or a druggist's pill, but a mother's kiss. Physical contact with those you love can create invaluable, spiritual bonding. Alice Bricklin, author of *Mother Love*, suggests that family members sleep in the same bed when the children are young, to create close family bonding. She points out that in many cultures, children often sleep with their parents up to ages three through six, whereupon they begin sleeping with older siblings. In Japan, children sleep with their parents until puberty. In our own culture, though, such constant, close contact—even between mother and child—is rarely encouraged.

However, as Ms. Bricklin writes, "For many, family sleeping together seems to be the ultimate key to a deeper, more spiritual growth, since the family bedroom offers greater family closeness in a way that heightens parental maturity and concern, the child's sense of contentment, and the security of each individual to an extent that she no longer feels so much of the aloneness or alienation that plagues many of us today."

While these sleeping arrangements may not be right for everyone, I nevertheless am impressed by the close family ties that can be formed under such circumstances. If you're interested in exploring this concept further, Ms. Bricklin discusses it in depth in *Mother Love*.

Movement and Exercise

One of the greatest sources of positive energy is your own body, as you fully and freely activate and animate it. The benefits of physical exercise are well-documented. In a sense, exercise is nature's most effective tranquilizer, for it provides a natural release for the anxieties and frustrations of daily life.

Think back to a recent, stressful situation. Perhaps you were tense, anxious, or in pain. Whatever the exact circumstances, it probably became very difficult for you to sit or lie still. It was almost as if your body were screaming out for movement. You may have even found yourself pacing the floor, as if responding to your body's inherent need.

I'm not a "physical fitness junkie," but I try to get as much exercise as I can. No matter what my mood or physical condition is at the start of the day, I always feel better after a hard game of basketball or a sprint along the beach. The human body seems to respond so well to a challenge of its capabilities. If you're not moving, not exercising every day, you're cheating yourself out of a wonderful source of positive energy.

I encourage my patients to get some kind of exercise every day. Not every second day, once a week, or just when they feel like it—but *every day* so that it becomes as much a habit as eating and sleeping.

Brisk walking is one of the most beneficial types of exercise. And there's no excuse for not finding time for a daily walk. Some of my patients get up a half hour earlier than they used to, and spend the first thirty minutes of their morning on foot, becoming reacquainted with their neighborhood. Others walk at night before going to sleep. One of my patients drives only part of the way to work each day, parking about two miles from his office and walking the rest of the way.

Walking gets you out into the world, and even if you walk the same path over and over, you can always spot something that you missed on previous days. Try it and see.

Remember to walk at as rapid a pace as is comfortable. An ideal rate is about three miles per hour. Begin with a ten-minute walk each day, and add five minutes each week until you have built up to a forty-five- to sixty-minute daily walk.

The benefits of walking for the individual with pain are well-documented. Few, if any, forms of exercise relieve tension so well, and thus help reduce the discomfort of tension-related disorders. One of my patients experienced a dramatic reduction in his back pain just two weeks after he began walking. A woman who suffered migraine headaches for most of her adult life stopped having them within three weeks of beginning her walking regimen.

Walking is not the only exercise that can start you on the road to better health. With your doctor's permission, try to engage in more strenuous activities that will raise your heart and breathing rates appreciably. Many of my chronic pain patients are getting into everything from jogging to bicycling to rope jumping to swimming to tennis. Some combine two or more forms of exercise—for instance, swimming three days a week, and jogging the other four. I advise patients to choose the exercises they enjoy that are also convenient (skiing is impractical if the nearest snowy slopes are a day's drive away).

But no matter what type of exercise you select, there will be days when you just don't feel up to it. On such occasions, exercise becomes just plain punishment. Well, don't despair. Even the best athletes in the world have days like that. If you miss a day occasionally, you won't do yourself any long-lasting harm. However, there are ways to combat those antiexercise feelings.

First, whenever possible, exercise with another person. Sociable exercising is more enjoyable than doing it alone. Also, knowing someone is waiting for you is usually enough to get you onto the exercise field when you'd rather be loafing on the couch.

After completing the Conditioned Relaxation exercise, some of my patients spend a couple of minutes envisioning themselves jogging, swimming, walking, or doing whatever other form of activity they've chosen. They may imagine themselves becoming physically stronger, with their heart beating lustily as their pain disappears. They may see themselves more alert, less depressed—truly enjoying the challenge of allowing their body to strive toward its peak performance level.

Try it yourself. Can you imagine how good it can feel to be so energized? Isn't there a real joy in observing the sustained movement of your body's muscles? Can you see the spring in your step, where once you could barely hobble? Use these images as a motivation to get your exercise program started each day.

Eventually, you may become addicted to exercise—but in a positive sense. As with negative addictions, if you decide to stop exercising, you may go through a withdrawal process—with the appearance of symptoms like anxiety, agitation, nervousness, and insomnia.

When I'm exercising, I understand just how positive this addiction can really be. I seem wonderfully in tune with the earth. As fresh air is inhaled into my lungs, I feel as though I am playing an important and active part in the flow of nature. I am very conscious of my own body—what it is doing and how good it feels. In short, exercise is a real joy and it can consistently increase your "serum fun level." Thus, why not give it an honest try?

Tasting the World

The world is brimming with pleasures that we miss because we simply are not sensitive to them or are unwilling to give them a try. There is so much around us to stimulate us, energize us, charm us, and give us pleasure. But because we do not fully use our minds and our senses, most of it passes us by.

Even if you have pain, the possibilities for restoring pleasure to your life are literally limitless. If you feel deprived of positive stimuli, you can change that. There is an exciting world out there that you probably haven't really looked at, touched, smelled, tasted, or listened to closely in years.

Why not expand your positive input by being as aware as possible of the environment? As Socrates said, "Not I but the city teaches." There's incredible beauty in the universe around us, but we've allowed our sensitivity to it to be smothered by the demands of day-to-day living. In a sense, it's time that you learned to live all over again, allowing your body to experience and respond to nature with the curiosity and spontaneity of a child.

People in pain often forget how good life tastes. Mark, a patient with severe low back pain, sat home every day, swallowed one pain pill after another, and barely did anything else because he was terrified that his pain would become even worse. By contrast, Alex, another victim of low back pain, took frequent walks, sat in the sun, practiced a few exercises, and listened to music. Although both had similar physical problems, their lives were totally different because Alex allowed himself to taste the world around him.

You, too, should start looking at and listening to the precious, enriching things that you had forgotten were part of the universe. Enhance your sensory awareness by letting yourself experience the "children's world" described by Victor Lowenfield in his book, *A Source Book for Creative Thinking*:

> You can make him [the child] conscious of the beauty of a row of tulips in a garden, of the difference between the long, flowing leaves of a weeping willow tree and the green-and-silver symmetry of a silver maple leaf. Encourage him to touch the rough, ridged bark of an old oak tree and the smooth, mottled bark of a sycamore. Let him feel the texture of wool and velvet and rayon in your clothes and in his own. Make him conscious of the way the cat's fur feels. . . . Even the sounds of the wind through the trees, the call of a robin in the early morning, the bubbling of brook water against smooth stones for a young child can be springboards to an expanding sensitivity which will enrich his entire life.

Take a day off to become reacquainted with the sensory magic of the universe we live in. There's never any need to be bored or depressed. I once spent an entire afternoon doing nothing but looking for four-leaf clovers, and it was wonderful. Recapture some of the child in you. If you allow the environment to enrich your life, you may be surprised at the positive impact it can have on the way you feel.

In their book, *Passages: A Guide for Pilgrims of the Mind*, Marianne S. Anderson and Louis M. Savary offer the following exercise, aimed at rediscovering the beauty of the world around you. Take a signal breath, relax yourself, and experience it as you read:

> Feel the earth beneath your bare feet, dig your toes into the rich, fertile soil. Go deeper: Beneath the soil is bed rock, layer upon ancient layer reaching to the molten center of the world. Go wider: As far as the eye can see there is earth stretching away to the mountains that edge the horizon, and beyond. Turn to the four directions, north, south, east, west. This is the great earth, mother earth from whose womb all life has emerged and still emerges. Lie down and embrace the earth, your earth, the earth from which every life force comes. Feel that life within yourself—a powerful indestructible force.
>
> Now the wind begins to rise, making waves over the grasslands. Rise and face the wind. Let it stream through your hair and feel its coldness on your body. A good coldness, clean and bracing . . . Air without which we die, air that feeds every living planet and creature and sculpts even the rocks into strange and beautiful shapes. Air that is the breath of life. Breathe in and out deeply . . .

SAMPLE

EXERCISE TWENTY-THREE:
Serum Fun Levels

DATE: May 4

TIME: 8:30 p.m.

		ACTUAL	POTENTIAL
Activities that *attract* positive energy	1	I run errands for Mrs. Jenkins	Help my spouse clean and polish the car
	2	I please my spouse sexually	Take Linda to a Saturday matinee once a month
	3	I help the kids with their homework	Buy a toy for Linda
	4		Take Linda and Mark to their favorite restaurant
	5		Build a sandcastle for Mark
	6		Teach Mark to throw a frisbee
	7		Do volunteer work for Muscular Dystrophy Assn.
	8		Take the family on a trip
	9		Watch the neighbor's children for her more often
	10		Buy a surprise present for my spouse

		ACTUAL	POTENTIAL
Activities that *generate* positive energy	1	Play the clarinet	Learn some magic tricks
	2	I please myself sexually	Buy and read a book on trivia
	3	Take a long, hot shower	Go to auctions
	4		Tour the local bakery and get "high" on the aroma
	5		Take long walks
	6		Splurge and buy myself a present
	7		Climb a tree
	8		Go horseback riding
	9		Get 4 hugs a day
	10		Take a night class

EXERCISE TWENTY-THREE:
Serum Fun Levels

DATE: _____

TIME: _____

		ACTUAL	POTENTIAL
Activities that *attract* positive energy	1		
	2		
	3		
	4		
	5		
	6		
	7		
	8		
	9		
	10		

		ACTUAL	POTENTIAL
Activities that *generate* positive energy	1		
	2		
	3		
	4		
	5		
	6		
	7		
	8		
	9		
	10		

Now face the sun where it rises like a ball of fire in the heavens . . . The sun, source of energy and of life . . . Let the sun's rays bathe your body, let its radiance penetrate deep into your spirit . . .

Far off the horizon clouds begin to rise from behind the mountains . . . The rain begins to fall, slowly at first, with warm, gentle drops, but quickly becoming a torrent drumming on the surface of the earth. The rain streams down your hair and face and bathes your whole body . . . Water without which all that lives would shrivel and wither away. Water of your life . . .

Drink deep of this experience that needs no words. When you are ready, return to your ordinary consciousness. Count from one to three and open your eyes. You are back in your usual reality state now, but the new dimensions of your spirit remain with you.

Creative Joy

The opportunities for enjoyment in your life are limitless. If you feel you are not experiencing enough joy, you have only yourself to blame. It is there if you want it. You have the chance to experience the world in a way no one else ever has. As Albert Szent-Gyorgyi has said, "Discovery is seeing what everyone has seen, but thinking what no one has thought."

Become a scientist. Find out what activities can bring you pure joy and incorporate them into your life. If you do, you may be surprised to see how little room is left for the negative things that once dominated your existence.

Exercise Twenty-Three: Serum Fun Levels

This exercise is designed to help you determine how much positive energy you are allowing into your life. That is, what are your serum fun levels?

First, list in decreasing order of importance up to ten activities you now engage in that *attract* positive energy. These are usually things you do for another person that make you, yourself, feel good. For instance, one of my patients does a lot of volunteer work for the American Heart Association. By helping others, he attracts positive energy, which makes him feel good. Another patient helps his wife clean the house on weekends—hardly an enjoyable task, but it makes him happy to be able to help his mate. Still another bakes bread and cookies for her friends, since she likes to bring them enjoyment through her homemade foods.

Next, list in decreasing order of importance up to ten activities that you now do which *generate* positive energy for yourself. In other words, what do you do solely because it makes you (and only you) feel good? Perhaps you have a hobby—something you've enjoyed doing for most of your life.

Some people collect stamps, others work in their garden, still others play tennis. What turns you on?

In developing these lists, don't be surprised if you have trouble thinking of ten activities for each one. It's a sad fact, but many chronic pain patients attract and generate very little positive energy in their lives.

Now let's move on to the next part of this exercise, which is even more important. List the *potential* activities you could be doing to attract and generate positive energy. What are the things you *could* be doing that would help you to be a more positive person? For instance, in listing the potential activities that attract positive energy, you might include increasing your share of household chores, taking the family on weekend trips, playing games like Monopoly or Scrabble with the children, or teaching crafts at the neighborhood Boys Club. When listing the potential activities that could *generate* positive energy, you might consider returning to a childhood hobby you used to love (like piano playing or painting), taking university continuing education classes, going to movies or to the theater, or bicycling. Or how about writing letters to friends, reading some of the novels on the best-seller list, collecting stamps or coins, or stargazing on a clear night?

If you wish, ask family members to help you complete these lists. Perhaps they have some valuable suggestions on what might improve the quality of your family life. Once you've completed this exercise, you should begin putting your "potential activities" into action—making as many of them as you can a part of your reality. Just because you have pain doesn't mean you can't enjoy life. And once you begin saturating your life with positive energy, that pain which you once thought was debilitating may not seem nearly so bad.

Looking at Life Through Rose-Colored Glasses

In her book, *Passages*, Gail Sheehy suggests that we all "must be willing to outgrow what no longer fits."

If you're a victim of a chronic pain problem that you could have overcome months or years ago, isn't it time to take the steps necessary to divest yourself of this dreadful burden? If your pain has outlived whatever usefulness that it might once have had, wouldn't you like to be healthy again?

As I've said before, the way you perceive the world significantly affects how you experience it. Too often, people who hurt see only darkness at the end of the tunnel. Many feel like victims of "planned obsolescence": beyond repair, wasted away, and permanently ravaged by their illness. Nothing can help them now or ever, they think. And consequently, nothing does.

SAMPLE

EXERCISE TWENTY-FOUR: Describing Your Pleasure

DATE: _____

TIME: _____

MAXIMUM +10	MINIMAL +1		MAXIMUM +10	MINIMAL +1	
		able			entranced
		affable			equanimous
		agreeable	✓		exalted
		amiable			exquisite
		amused			exulted
✓		beaming			fascinated
		beautiful			felicitous
		beguiled			festive
		blissful			fresh
		blithe			frolicsome
		boisterous			fulfilled
		bright	✓		funny
		buoyant			gay
		calm	✓	✓	genial
		captivating			giggly
		carefree		✓	glad
		charming			gleeful
	✓	cheerful	✓		good-humored
		cheery			good-natured
		comfortable			grateful
		comical			gratified
		concentrated		✓	grinning
		congenial		✓	happy
		content			harmonious
✓		delectable	✓		healthy
✓		delicious	✓		heavenly
		delightful	✓		hilarious
		diverting		✓	hopeful
		droll			inexhaustible
		dynamic			invincible
		easy			inviting
		ebullient			irresistible
✓		ecstatic			jaunty
✓		energetic			jocular
		engaging			jocund
	✓	enjoyable			jolly
✓		elated			jovial
		enchanted			joyful
		enlivened			joyous
		enraptured	✓		jubilant
		enravished			keen

EXERCISE TWENTY-FOUR: Describing Your Pleasure

DATE: _____

TIME: _____

MAXIMUM +10	MINIMAL +1		MAXIMUM +10	MINIMAL +1	
		able			entranced
		affable			equanimous
		agreeable			exalted
		amiable			exquisite
		amused			exulted
		beaming			fascinated
		beautiful			felicitous
		beguiled			festive
		blissful			fresh
		blithe			frolicsome
		boisterous			fulfilled
		bright			funny
		buoyant			gay
		calm			genial
		captivating			giggly
		carefree			glad
		charming			gleeful
		cheerful			good-humored
		cheery			good-natured
		comfortable			grateful
		comical			gratified
		concentrated			grinning
		congenial			happy
		content			harmonious
		delectable			healthy
		delicious			heavenly
		delightful			hilarious
		diverting			hopeful
		droll			inexhaustible
		dynamic			invincible
		easy			inviting
		ebullient			irresistible
		ecstatic			jaunty
		energetic			jocular
		engaging			jocund
		enjoyable			jolly
		elated			jovial
		enchanted			joyful
		enlivened			joyous
		enraptured			jubilant
		enravished			keen

SAMPLE

EXERCISE TWENTY-FOUR—_Continued_

MAXIMUM +10	MINIMAL +1		MAXIMUM +10	MINIMAL +1	
	✓	laughable			rosy
✓		lighthearted			satiated
		likable			satisfied
✓		lively			savory
		lovable			secure
		lovely			sensual
		luscious		✓	serene
		luxurious			settled
	✓	mellow			sidesplitting
		melodic		✓	smiling
		merry	✓		soaring
		mighty			spicy
		mirthful			sportive
	✓	nice			sprightly
		omnipotent			strong
		overjoyed		✓	sunny
		overpowering			sweet
		palatable	✓		thrilled
		peaceful		✓	tickled
		placid			titillated
✓		playful			together
		pleasant			tough
	✓	pleasing		✓	tranquil
	✓	pleasurable			triumphant
		powerful			unanxious
✓		rapturous			unfailing
		ravishing	✓		uproarious
		recreative	✓		vibrant
		refreshed			vigorous
		regaled			virile
		rejoicing			vital
		relaxed			voluptuous
		relieved		✓	warm
		rested			well-being
		rhapsodic			welcome
		riant			winning
		riotous			winsome
		rip-roaring	✓		witty
✓		robust	✓		zestful
✓		rollicking			zesty

EXERCISE TWENTY-FOUR—*Continued*

MAXIMUM +10	MINIMAL +1	
		laughable
		lighthearted
		likable
		lively
		lovable
		lovely
		luscious
		luxurious
		mellow
		melodic
		merry
		mighty
		mirthful
		nice
		omnipotent
		overjoyed
		overpowering
		palatable
		peaceful
		placid
		playful
		pleasant
		pleasing
		pleasurable
		powerful
		rapturous
		ravishing
		recreative
		refreshed
		regaled
		rejoicing
		relaxed
		relieved
		rested
		rhapsodic
		riant
		riotous
		rip-roaring
		robust
		rollicking

MAXIMUM +10	MINIMAL +1	
		rosy
		satiated
		satisfied
		savory
		secure
		sensual
		serene
		settled
		sidesplitting
		smiling
		soaring
		spicy
		sportive
		sprightly
		strong
		sunny
		sweet
		thrilled
		tickled
		titillated
		together
		tough
		tranquil
		triumphant
		unanxious
		unfailing
		uproarious
		vibrant
		vigorous
		virile
		vital
		voluptuous
		warm
		well-being
		welcome
		winning
		winsome
		witty
		zestful
		zesty

SAMPLE

EXERCISE TWENTY-FOUR—*Continued*

At its least (+1), pleasure is

a very happy experience. It's nice feeling joy in my life. At times it feels like I'm being tickled, and I just want to laugh because I feel warm and happy.

At its best (+10), pleasure is

a totally rapturous feeling. I feel totally zestful, full of the most exciting parts of life. It's absolutely luscious. And I'm healthy again!

EXERCISE TWENTY-FOUR—*Continued*

At its least (+1), pleasure is

At its best (+10), pleasure is

Don't let yourself become trapped like this. Take an eternal sabbatical from the tired beliefs that may be perpetuating your illness. If you begin looking at life through rose-colored glasses—seeing the joys and pleasures that you could be experiencing—you may be surprised to find how easy it can be to take the hurt out of your life.

Exercise Twenty-Four: Describing Your Pleasure

In Exercise Four, I asked you to select words that best described your discomfort. In this exercise, we'll approach things from the opposite direction. This time, review the following list of words that people use to describe pleasure. Check those words that apply when you experience *maximum* pleasure (+10 rating in your Daily Comfort Log and Progress Chart), and *minimal* pleasure (+1 rating).

When you have completed this part of the exercise, write a few sentences or a short paragraph that encompasses your experiences of pleasure at the +1 and +10 levels. If you try very hard to move from the +1 level toward the +10 level, your life can be filled with joy. So loosen up, laugh, and start living!

Oasis

Time to take another break. You are now about to begin one of the most ambitious sections of the book, dealing with the power of imagery in the healing process. But before you do, take a moment to review any information or exercises in the previous chapters that you feel would be particularly worthwhile to examine again.

When you're ready to proceed, move on to Chapter 10.

IV
Getting Help from Within

10 *Expanding Your Mind's Eye Through Guided Imagery*

Imagination is more important than knowledge.

—Albert Einstein

So how are you progressing?

As you have moved through the previous chapters, I hope that you have incorporated some of the ideas I've presented into your daily life. If so, you may have already noticed significant improvement in how you feel. But some of the most powerful pain-relieving techniques are still yet to come.

Up to this point, I have concentrated on how you can improve your relationship with the outside world by learning to relax in the face of stress, eat more sensibly, and raise your serum fun levels. Hopefully, you have started to replace pain-promoting habits with positive behaviors that can make your life fulfilling, meaningful, and enjoyable once again.

But there are other habits that may also need to be changed—habits related to the way you think and feel about yourself. For deep inside, a part of your nervous system may be working against you, sabotaging every attempt to achieve pain relief. Remember, the natural state of the organism is to be pain-free (except in situations of short-term danger). Why, then, is a part of you getting in the way? What message is it trying to communicate?

To find out, you must first learn to speak its language, the nonverbal language of symbolism and imagery. Only through a process of self-discovery can you learn to communicate with the deeper parts of yourself that cry out for change. No doctor or therapist can do it for you. The land of imagery is largely neglected, and its language is often as unfamiliar as one spoken in a faraway country. During most of your exploration of this part of yourself, you'll be on your own, but perhaps I can help you to get started.

This chapter will present my own personal theory concerning the nature of inner communication. In addition, I'll describe several imagery techniques that many of my patients have found helpful. In Chapter 11, you will meet an inner adviser who can help to guide you the rest of the way.

The Languages of Your Nervous System

The human body is an enormously complex organism. Its nervous system contains at least seven to ten billion neurons (nerve cells), and an average cell has approximately five thousand interconnections. Thus, according to neurophysiologist Charles Herrick, there are at least $10^{2,783,000}$ possible connections for receiving, storing, correlating, and transmitting data. How is this incredibly complex system regulated?

In the discussion of guided imagery in Chapter 5, I suggested that there are two fundamentally different "higher-order" languages used by the nervous system for inner communication. The control language used by the conscious mind is a verbal one, consisting of words that form verbal thoughts. This language has direct access to the *somatic* nervous system, the part that controls your muscles and mediates voluntary movement. Thus, if you want to stand up, all you need do is think Stand up, now, and your nervous system will coordinate all the muscular activity required to perform this action.

Yet, verbal thoughts are a foreign tongue to your unconscious mind, for it communicates through imagery and symbolism. The language of imagery directly accesses the autonomic nervous system (ANS), which regulates breathing, the heartbeat, blood chemistry, digestion, tissue regeneration and repair, immune and inflammatory responses, and many other bodily functions essential to life. The lungs breathe in fourteen pints of air each minute, the heart pumps two thousand gallons of blood a day, and the body perspires between one and two pints daily. All of these "involuntary" processes are relatively unaffected by verbal commands from the conscious mind, but they immediately respond to imagery.

To illustrate the powerful control that imagery has over "involuntary" functions, try the following experiment:

First, using verbal language, order yourself to "manufacture and secrete saliva." By thinking about this command, see how much saliva you can generate.

Did you have much success? If you're like most people, you probably produced a little, but not much. It's not easy to do, because the parts of you that produce saliva do not respond to verbal commands.

So let's try a different approach:

Imagine that you have in your hand a big, yellow, juicy lemon. Can you see it? Can you smell its fresh tartness?

Now imagine taking a knife and slicing into the lemon. Carefully cut out a thick, juicy section. In just a moment, I'm going to ask you to bite into that slice of lemon, using your teeth to squirt the sour, bitter juice into your mouth and down your throat.

All right, take a deep bite of your imaginary lemon. . . . Can you sense that tart, sour lemon juice splashing in your mouth, saturating every taste bud of your tongue so fully that your lips and cheeks curl? Swirl it in your mouth for another fifteen to twenty seconds, bathing every corner of your mouth with its acrid taste. . . .

Well, how much saliva did you create this time? If you were able to paint the picture vividly in your mind's eye, the image probably produced substantial salivation, for the autonomic nervous system easily understands and responds to the language of imagery.

The Brain's Two Hemispheres

Recent research studies suggest an anatomical explanation for the two languages used by the nervous system. This explanation may lie within the brain itself, which has two separate hemispheres. When viewed by the naked eye, these hemispheres appear identical, but functionally they could hardly be more different.

In most individuals, the left hemisphere is the seat of the conscious mind, for it is involved in the process of rational, logical, analytic, and evaluative thinking. Most importantly, the nerve centers that control speech are localized primarily in the left hemisphere, so its major communication system is a verbal one. It is the seat of the little voice in your head that constantly talks to you.

The right hemisphere, on the other hand, processes the information it receives in an abstract, symbolic manner, and appears to be involved in creative, artistic, intuitive, impulsive, and instinctual thought processes. Its linguistic abilities are quite limited, so it communicates primarily through the language of imagery—most notably in dreams, daydreams, and intuitions.

In a sense, dreams are a form of communication between the two hemispheres of your brain. While part of these nighttime minidramas may have some verbal content, they are also highly symbolic. Dreams, then, are an important way that the nervous system communicates with itself, and they represent a vital link between the conscious and unconscious minds.

Although your unconscious mind cannot talk to you in your native tongue (for example, English), don't ever assume that it is stupid or uninformed. Remember, "a picture is worth a thousand words," and the language of imagery is incredibly informative.

As an illustration of the difference between the logical, problem-solving ability of the left hemisphere, and the creative, intuitive approach of the right, try solving this puzzle:

> A father and his son, driving together in their car, are involved in a horrible accident, in which the father is killed instantly. The son is rushed to an emergency hospital, where a surgeon is summoned to perform immediate, life-saving surgery. However, after looking at the boy, the surgeon turns away, muttering, "I can't operate. That's my son."

How is this possible? Think about it for a few moments.

When I present this same problem to my students, they typically analyze it very logically, arriving at well-reasoned conclusions, like:

"Obviously, the surgeon must be a *step*father," or

"The boy's body must be so disfigured by the accident that the surgeon is guilty of a case of mistaken identity."

Very logical. Very left hemispheric. But also very inaccurate. The correct answer is that the surgeon is a woman—the boy's mother.

If you answered the question correctly, where did that solution come from? The answer was inside you, well within reach of your intuitive, creative right hemisphere, which holds the solution to thousands of other problems if you can just liberate yourself from the constraints of the rational, straightforward thinking of your left hemisphere. You may feel trapped and helpless, drowning in the pain experience, while the answer may be close at hand—there for the taking if you would just stop and listen, believe in your intuition and instincts, and trust the inner wisdom of your organism.

Consciousness and the Brain

Although no one really knows what "consciousness" is, I believe that it is nearly identical to "attention"—what we attend to is what we experience. Your attention is one of your most coveted possessions, and few things are more valuable to give to a child or loved one.

Over the years, we have learned to give most of our attention to our conscious mind, the left hemisphere. We listen endlessly to the chatter of the little voice that maintains a logical, rational, analytic monologue in

Left Hemisphere	Right Hemisphere
speech	images
words	symbols
analytic	synthetic
rational	impulsive
logical	creative
sequential	synchronous
active	receptive
evaluative	intuitive
cognitive	emotional
wordly	spiritual
somatic control	autonomic control

Fig. 14 *Specializing functions of the brain's hemispheres.*

our head. We quickly become lost in it, forgetting that any other part of us exists. In short, our consciousness becomes imbedded almost exclusively in the activities of the left hemisphere.

Nothing could be more counterproductive. You are *not* solely your conscious mind, for it is no more (or less) important than any other aspect of your being. Your left hemisphere is just one part of your brain, and like other vital organs, it has a specialized function that aids survival—that is, it makes logical associations from Thought A to Thought B to Thought C, and so on.

Have you ever stopped yourself to ask, "Now what made me think of that? Well, first I was thinking of (something) which reminded me of it. And before that, I was thinking of (something else), and even before that, I guess I was thinking about (something else)" . . . The conscious mind can race through a series of associations in a flash, and when you allow your attention to reside solely there, your total experience becomes that chain of thoughts.

However, you are much more than your conscious mind. You are also your intuitions, emotions, and feelings; your drives and motivations; your goals and aspirations; your values and beliefs; your personality; and, of course, your physical body. To me, it makes no more sense to believe that you are primarily your conscious mind than to believe that you are primarily your liver (or your anger, your appetite, and so forth).

How do you get in touch with the other parts of yourself? Simply give them your attention. Unfortunately, most of us do this only under strong coercion. When a part of us desperately needs to be heard, it will briefly capture our attention. For example, when we injure ourselves, the alarms go off and our attention is temporarily shifted to the body. But shortly thereafter, we wander back to the conscious mind, and the inner voice begins again—"What am I going to do about this injury? Should I call the doctor? Should I lie down for the rest of the day? How can I cancel my plans for tonight?"

Why do we allow the conscious mind to dominate our attention so thoroughly? Because most of us have been trained and rewarded for doing so. In the Western world, the accomplishments of the left hemisphere— our rational, logical side—are usually respected over all others. Our educational, social, and vocational systems offer great recognition, honor, and advancement to people who are analytic, logical, and articulate. True, athletes are rewarded for the accomplishments of their physical bodies (and as a result, their bodies receive much of their attention). In a similar manner, actors, writers, or artists may rely primarily on their intuitions and emotions.

But most of us receive little, if any, positive recognition for the achievements of the right hemisphere—our creative, intuitive, instinctive side. In fact, we are usually discouraged from "wasteful" and "petty" activities like daydreaming. Consequently, we suppress the most creative part of our nervous system and literally forget how to use it. As Roger W. Sperry wrote in *Mosaic*, "Our educational system and modern society generally (with its heavy emphasis on communication and on early training in the three Rs) discriminate against one whole half of the brain." Thus, identifying exclusively with the conscious mind becomes a bad habit—one that seems very much unmanageable. If you think it's *not* difficult to control it, try these simple experiments:

Stop your conscious mind from thinking for one minute. Can you do it? How about for ten seconds? One second?

Tell your conscious mind to give you any *wrong* answer to the equation $2 + 2 = (\ )$. *Don't* think of the number "4."

These experiments illustrate the notion that the conscious mind is nothing more than a complex biocomputer, totally programmed by the rewards and punishments in your life experience. In many ways, it is inflexible, rigid, and automatic. Like Pavlov's dogs, certain stimuli will almost invariably produce stereotyped patterns of thinking. When discomfort flares up, a pain patient might think, Oh, no. Now what will I do about tonight? How will my friends ever forgive me for missing the party? Why did this ever have to happen to me? Lost in thought, this patient may be oblivious to the nonverbal messages that the right hemisphere is trying to communicate.

The Unconscious Mind

For years, you may have relied on your left hemisphere to analyze and conquer your pain problem, with no success. Thus, by now, you should be willing to recognize that you can't depend solely on the dominant side of your brain, with its limited language of thoughts and words. You must now begin to communicate with the nondominant hemisphere, and on its own terms—in the language of imagery.

I believe that the mobilization of the right hemisphere is critically important for the individual with chronic pain. The right hemisphere provides access to the autonomic nervous system (ANS), which, according to some investigators, regulates the experiences of both pleasure and pain. To help you learn to maximize your ability to control your discomfort, a brief explanation of autonomic functioning may be appropriate.

The ANS has two complementary branches. The first, the *sympathetic nervous system* (SNS), is designed to prepare the body for action, and when it does, it accelerates the breath and the heartbeat, and constricts the major blood vessels, causing a subsequent rise in blood pressure. Concurrently, processes less critical to the organism's immediate survival, like digestive activities, decrease.

The second branch, the *parasympathetic nervous system* (PNS), is designed to rest the body. When activated, the PNS slows the breath and the heartbeat, and dilates the major blood vessels, lowering the blood pressure. Simultaneously, digestive activities increase.

In terms of pleasure and pain, I believe that SNS activation is typically experienced as a feeling of power, control, confidence, and excitement. By contrast, decreased SNS activity is manifested as helplessness, futility, worthlessness, and lethargy.

Conversely, activation of the PNS is experienced as security, tran-

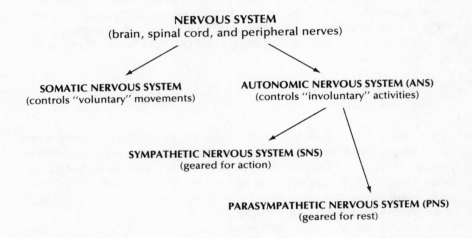

Fig. 15   *Divisions of the nervous system.*

quillity, safety, and serenity, while low PNS activity produces feelings of tension, agitation, anxiety, and hypersensitivity.

Thus, each of the emotional states we experience represents a unique blend of various levels of SNS and PNS activation. The fight-or-flight response, for example, is correlated with extremely high SNS and very low PNS activation.

In my opinion, most chronic pain patients have exhausted both their SNS and PNS. Not only do they feel helpless and/or hopeless, but they are also victimized by feelings of tension and anxiety.

Because the experiences of pleasure and pain are related to autonomic nervous system functioning, I insist that my patients learn how to communicate more directly with their ANS, using the higher-order language of the unconscious mind—the language of imagery and symbolism. It is a difficult process for many people, simply because they have been preoccupied with their conscious mind for so long. However, like other habits, this one can be broken by creating a new habit incompatible with the old.

An important first step is to practice dissociating yourself from the thoughts of your conscious mind. And what is the best way to accomplish this? Initially, by using the same approach you did in Chapter 6, when you learned to detach yourself from your emotions. Observe your conscious mind, allow yourself to be aware of its thoughts, but choose not to identify with them.

One way to achieve this type of dissociation is to allow yourself to relax, using the Conditioned Relaxation exercise. Not only can this exercise be an effective tool for easing tension and the pain that accompanies it, but it is also a means for quieting down the dominant, rational, verbal part of your nervous system. By relaxing the muscles controlled by the somatic nervous system, you quiet the conscious mind so you can get in touch with your nondominant self, and take fullest advantage of the power of your imagination.

Once you're relaxed, then spend a few minutes simply daydreaming. If you carefully pay attention to the images, and not to random verbal thoughts, you will find yourself gaining access to your right hemisphere— your intuitive, creative, instinctive side.

As you become more familiar with your right hemisphere, aided by the techniques presented over the following pages, you may find it to be the source of the following benefits:

—Through the language of the right hemisphere, you may uncover new insights and new information that will lead to improvement not just in your pain problem, but in your entire life.

—You may also discover unconscious misconceptions that need to be corrected in order for the healing process to occur. For example, you may find that your right hemisphere is brimming with negative expectations which, in turn, are responsible for many or most of your negative experiences. These inappropriate expectations must first be identified before they can be changed.

—Finally, you may be able to actively promote the healing process through the language of the right hemisphere. Keep in mind that the autonomic nervous system, which regulates pain and pleasure, is controlled by the unconscious mind. By communicating effectively with the right hemisphere, you may be able to produce dramatic changes in your body, as easily as the ones you accomplished in your experiment with the lemon.

Imagination and the Disease Process

Your nondominant hemisphere knows precisely what to do when presented with various images. When you imagined biting into a lemon slice, for example, what action did it take? It activated the autonomic nervous system centers responsible for producing saliva, didn't it?

Bringing things into the realm of the pain experience, think for a moment of how you envision yourself. If you're like many other patients with pain, you may picture yourself as a helpless, hopeless victim of an incurable illness. And with that kind of a picture before it, your right hemisphere may be saying, "Prepare the body to be helpless. Don't even bother mobilizing the immune and inflammatory defenses that might facilitate healing. Just give up." It's not surprising, then, that you don't get better.

Why give your right hemisphere such counterproductive information? You are only making your pain worse when you focus on thoughts like, "I hurt so much . . . I am so limited by this pain . . . I feel terrible . . . No doctor can help me."

The right hemisphere is very literal. If you picture your discomfort as "a sizzling hot poker that is constantly being stabbed into my neck," or as "a lion gnawing on my back, tearing deeper into the nerves with every bite," or as "wringing out the nerves like they're a wet washcloth"—then you can expect to feel it in just that way.

The right hemisphere also picks up cues that it interprets very strictly. A child who is told that he or she is a "pain in the neck" may develop arthritis in the neck as an adult. A man or woman can die of a "broken heart." An individual who feels as though he is "eating himself up inside" may develop cancer.

A single picture, then, can be more potent that a dictionary of words. So why not use one to help your body heal itself? For example, while sitting in a dentist's chair, you may be able to stop your gums from bleeding by creating a vivid image of it actually happening. Several dentists have told me that when they have asked their patients to imagine that freezing-cold ice was being applied to their bleeding gums, the patients reported that the area soon became numb. In addition, the blood vessels constricted, and the bleeding stopped.

In a similar way, the effectiveness of medication can often be enhanced through imagery. Let's assume, for instance, that you are suffering from an ear infection, for which you are taking antibiotics. Well, why not imagine that the blood vessels which nourish your ear are becoming dilated? This may permit more blood—and a greater concentration of the antibiotic—to flow into the ear, thus hastening the healing process.

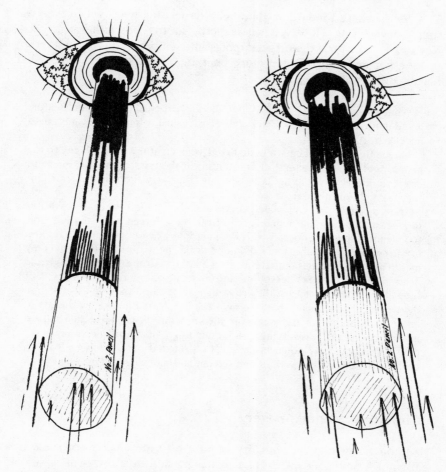

Fig. 16 *This vivid picture was drawn by a patient who experiences severe headaches.*

Carl Simonton, M.D., and Stephanie Matthews-Simonton have pioneered the use of imagery techniques that have often significantly extended the life spans of their cancer patients. In addition to conventional therapy, the Simontons' technique encourages these patients to visualize their cancer as broken-up hamburger meat, and their white blood cells as dogs or white knights devouring and destroying the hamburger.

True, it sounds a little bizarre. But I am open to any safe technique that will maximize your chances of regaining your health. It's also clear to me that a vivid image can be incredibly potent. Refer back to the beginning of

Chapter 1, where Linda described her excruciating pain, which then was simply devastating. However, when she began to work with imagery, she was able to transform the original image into a more positive one, thereby making her discomfort much more bearable. Here's how she described her discomfort at its best:

> What a strange way to put it. When the unsharpened bread knife cuts the bread lumpy, when the razor nicks but doesn't slice, when the screams are in the closet.
>
> Maybe this is a good day to write this. I've been at the office all day so the pain cannot be "at its worst." I'm squinting at the typewriting, the blackout draperies are closed, the lights are off, and I'm sorry, President Carter, but the air conditioner is on. At least I'm here.
>
> The cars outside this air-sealed building are the loudest cars in the world. I think I can hear the traffic lights snap from red to green to mostly red. But red means stop and it doesn't. It is the pain in my head, loud and bright and brash, sending out sparks like a diamond drill. The dentist has the drill in my mouth and my mouth is sealed shut. It would be a drone except for its triple heads—one on my back teeth, one into my ear, one into my eyebrow. But they all go at once; at least they're not separate. And they don't shake me the way the bad ones do, because my neck is stiff, my head is held exact in an iron cap, and as the day wears on, the screws in the cap tighten. The pain is hard, consistent, unswerving, solid, unending. All the way down my neck, down my back, now down my arm. It's stretched out, yowling, droning, drilling. It's the difference between scream and screech. And it's endurable.

The Art of Mental Imagery

Although this may be your first exposure to the imagery process, it is really not a new concept. In fact, it has existed in a surprisingly similar form for many centuries. In pre-Cartesian times, Agrippa (1510) proclaimed, "So great a power is there of the soul upon the body, that whichever way the soul imagines and dreams that it goes, thither doth it lead the body."

For many years thereafter, doctors talked about the relationship between imagery and disease. As recently as the seventeenth century, imagination was thought to be so potent in stimulating bodily changes that it could even imprint characteristics on embryos in the womb. In his *Oratio de Imaginatione* (1593), Nymannus wrote about the therapeutic effects of music, whose soothing and excitatory potential could be used to treat painful ailments like arthritis.

In the post-Cartesian era, medicine began to emphasize a more mechanistic, physiological approach to disease. No longer were medical students taught the role that the mind can play in disease. Consequently, imagery techniques laid dormant for many years, only to be revived in the late twentieth century—because they work.

Even so, many patients now approach the imagery process with skepticism. Initially, they typically say that they feel silly creating make-believe images in their heads.

However, I'm not asking you, even in your mind's eye, to create totally unrealistic pictures. I'm not encouraging you to envision something that is impossible. If you have a ruptured disk, for example, it's probably senseless to imagine that you'll be playing football by week's end. But it's very realistic to assume an attitude like, "Maybe I have the chance to extricate myself from the situation in which I find myself. Maybe I can help myself to function more effectively, and lead a more fulfilling life."

Your autonomic nervous system will react much more positively if you present your unconscious mind with a strong image of how you'd like your body to become. If you start to *see* yourself that way, your ANS may help you to *be* that way.

Within you is a creativity that desperately wants you to survive. Mother nature, in her wisdom, gave you a powerfully intuitive, instinctual ability, and if you learn how to speak its language of imagery, you may discover the road to long-awaited relief from your chronic pain.

Guided Imagery Training Techniques

For many people, their power of imagination has not been tapped since childhood. Getting in touch with images in the mind has become a difficult and awkward process, for their creative and intuitive abilities have long been ignored.

If this description fits you, don't despair. Yes, your ability to imagine will be very important as you proceed through the following pages. But you can strengthen your skills through diligent and conscientious practice. The next four exercises are designed to help you do just that. Use your creativity and see what happens.

Exercise Twenty-five: The Negative Afterimage

For this exercise, take a piece of plain white paper, and with a pen or pencil, draw a solid black circle about the size of a pea in its center. Place the paper in front of a dark background in a well-lit room. Then, standing about three feet away from the paper, stare intently at the circle. Focus all of your attention and concentration on the circle for about sixty seconds, without letting your eyes drift away from it. Soon, you will begin to see a

SAMPLE

**EXERCISE TWENTY-FIVE: The Negative
Afterimage**

Session No.	1	2	3	4	5
Date	5/14	5/15	5/16	5/17	5/18
Moving the image	I had difficulty moving it	The image moved a little	I moved the image a lot	Easy to move the image	Easy to move the image
Changing its color	Changed color to blue and red	Changed color to blue and red	Changed color to all shades in the rainbow	Changed color to all shades in the rainbow	Changed color to all shades in the rainbow
Changing its shape	Changed shape easily to square and oval	Shape-changing is easy to all shapes	Shape-changing is easy to all shapes	Shape-changing is easy to all shapes	Shape-changing is easy to all shapes
Making it disappear	I can't do it	I can't do it	I did it once	I did it once	I can do it at will
Making it reappear	—	—	It didn't reappear	It didn't reappear	It reappeared
Creative imagination	—	The image danced	The image danced	The image developed facial features	The image bounced and developed legs

EXERCISE TWENTY-FIVE: The Negative Afterimage

Session No.	1	2	3	4	5
Date					
Moving the image					
Changing its color					
Changing its shape					
Making it disappear					
Making it reappear					
Creative imagination					

halo around the paper. This will simply mean that you have saturated the visual pigments in your retina.

Next, close your eyes and count slowly to ten. A dark, negative afterimage will appear identical in size to the image of the piece of paper. The contrasting background will now be light-colored. A few seconds later, the image will begin to fade. As it does, start to play with it. Move it around your visual field to the left side, the top, the right side, the bottom.

Change its color to deep purple, to blue, to green, to yellow, to orange, to red. Change its shape to a square, a circle, an oval, a triangle, then back to a circle.

Make it disappear, then reappear.

Next, allow your imagination to flow creatively, and to do whatever it wants with the circle. Is it becoming a bouncing ball? Does it have the features of a face? Is it growing legs and assuming the shape of a spider? Be creative, and have fun with the image.

When you are ready to end the exercise, simply open your eyes. Repeat this exercise on at least five separate occasions, and record the results. The following chart will help you to keep track of your progress.

How did you fare? Some people are able to perform this exercise very easily. Others aren't so fortunate. No matter how hard they try, they can't seem to visualize the image, nor anything else, for that matter. Once their eyes close, all they see is black. And they feel like utter failures.

If this sounds familiar, don't be alarmed. Some people need more practice to rediscover their imaginative abilities than others. Keep experimenting with your imagination. Repeat Exercise Twenty-five as often as you want to or need to. As you proceed, keep in mind that it is not necessary to literally *see* things; rather, try to *sense* and *experience* them in your imagination. The goal is to see with your *mind's* eye, not with your body's eyes.

Much of your memory is coded and stored, using images and symbols. Thus, learning the language of imagery can unlock the door to a veritable storehouse of information about your past. In addition, it can provide vital information concerning the beliefs, expectations, and intuitions of your unconscious mind. The next two exercises will illustrate these points.

Exercise Twenty-six: Reexploring a House

For this exercise, sit upright in a comfortable chair, feet flat on the floor. Close your eyes and spend a few moments getting in touch with your breathing. . . . Now take a signal breath, and enjoy the wonderful feelings of relaxation you experience. . . .

In a state of gentle relaxation, think about a house you once lived in—preferably, one associated with many positive memories. Can you recall what the outside of it looked like? Can you remember the front and backyards? . . .

In your imagination, enter through the front door and look around. Reexplore the house at your leisure in your mind's eye. . . Can you remember the kitchen? Your bedroom? Look around carefully and see what other things you can recall. . . . Pay attention to details. . . .

To end the exercise, simply take a signal breath and open your eyes. Then try to draw a floor plan of the house you explored, adding as many details as you can.

This exercise demonstrates how easily imagery can be used to explore your past. Anytime you wish to examine earlier life events, simply take yourself back to them in your mind's eye, and have a good look.

Exercise Twenty-seven: Beyond the Door

Sit upright in a comfortable chair, feet flat on the floor. Get in touch with your breathing, close your eyes, and relax . . .

When you are comfortably settled, take a signal breath and allow your conscious mind to quiet itself . . . Now imagine that you are standing before a serene, stately, three-story mansion. It is a beautiful structure, and you are awed by its grandeur.

Walk slowly through the gardens to the front door and enter the antechamber. The furnishings of the house are magnificent. Directly in front of you is a sign instructing you to climb the stairway to your right, and to open the door at the top of the stairs.

Imagine yourself climbing the stairs . . . one step at a time . . . As you near the top, you can see the door for the first time . . . At the top step, pause for a moment, then reach for the door handle . . . Slowly turn it and gently open the door . . .

What do you see? Examine every detail very closely.

To end the exercise, simply take the signal breath and open your eyes. Repeat the exercise on at least five separate occasions, and record your observations. Describe what you saw as vividly as possible. Then interpret its symbolic meaning as best you can. Often it will provide amazingly accurate information about your beliefs, future expectations, and intuitions. Try it and see.

Now, do you have a better sense of what imagery is all about? Remember, imagery is *not* exclusively visual; in fact, the richest imagery may involve other senses as well. For example, can you reexperience the invigorating taste of a cold glass of freshly squeezed orange juice on a

SAMPLE

**EXERCISE TWENTY-SIX: Reexploring
a House**

DATE: _May 19_

TIME: _6 p.m._

The floor plan of my house

Back yard

Bathroom	Bedroom #3
Bedroom #2	Bedroom #1
Kitchen	Den

Hallway

Garage

Driveway

Dining room

Living room

Entrance hall

front yard

Other aspects of this experience

The house was so vivid in my
mind that I felt like I was
actually visiting it in reality.

EXERCISE TWENTY-SIX: Reexploring a House

DATE: _____

TIME: _____

The floor plan of my house

Other aspects of this experience

SAMPLE

EXERCISE TWENTY-SEVEN:
Beyond the Door

Session	Date Time	Behind the Door Was	This Can Be Interpreted as
1	May 21 2 p.m.	A line of doctors with stethoscopes around their necks.	I am obsessed with doctors and illness. Why can't I think of anything else?
2	May 23 8:30 p.m.	Nothing at all except empty space.	I don't know.
3	May 24 8:30 p.m.	My entire family. They were all happy to see me.	I must make more efforts to see my family.
4	May 26 12 noon	The doctors (again).	same explanation as session #1.
5	May 27 8:30 p.m.	A beautiful room with elegant furniture and beautiful music playing.	This is a peaceful, pleasant place that makes me feel content.

EXERCISE TWENTY-SEVEN:
Beyond the Door

Session	Date Time	Behind the Door Was	This Can Be Interpreted as
1			
2			
3			
4			
5			

warm summer's morning? Can you remember the smell of freshly baked bread as you walked past a bakery? Can you recall a favorite melody, and hear it from beginning to end?

When using the language of imagery, try to recruit and involve as many of your senses as possible. Experience what you are imagining as fully as you can—the way you would if it were real. The next exercise will illustrate this point.

Exercise Twenty-eight: A Walk in the Country

Again, sit upright in a comfortable chair, feet flat on the floor. Close your eyes, get in touch with your breathing, and relax . . .

When you are comfortably settled, take a signal breath and allow your conscious mind to quiet itself . . .

Now imagine that you are walking down a quiet country road. The golden sun's warmth beats down upon your body. Can you feel it?

The foliage is green and alive, and the sky is a brilliant blue, with white, puffy clouds floating by. Can you see them?

The air is fresh and clean, filled with the sweetness of honeysuckle and wild flowers. Can you smell them?

Next to the road is a mountain stream, gently winding its way through the countryside. Stop for a moment and take a long refreshing drink of the cool, sparkling mountain water. Can you taste it?

The birds are perched lazily around you, oblivious to any intrusion, as they freely warble and chirp. Can you hear them?

Spend a few minutes continuing your journey down the country road on your own. Explore whatever you wish. Experience all of your senses as fully as you can. Enjoy it.

To end the exercise, simply take a signal breath and open your eyes. Record as completely as you can what you experienced through each of your senses.

Mind-Controlled Analgesia

Now that you've progressed through the practice exercises, let's proceed with some techniques designed specifically for pain alleviation. The first one—Mind-Controlled Analgesia (MCA)—is an extension of the Conditioned Relaxation exercise, incorporating various aspects of guided imagery.

How effective can MCA be? I recall introducing it to Marie, a forty-two-year-old homemaker who suffered from severe facial pain. Marie had already been practicing Conditioned Relaxation for about three weeks and had obtained some positive results. "Sometimes, during the relaxation exercise, the pain really does decrease a lot," she told me. "But at other times, it doesn't seem to help much at all."

However, when Marie began working with MCA, more dramatic relief occurred very quickly. After practicing MCA three times a day for only a week, Marie reported:

"I can actually turn off my pain whenever I want to. And amazingly, the discomfort stays away for a long time. Oh, I've had a few relapses and some flare-ups, but this has worked better for me than anything I've tried before. It's absolutely wonderful."

The credit for Marie's success belongs solely to her. Like the other pain-alleviation techniques described in this chapter, MCA involves purely psychological processes. It is something you can do for yourself, without having to rely on a doctor or anyone else. All it requires is dedicated, diligent practice. Work with it three times a day for one week, and see what happens. All you stand to lose is your discomfort.

Exercise Twenty-nine: Mind-Controlled Analgesia

Mind-Controlled Analgesia (MCA) is a guided imagery technique that uses the language of the unconscious mind to transform your pain experience from the way it is now to the way you want it to be.

Before beginning MCA, it is important that you prepare three pictures to utilize in this exercise. As a starting point, refer back to Exercise Five in Chapter 2, where you drew pictures of your discomfort at its worst and at its best. Examine these pictures closely. Are they still accurate? If not, how would you change them? If the suggestions offered in this book have been helpful to you, you may experience your discomfort quite differently now. The new pictures you are about to draw should reflect that difference.

In the space provided on the following pages, draw two new pictures of your discomfort as you now experience it—one of your pain at its worst (Pain/Pleasure Level = −10), and the other of your pain at its best (Pain/Pleasure Level = −1). As you did in Exercise Five, let your imagination run free, and incorporate the entire pain experience into your drawings, using the input of all your senses.

Next, take a few moments to imagine how you'd feel if you were experiencing the most intense pleasure possible. Close your eyes, take a signal breath, and vicariously experience what your area of discomfort would feel like if your Pain/Pleasure Level was +10. When you have a clear image of this experience in mind, draw a picture of it in the space provided. Once again, make it as vivid and detailed as possible.

After you have finished drawing all three of these pictures, study them

SAMPLE

EXERCISE TWENTY-EIGHT: A Walk in the Country

DATE: _May 30_

TIME: _8 p.m._

During my imaginary walk in the country
I felt the sun beating down on my skin and a light breeze blowing against my skin. I also felt the dirt touching the bottom of my feet.
I saw beautiful yellow and white flowers. The sky is blue, with some dark clouds in the distance. Birds are flying in a group overhead.
I smelled the flowers and the fresh air.
I tasted the freshness and coldness of the spring water.
I heard the birds chirping, leaves crunching under my feet, the bubbly brook.
Other experiences

EXERCISE TWENTY-EIGHT: A Walk in the Country

DATE: _____

TIME: _____

During my imaginary walk in the country
I felt
I saw
I smelled
I tasted
I heard
Other experiences

very carefully, or even better, memorize them. They will play a very important part in MCA, for your goal will be to transform your pain experience from that of the first picture (-10 rating) to the second (-1), and then to the third ($+10$). You are going to attempt to unlock your creative energies literally to turn off your discomfort in your mind's eye, and simultaneously in your body. If you have been practicing the relaxation exercise regularly, you may even obtain complete relief the very first time you try it.

As with the Conditioned Relaxation exercise, I strongly recommend that you record the MCA text on a cassette tape or purchase a prerecorded version (see Appendix), so that you can simply listen to it as you perform the technique.

Now let's get started.

Mind-Controlled Analgesia

This tape contains a Mind-Controlled Analgesia technique which you can use to help transform your current pain experience into what you want it to be . . .

Before beginning, take a moment to get comfortable and relax . . . Sit upright in a comfortable chair, close your eyes, and loosen any tight clothing or jewelry or shoes that might distract you. Make sure you won't be interrupted for a few minutes . . . Take the telephone off the hook if necessary . . . Now take a few slow, deep abdominal breaths . . . Inhale . . . Exhale . . . Inhale . . . Exhale . . .

Focus your attention on your breathing throughout this exercise, and recognize how easily slow, deep breathing alone can help to produce a nice state of deep, gentle relaxation . . . Let your body breathe itself, according to it's own natural rhythm . . . Slowly . . . easily . . . and deeply . . .

Now let's begin the exercise with the signal breath, a special message that tells the body that you are ready to enter a state of deep relaxation . . . Exhale . . . Breathe in deeply through your nose . . . And blow out through your mouth . . . You may notice a kind of tingling sensation as you take the signal breath . . . Whatever you feel is your body's way of acknowledging the experience of relaxation, comfort, and peace of mind . . .

Remember your breathing . . . Slowly and deeply . . . As you concentrate your attention on your breathing, give your body a few moments to relax deeply and fully . . . Feel all the tension, tightness, pain, or discomfort draining away, down your spine, down your legs, and into the ground . . . With each breath, you may be surprised to feel yourself becoming more and more deeply and fully relaxed . . . comfortable . . . and at ease . . . Enjoy this nice state of relaxation for a few minutes . . .

Remember your breathing, slowly and deeply from the abdomen . . . Now take a brief inventory of your body, starting at the top of your head, working down to the tips of your toes . . . Is every part of your body totally relaxed and comfortable? If so, wonderful. Enjoy how good it feels . . .

However, if there is still any part of your body that is not yet fully relaxed and comfortable, simply inhale a deep breath, and send it into that region, bringing soothing, relaxing, nourishing, healing oxygen into every cell of that area, comforting it and relaxing it . . . As you exhale, imagine blowing out—right through your skin—any tension, tightness, pain, or discomfort from that area . . . Again, as you inhale, bring relaxing, healing oxygen into every cell of that region, and as you exhale, blow away—right through the skin and out into the air—any tension or discomfort that remains in that area . . .

In this way, you can dispatch your breath to relax any part of your body which is not yet as fully relaxed and comfortable as it can be . . .

Breathe slowly and deeply, and with each breath you may be surprised to find that you have become twice as relaxed as you were before . . . and that you are able to blow away twice as much tension and discomfort as you did with the previous breath . . . Inhale . . . Exhale . . . Twice as relaxed . . . Inhale . . . Exhale . . . Twice as comfortable . . .

Now, paint a picture in your mind's eye of your discomfort at its very worst . . . Recall the symbolic picture you drew as fully and as clearly as you possibly can . . . (Try to remember this image, since it will soon become a thing of the past . . .) Can you vicariously experience the agony that was once associated with it?

Now . . . watch how quickly your discomfort passes as you transform this image to the one of your discomfort at its best . . . See how powerfully the mind's eye affects what you experience . . . As you carefully examine this second picture in your imagination, notice how different you feel . . . Fully sense the experience of your discomfort at its best, and allow this image to become strong, natural, and real . . .

An even more powerful way to stimulate the body's healing abilities is to transform the second picture to the third one . . . Unlock your creative potential, and dissolve any remaining pictures of discomfort into the image of how you most want to be . . . Use your imagination to see yourself exactly as you want to be . . .

You don't have to tell your body *how* to heal itself, for it already knows . . . All you need to do is to tell your body what you *want* it to do, how you want it to be . . . then watch what happens through your mind's eye . . .

If a part of your body has been injured, for example, you may see and experience a rush of new blood to that area, carrying with each heartbeat the oxygen and vital nutrients essential to the healing process . . . In your imagination, you may see your body's immune system spring to life—the white blood cells racing to the injured area to metabolize and carry away any damaged tissue . . . Watch closely as the areas of irritation, inflammation, or infection are replaced by the formation of new, healthy tissue . . . See in your mind's eye what happens as the area of discomfort becomes healed and restored . . .

By focusing your attention on the experience of being as you want to be, you help your body make it a reality . . . You may continue to work with

SAMPLE

EXERCISE TWENTY-NINE: PART ONE:
Mind-Controlled Analgesia

DATE: June 1.

TIME: 10 a.m.

My Current Discomfort at Its Worst (Pain/Pleasure Level = −10)

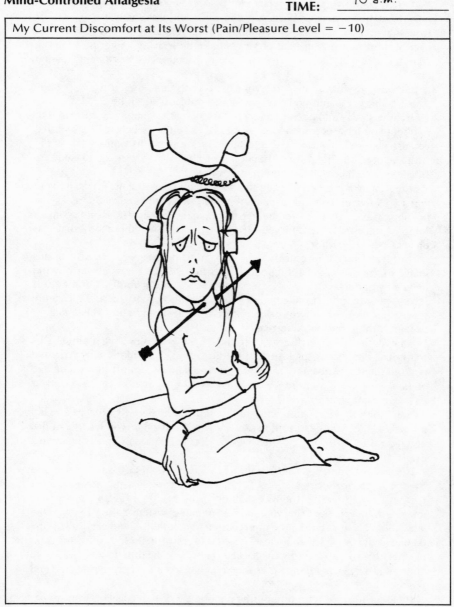

EXERCISE TWENTY-NINE: PART ONE:
Mind-Controlled Analgesia

DATE: _____

TIME: _____

My Current Discomfort at Its Worst (Pain/Pleasure Level = −10)

SAMPLE

EXERCISE TWENTY-NINE: PART ONE—
Continued

DATE: _June 1_

TIME: _10:30 a.m._

My Current Discomfort at Its Best (Pain/Pleasure Level = −1)

EXERCISE TWENTY-NINE: PART ONE—
Continued

DATE: _____

TIME: _____

My Current Discomfort at Its Best (Pain/Pleasure Level = −1)

SAMPLE

EXERCISE TWENTY-NINE: PART ONE—
Continued

DATE: June 1

TIME: 10:45 a.m.

How I'd Most Like My Area of Discomfort to Feel (Pain/Pleasure = +10)

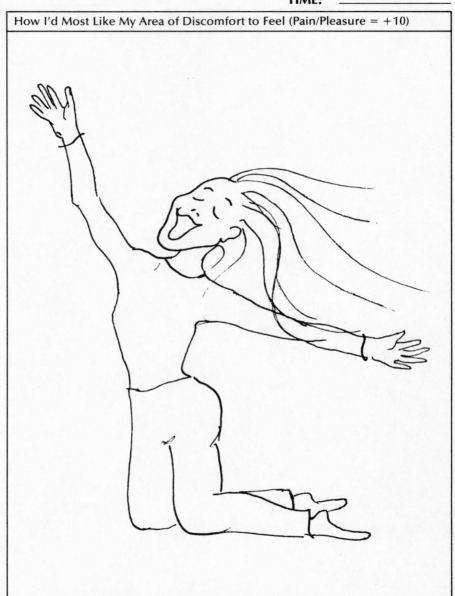

EXERCISE TWENTY-NINE: PART ONE—
Continued

DATE: _____

TIME: _____

How I'd Most Like My Area of Discomfort to Feel (Pain/Pleasure = +10)

this image for as long as you like . . . Breathe slowly and deeply, and sense the healing process in action . . .

When you end this exercise, you may be surprised to notice that you feel not only relaxed and comfortable, but energized with such a powerful sense of well-being that you will easily be able to meet any demands that arise . . .

To complete the exercise, open your eyes and take the signal breath . . . Exhale . . . Inhale deeply through your nose . . . Blow out through your mouth . . . And be well . . .

© 1976 by David E. Bresler, Ph.D.

Practice this Mind-Controlled Analgesia technique over and over again. Each time you do, record how effective the technique has been. How much pain relief are you able to gain? Does your discomfort ease up a little more each time you do the exercise?

A simple way to keep track of your progress is to plot the changes in how you feel on a graph. Each time you begin the exercise, assess your Pain/Pleasure Level, using a scale from −10 to +10, and enter it on the graph. When you complete the exercise, evaluate and chart your Pain/ Pleasure Level once again, using the same −10 to +10 scale. This will allow you to evaluate the effectiveness of MCA over time.

Glove Anesthesia

I am eternally grateful to William Kroger, M.D., for teaching me Glove Anesthesia—a two-step imagery exercise in which you first learn to develop feelings of numbness in your hand, as if it were in an imaginary anesthetic glove. Next, you learn to transfer these feelings of numbness to any part of your body that hurts, simply by placing your "anesthetized" hand on it.

Glove Anesthesia is a symptomatic technique—that is, it reduces the physical symptoms of pain without concern for its cause. It is a useful alternative to analgesic medications, particularly when discomfort is so intense that the patient cannot concentrate enough to use other guided imagery approaches. Glove Anesthesia often helps to "take the edge off" the pain sensation, thus permitting the patient to explore other aspects of the pain experience more fully.

In addition, Glove Anesthesia provides a dramatic illustration of the power of self-control. When patients realize that they can produce feelings of numbness in their hands at will, they also recognize that they may be able to control their discomfort, too. This is profoundly therapeutic for pain sufferers who feel totally helpless and unable to affect their discomfort.

I recall one of my patients, Jerry, who was able to achieve a significant degree of pain relief in his shoulders using Glove Anesthesia. Jerry, an elderly retired widower, had little positive input to distract him from the arthritic pain that so often afflicted him. He was a classic complainer, eager to tell his problems to anyone who would listen for even a moment. None of the doctors that he had seen could offer him any help, and Jerry strongly believed that there was absolutely nothing he could do to alleviate his discomfort.

After practicing Conditioned Relaxation for two weeks, Jerry was taught Glove Anesthesia. First, I instructed him to relax himself for a few moments, and then to close his eyes and imagine that a bucket filled with a deeply penetrating anesthetic solution was being placed in front of him. At my suggestion, Jerry dipped his hand into the imaginary bucket, and soon began to experience a numbing sensation in his hand and fingers. Over the next few minutes, the sensation of numbness progressively increased.

Once Jerry reported that his hand felt totally numb, I directed him into the second stage of this exercise. I asked him to rub his pain-racked left shoulder with his "numb" hand, transferring some of the anesthetic feelings into the painful area. As he rubbed his hand on his shoulder, he sighed several times, as a half-smile came over his face. "It feels much better, much better," he said in amazement.

The imagined numbness that he was able to bring to his painful shoulder reduced his discomfort more significantly than any pain medication he had ever taken. And it unmistakably demonstrated that *he* had the power to control his discomfort. With his increased self-confidence, Jerry soon began to emerge from his shell, and assume a more active life-style. When I saw him a year later, he reported that he could hardly find enough time to pursue his many activities. And with the help of Conditioned Relaxation and Glove Anesthesia, he was able to keep his arthritic shoulder pain well under control.

Exercise Thirty: Glove Anesthesia

Glove Anesthesia is a guided imagery technique using the language of the subconscious mind to help suppress the symptoms of pain. As with the previous exercises, I strongly recommend that you record or purchase a cassette tape, so that you can simply listen to it as you perform the technique.

Glove Anesthesia

This tape contains a Glove Anesthesia technique which you can use to help suppress any pain symptoms that you may experience . . .

SAMPLE

EXERCISE TWENTY-NINE: PART TWO:
Mind-Controlled Analgesia

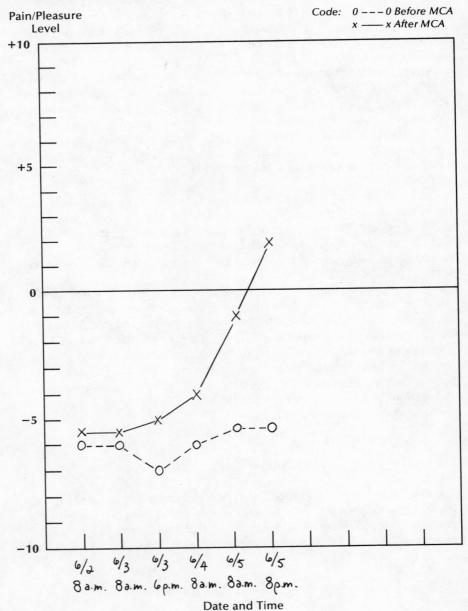

Pain/Pleasure
Level

Code: 0 – – – 0 *Before MCA*
        x —— x *After MCA*

Date and Time

EXERCISE TWENTY-NINE: PART TWO:
Mind-Controlled Analgesia

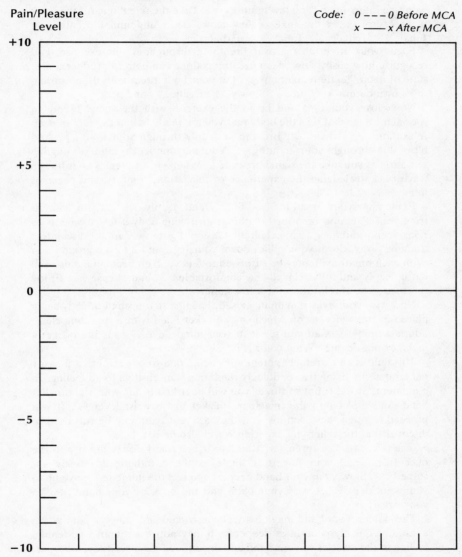

Pain/Pleasure
Level

Code: 0 – – – 0 *Before MCA*
        x —— x *After MCA*

+10

+5

0

−5

−10

Date and Time

Before beginning, take a moment to get comfortable and relax . . . Sit upright in a comfortable chair, feet flat on the floor, and loosen any tight clothing or jewelry or shoes that might distract you . . . Make sure you won't be interrupted for a few minutes . . . Take the telephone off the hook if necessary . . . Now take a few slow, deep abdominal breaths . . . Inhale . . . Exhale . . . Inhale . . . Exhale . . .

Focus your attention on your breathing throughout this exercise, and recognize how easily slow, deep breathing alone can help to produce a nice state of deep, gentle relaxation . . . Let your body breathe itself, according to its own natural rhythm . . . Slowly . . . easily . . . and deeply . . .

Now close your eyes and begin the exercise with the signal breath, a special message that tells the body that you are ready to enter a state of deep relaxation . . . Exhale . . . Breathe in deeply through your nose . . . And blow out through your mouth . . . You may notice a kind of tingling sensation as you take the signal breath . . . Whatever you feel is your body's way of acknowledging the experience of relaxation, comfort, and peace of mind . . .

Remember your breathing . . . Slowly and deeply . . . As you concentrate your attention on your breathing, give your body a few moments to relax deeply and fully . . . Feel all the tension, tightness, pain, or discomfort draining away, down your spine, down your legs, and into the ground . . . With each breath, you may be surprised to feel yourself becoming more and more deeply and fully relaxed . . . comfortable . . . and at ease . . . Enjoy this nice state of relaxation for a few minutes . . .

Now with your eyes remaining closed, imagine that a small table is being placed in front of you, on which sits a bucket filled with a sparkling clear, odorless fluid . . . Can you see it in your mind's eye? . . . Is the bucket a metal or plastic one? What color is it? . . .

This fluid is an extremely potent anesthetic, one so powerful that it easily penetrates any living tissue, quickly rendering it insensitive to all feeling. In a moment, at the count of three, you will be asked to lift your right or left hand, and dip it into the imaginary bucket up to wrist level . . . If you proceed through these actions as if they are real, you may be surprised to discover that the relief you experience will also be real . . .

One . . . two . . . three . . . Raise your hand and slowly dip it into the bucket . . . Feel your fingertips tingle as the anesthetic is quickly absorbed . . . Slowly dip your hand deeper, and feel the numbness move up to your knuckles . . . Across your palm and the back of your hand . . . To your wrist . . .

The skin on your hand may now feel constricted and "tingly," and as the anesthetic quickly penetrates deeper, you may notice a numb, woodenlike feeling in the muscles of your hand and fingers . . . As it seeps even deeper, the bones themselves may lose all feeling . . .

Gently swirl your hand around in the bucket to ensure the deepest possible penetration of the anesthetic solution . . . Sense any remaining feelings in your hand moving out the tips of your fingers, floating down softly to the bottom of the bucket . . . Continue to swirl your hand around for as long as it takes to achieve total anesthesia—a deep feeling of tingly numbness.

In a moment, at the count of three, I will ask you to remove your hand from the bucket and gently to place it directly on the part of your body that hurts . . . This will permit you to transfer the feeling of numbness from your hand into the area of your discomfort, and in exchange, any tension, tightness, pain, or discomfort will flow from this area back into your hand . . . You can then dip your hand into the bucket once again to repeat the exercise . . .

One . . . two . . . three . . .

Now remove your hand from the bucket and place it directly on the part of your body that hurts . . . Imagine all the deep feelings of numbness from your hand streaming into your body, and simultaneously, picture your hand beginning to absorb your body's discomfort . . .

Gradually, the same numbness that quickly developed in your hand is now permeating the affected part of your body . . . Can you sense the skin constricting? . . . And the muscles losing all feeling as the numbness penetrates even deeper? . . . Can you experience your hand becoming filled with the sensations you once experienced only in that affected area? . . . Slowly rub your hand around the once-painful area until you feel you have transferred as much anesthesia (and absorbed as much of the discomfort) as you can. Allow yourself to be surprised to notice what an immediate difference this has made . . .

Then, dip your hand once again into the bucket to repeat the exercise . . . Swirl your hand around in the anesthetic solution, and allow the transferred feelings of discomfort to move out through your fingertips, and float gently down to the bottom of the bucket . . .

At the same time, feel your hand once again react to the anesthetic, deeply absorbing it through the skin, into the muscles and bones . . . Fill your hand once more with the feeling of total numbness . . . It will probably take much less time to achieve this state than it did the last time, but continue to swirl your hand around for as long as it takes, whether that be a few seconds, or even a minute or more . . . Soak up as much numbness as your hand possibly can . . .

When you're ready, put your hand back on your area of discomfort . . . Once again, transfer the numb, relaxed feeling deeply into the area, and if there is any remaining discomfort, take away as much of it as you can . . . Gently rub your hand over the area until you are ready to dip it another time . . .

Repeat the transfer process as many times as you wish . . . For each time you repeat it, you will be able to experience an even greater amount of comfort and relief in the affected area . . . And each time you repeat it, it will become easier and easier . . .

When you are ready to end this exercise, simply shake your hand briskly to return quickly all the feelings to it that existed before the exercise began.

After completing this session of Glove Anesthesia, you may be surprised

SAMPLE

EXERCISE THIRTY: Glove Anesthesia

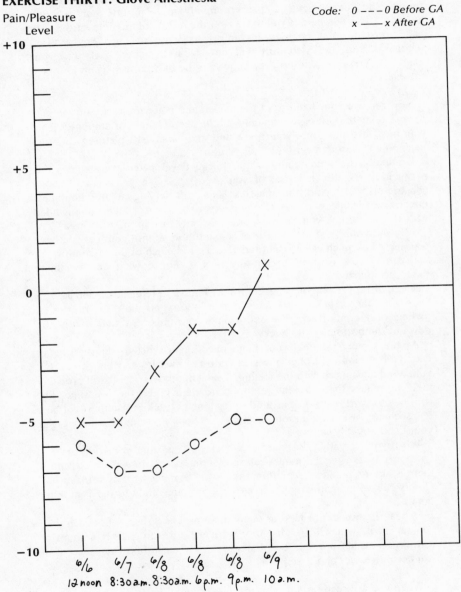

Pain/Pleasure
Level

Code: 0 – – – 0 Before GA
       x ——— x After GA

Date and Time

EXERCISE THIRTY: Glove Anesthesia

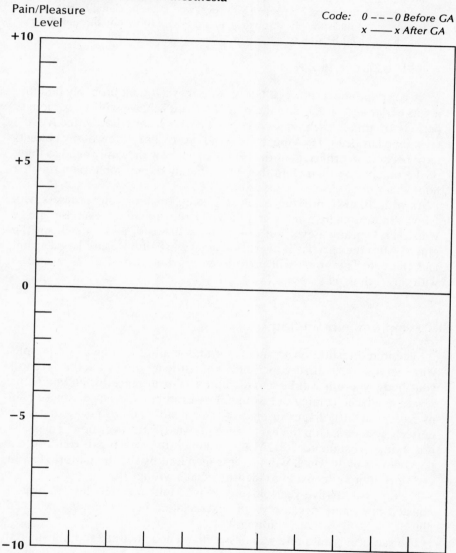

Pain/Pleasure
Level

Code: 0 – – – 0 *Before GA*
        x ——— x *After GA*

+10

+5

0

−5

−10

Date and Time

to notice that you will feel not only relaxed and comfortable, but energized with such a powerful sense of well-being that you will easily be able to meet any demands that arise . . .

To complete the exercise, open your eyes and take the signal breath . . . Exhale . . . Inhale deeply through your nose . . . Blow out through your mouth . . . And be well . . .

© 1976 by David E. Bresler, Ph.D.

As you continue to practice Glove Anesthesia, you'll probably find that it gets easier and easier, and the relief that you achieve will last for longer periods of time. Each time you practice it, record how effective the technique has been. How much relief did it provide? A few of my patients have become so proficient at the exercise that now they only need to think of the potent anesthetic and they immediately obtain some pain relief. I hope this will be true for you, too.

As with Mind-Controlled Analgesia, keep track of your progress with Glove Anesthesia by using a graph. Before beginning the exercise, gauge your Pain/Pleasure Level, on a −10 to +10 scale, and enter it on the graph. After the exercise is over, evaluate your Pain/Pleasure Level again, and chart it. The graph will provide an ongoing record of your success with this technique.

Symptom Substitution

Symptom Substitution is another symptomatic technique that permits your nervous system to experience your discomfort in another area of your body where it will be less disruptive. For instance, when you feel a severe headache coming on, wouldn't you rather experience intense pain in, say, your little finger instead of your head? You're not asking your nervous system to stop the experience of pain (or to cover up the message it is trying to communicate). You're asking it to move the discomfort to a part of your body which will feel less menaced by the discomfort, so you can work more effectively to identify what's wrong.

Fred, a twenty-five-year-old electrician, told me that his life was a nonstop nightmare because of the excruciating headaches that attacked him periodically without warning.

The physical pain alone was destructive enough. But Fred also feared that he was seriously ill, perhaps with a brain tumor. Although a comprehensive series of medical tests established that no tumor existed, Fred was not convinced, for he was certain that his headaches would somehow eventually kill him.

With the help of Conditioned Relaxation and Symptom Substitution, Fred learned how to transfer his headache pain to his little finger. This displaced pain was equal in intensity to what it had been in his head. But he found that when the pain was located in his finger, it was much more bearable, since it did not seem nearly as threatening there.

Fred was able to accept the pain in his little finger quite well, leading a much more normal life than he ever had when the discomfort was localized in his head. Eventually, he realized that his fear of a tumor (or other illness) was a major stressor that, in fact, frequently triggered his headaches. As is often the case with headache patients, Fred's discomfort was primarily stress-related, but this was not apparent to him until he began to experience it in his little finger.

The strategies for pain reduction through Symptom Substitution can vary considerably. For instance, some of my patients suffer from stress-related bruxism (grinding of the teeth), which can result in terrible jaw pain. After grinding their teeth throughout the night, they awaken with excruciating discomfort in their jaws, often accompanied by headaches, ringing in the ears, and tension in the neck and back.

I recently treated Herbert, a victim of this syndrome, using a form of Symptom Substitution that centered around a tennis ball. I instructed Herbert to hold the ball in his hand and to practice moving any excess tension from his jaw into his hand. When this tension reached his hand, he would then squeeze the tennis ball rather than clenching his teeth. Yes, the tension was still there, but it felt more manageable and tolerable in his hand, while he was learning to deal more effectively with the stress itself.

Sometimes, instead of moving the discomfort to another part of the body, patients use Symptom Substitution to change the character of their pain. With a little creativity, and a lot of practice, I have seen patients transform "an agonizing burning sensation" into a "feeling of strongly localized pressure," or they have changed "jolting electric shocks" into a "tingling itch." Why not see what *you* can do?

Exercise Thirty-one: Symptom Substitution

At this point, you are probably ready to work with guided imagery on your own. Use your creative abilities to invent an original exercise that is designed exclusively for you.

You might wish to follow the format I have recommended for previous exercises: Begin with the first part of the Conditioned Relaxation technique, then write your own script. What other part of your body do you want to send your discomfort to? What type of sensation might be an acceptable alternative to pain?

Tie your script to your breathing, so that with each breath, the image is programmed to become stronger. End your exercise using the last part of Conditioned Relaxation, or in any other way you choose.

SAMPLE

EXERCISE THIRTY-ONE:
Symptom Substitution

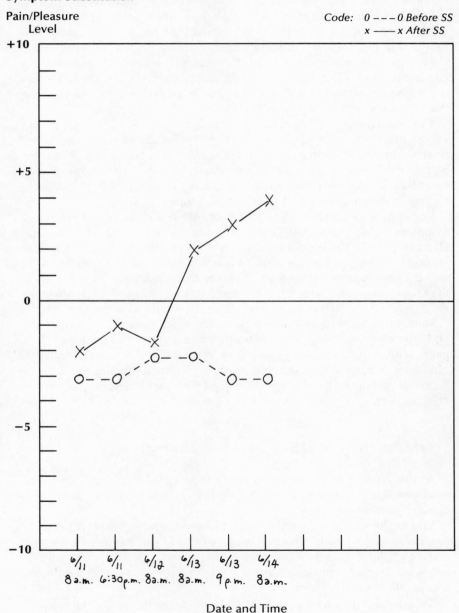

Pain/Pleasure
    Level

Code: 0 – – – 0 *Before SS*
       x ——— x *After SS*

Date and Time

EXERCISE THIRTY-ONE:
Symptom Substitution

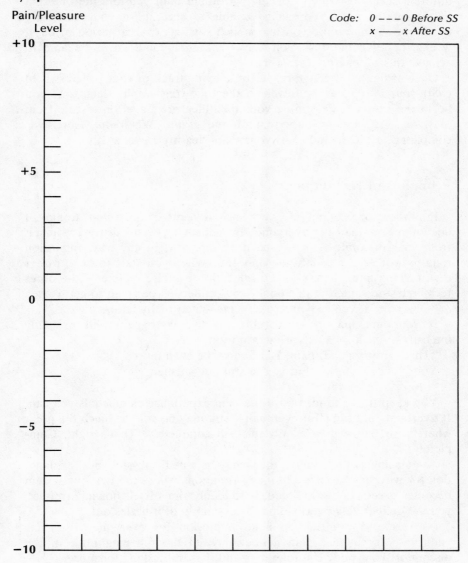

Pain/Pleasure
Level

Code: 0 – – – 0 Before SS
        x —— x After SS

+10

+5

0

−5

−10

Date and Time

As I have previously suggested, record your text onto a cassette tape, so that you can participate in it more fully as you listen. Try writing several different scenarios. Keep working with them until you find the one that helps you the most. You may be able to accomplish your goal very quickly, or it may take you many such sessions over a period of days, weeks, or even months. You may think that you'll never be able to achieve this state. But at least try.

Once again, an effective means of keeping track of your progress is to chart your Pain/Pleasure Level on the following graph. Each time you begin the exercise, determine your Pain/Pleasure Level on a scale from -10 to $+10$, and indicate that on the graph. When the exercise is completed, evaluate and chart your Pain/Pleasure Level again.

Implosion Techniques

Implosion, or flooding, is a very ancient Zen technique that, frankly, I do not recommend for everyone. Instead of trying to distract yourself from your discomfort, or escape it or reduce it in any way, implosion requires you to do exactly the opposite. When you start to hurt, rather than turning immediately to the relaxation exercise or one of the other techniques presented in this book, you challenge your pain to get worse:

"OK, pain, if you're going to hurt me—then really let me have it."

If your imagination is working vividly, your pain will probably intensify—which is exactly what you want:

"That's pretty good, pain. But I can take even more."

Your pain intensifies, but you're still not satisfied:

"More. More. More."

You keep trying to maximize the pain experience as much as you can. It's certainly not fun. But eventually, you may be able to reach the point where your pain will suddenly turn off completely. That's right. Completely.

As amazing as this sounds, there may be a neurophysiological explanation for why this happens. In many situations where the nervous system becomes excessively stimulated, it suddenly shuts itself down. In effect, you are deliberately overloading the system until it fizzles out.

As I said, I don't recommend implosion for everyone. It means enduring very intense pain deliberately, to the full magnitude of the discomfort your body can tolerate—and then still asking for more.

Some people are willing to participate in the implosion technique because they feel it reduces the duration of their painful experience. Instead of feeling a moderate amount of pain over a long period of time, they endure an intense amount of pain for only a few minutes. Then the pain is gone.

One of my patients, a twenty-nine-year-old secretary named Debbie, recently used this technique while horseback riding. She began to feel a migraine headache coming on, and she was so distressed about having her afternoon of recreation ruined, she "ordered" the pain to run its course as quickly as possible. "It hurt so much I almost cried," she later told me. "But in a few minutes it was over."

Should you try it? It's your decision. To me, it's like taking a freezing cold shower. It's a most unpleasant experience, but when it's over, you often feel amazingly better.

Exercise Thirty-two: Implosion

If implosion is something that you'd like to try, I encourage you to use your own creativity to design an implosion exercise specifically for you. Rely on your imagination in creating a text which you can transfer to a cassette tape before you begin working with it.

In fashioning your exercise, keep in mind that it should *not* begin with the first stages of Conditioned Relaxation, as was the case with Glove Anesthesia and Symptom Substitution. After all, with implosion, your intention is not to relax the body, but to create excruciating pain, with the ultimate goal of shutting down the nervous system's pain centers.

As with earlier exercises in this chapter, plot your progress using implosion on a graph like the one below, charting your Pleasure/Pain Level both before and after the exercise.

Imagery and Self-Healing

Since childhood, you've probably ignored and disowned the intuitive side of your brain. In the upcoming weeks, try listening to your intuitions, and communicating with an aspect of yourself that has been largely neglected.

When I examine cases of "spontaneous remission," and the successes of the unorthodox therapies discussed in Chapter 5, many of them seem to depend upon the patient's ability to recruit positive expectations. Each individual believed it was *possible* for him or her to get better.

That's an important attitude for you to assume. So fire up your left and right hemispheres. Give yourself an honest chance to use all your inner resources. Perhaps these techniques will help you; perhaps they won't. But open yourself up to the possibility and find out how well your body can respond to the power of suggestion through imagery.

Be as creative as you can, not only in visualizing your pain, but also in developing your own imagery exercises. One woman visualized her

SAMPLE

EXERCISE THIRTY-TWO: Implosion

Pain/Pleasure
    Level

Code: 0 – – – 0 *Before Implosion*
          x ——— x *After Implosion*

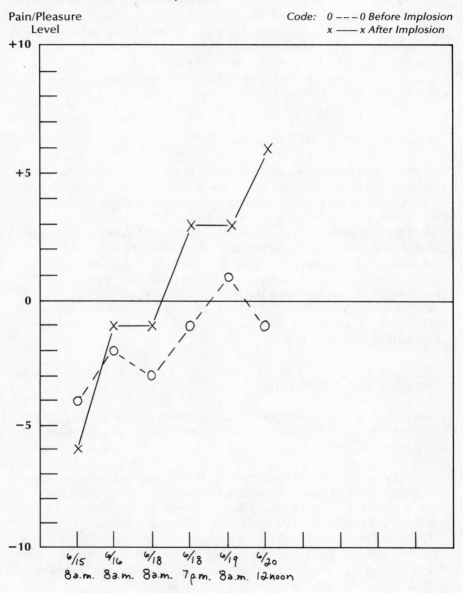

Date and Time

EXERCISE THIRTY-TWO: Implosion

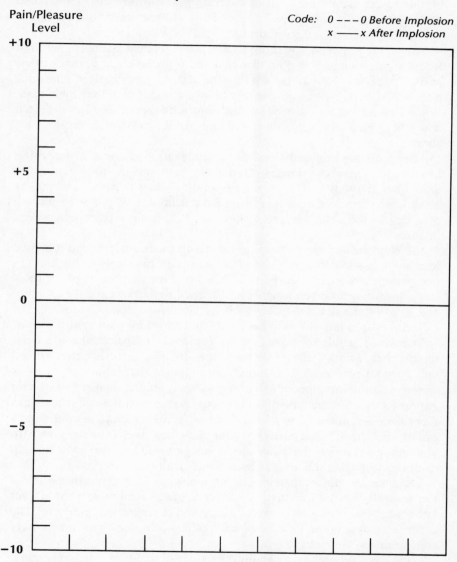

Pain/Pleasure
    Level

Code: 0 – – – 0 *Before Implosion*
          x ——— x *After Implosion*

Date and Time

discomfort as a cement truck parked on her shoulders, dropping a thousand pounds of cold, wet cement on her neck. Another envisioned a blazing forest fire burning out of control on her lower back. How could you work with either of these images? How will you work with the image you have of your own discomfort?

One of my patients, a man in his late fifties named Leonard, suffered from excruciating angina pain that radiated from his chest to many other parts of his body. He had been hospitalized thirty-one different times, for a total of 193 days, but no conventional treatment could ease his pain. When I asked him how he saw his discomfort, he replied that he visualized it as a huge elephant sitting on top of him, with its full weight crushing his chest.

After teaching Leonard Conditioned Relaxation, I advised him to use his imagination in working with the elephant image, to see how his autonomic nervous system might respond to some positive thinking. A week later, he told me he had imagined putting the elephant on a crash diet, and as the animal began to lose weight, his chest pain became less intense.

The elephant ultimately became Leonard's inner adviser, and it helped him in many ways to deal more effectively with the stress in his life. On one particularly happy occasion, Leonard told me that the elephant (now tiny after losing so much weight) had learned to flap its ears like Dumbo, and had, for the first time, flown off his chest for a few minutes. As the elephant soared into the sky, Leonard felt most of his pain vanish with it.

In essence, guided imagery is the formation of personalized mental images that facilitate the healing process. Its use, then, is not restricted only to pain problems. Because it can mobilize the autonomic nervous system and the immune/inflammatory system, guided imagery can be an important tool for any type of self-healing. So the next time your body has a problem—from the flu to a broken arm—create a picture in your mind's eye of what the afflicted part(s) of your body look like. Then working with your mind—through the language of imagery—help your body to help itself by visualizing the area as healed and healthy.

Some people, unfortunately, give up too soon. They typically say, "I'm too severely injured for this type of technique." However, we don't yet know what the limitations of self-healing and regeneration really are. The absence of data doesn't disprove a hypothesis. So don't put unnecessary constraints on yourself.

What I've said previously about the nature of reality is worth repeating. Reality is vague and ambiguous. If you see your pain as a ton of bricks hanging around your neck, that is how you will experience it. But if you can realistically see yourself in your mind's eye as being totally healed, restored, and fully functional, perhaps that is what you will soon experience.

11 *Your Inner Adviser*

Julie's life changed dramatically on a Thursday afternoon not long ago.

Until then, she had been miserable and confused, and tormented by a grinding, throbbing pain in her lower back that had persisted for nearly six years. At its worst, the discomfort radiated into other parts of her body as well—like razor-sharp bullets fired into her shoulders, chest, and buttocks. To aggravate things even further, her marriage had collapsed, and she felt ravaged by the strain of raising her teenage sons by herself.

But one afternoon, during a period of relaxation, Julie learned how to contact her inner adviser—an imaginary living creature—in her unconscious mind. This technique—perhaps the most fascinating form of guided imagery—allows patients to communicate actively with the nondominant part of their brain, and in turn reach a more complete understanding of their pain experience.

During Julie's first experience with this technique, she imagined she was in a beautiful wooded forest, and soon made contact with an imaginary hummingbird.

Doctor: What is the hummingbird's name?
Julie: Sam.
Doctor: Tell Sam you mean him no harm, that you would just like to meet with him occasionally to talk things over with him. Would that be OK?
Julie: He says he'd be willing to do that.
Doctor: Good. Tell him you have brought some honey and water for him

	today. And ask him if there is any advice he'd like to give you in return.
Julie:	He says yes.
Doctor:	What does he want to tell you?
Julie:	He says he wants me to start liking myself more, and filling my life with more fun.

Later in the exercise, I told Julie to try the following experiment:

Doctor:	Ask Sam, as a demonstration of his friendship and good faith, if he is willing to take away your pain *right now,* even for just a moment. . . . Will he do that?
Julie:	Yes, he says he will.

Within seconds, Julie's pain was gone. Completely gone. And it stayed away for several hours. Those sore and aching muscles that had plagued her for so long were finally free of discomfort.

Yes, Julie's pain did return later that day. But by then her disposition had improved remarkably. For the first time in years, she realized that it was possible for her to be pain-free.

In the ensuing weeks, she continued to communicate with her adviser, who helped her to start thinking more positively about her own future. When we most recently talked, she was progressing very well toward completely controlling her pain.

The advisers that people like Julie create are able to search the inner recesses of the unconscious mind. As I explained in Chapter 10, the right hemisphere is a vast storehouse of information that can be tremendously useful to us.

The adviser can also help change unconscious belief systems. I've talked earlier about how people become imprisoned by their own inappropriate belief systems. Well, this not only happens on the conscious level, but unconsciously as well. So if quite unknowingly you envision yourself as a hopeless, helpless victim of your pain, it's essential for you to become aware of that and adopt a new belief system that will facilitate healing. Your adviser can keep you intimately connected with your unconscious mind and can tell you how well you are incorporating new beliefs, new expectations, and new habits.

In the process, communication with your adviser also fosters a "centering process," in which your ability to observe your intuitive side becomes very sophisticated. Long after your most immediate problem—your pain, for example—has been resolved, your sensitivity to your unconscious mind will continue. Once you've learned to make conscious contact with your right hemisphere, it's a skill that you should never allow to deteriorate.

The Friend Inside

When I was first introduced to the adviser technique by Dr. Irving Oyle, I was as quick to challenge it as anyone. How could it do all the things he claimed? Also, it was so unorthodox that I doubted if the typical patient would accept it. After all, what would be your initial reaction to a doctor who encouraged you to start talking to little animals in your head?

However, I have been surprised, not only by the immense value of guided imagery, but at how receptive most pain sufferers are to the technique. In retrospect, maybe this open-mindedness on the part of patients is not as amazing as I had originally thought. Guided imagery is basically just a way of talking to ourselves, which is hardly a new concept.

Haven't you sometimes found yourself reacting to a particular event by saying, "Damn, I knew that was going to happen!" Well, *how* did you know? Who told you? Of course, it was the intuitive part of your nervous system—in essence, an inner adviser—that told you. And you should have listened to it.

Interestingly, children are not as negligent of their unconscious mind as adults. They naturally communicate with that part of themselves and are constantly creating their own imaginary playmates. But unfortunately, parents often discourage such behavior ("It's not real, don't daydream, stop talking to imaginary things"). As a result, they unknowingly disconnect their offspring from this vital part of themselves. I think this situation is tragic. For when a child communicates with his intuitive side, it's a very normal, healthy activity. How sad it is when children are outrightly told not to be impulsive, spontaneous, or creative.

Through guided imagery, however, people can once again make contact with inner "playmates" who are able to provide important insights about their lives. My patients have created advisers like Rocky the Dog, Mary the Tiger, Pitu the Bird, Bambi the Deer, and Charlie the White Rat. These imaginary creatures have helped them to accomplish what many doctors thought was impossible—a life free of agonizing pain.

Exercise Thirty-three: Finding a Personal Place

As a prerequisite for finding your own adviser, it is important to remove yourself from the intrusions of day-to-day life. Perhaps the best way to accomplish this is to find a favorite place in your mind's eye—one that you can visit at any time—where you can truly be yourself.

As with the previous exercises, I suggest that you record or purchase a cassette tape, and play it back as you proceed through the technique.

Now, let's begin.

Finding a Personal Place

This tape contains a guided imagery exercise which will help you to find a favorite place in your mind's eye that you can visit anytime you wish.

Before beginning, take a moment to get comfortable and relax . . . Sit upright in a comfortable chair, feet flat on the floor, and loosen any tight clothing, jewelry, or shoes that might distract you . . . Make sure you won't be interrupted for a few minutes . . . Take the telephone off the hook if necessary . . . Now take a few slow, deep abdominal breaths . . . Inhale . . . Exhale . . . Inhale . . . Exhale . . .

Focus your attention on your breathing throughout this exercise and recognize how easily slow, deep breathing alone can help to produce a nice state of deep, gentle relaxation . . . Let your body breathe itself, according to its own natural rhythm . . . Slowly . . . easily . . . and deeply . . .

Now close your eyes and begin the exercise with the signal breath, a special message that tells the body you are ready to enter a state of deep relaxation . . . Exhale . . . Breathe in deeply through your nose . . . and blow out through your mouth . . . You may notice a kind of tingling sensation as you take the signal breath . . . Whatever you feel is your body's way of acknowledging the experience of relaxation, comfort, and peace of mind . . .

Remember your breathing . . . Slowly and deeply . . . As you concentrate your attention on your breathing, imagine a ball of pure energy or white light that starts at your lower abdomen and as you inhale, it rises up the front of your body to your forehead . . . and as you exhale, it moves down your spine, down your legs, and into the ground . . .

Again . . . imagine this ball of pure energy or white light rise up the front of your body to your forehead as you inhale . . . and as you exhale, it goes down your spine, down your legs, and into the ground . . . Circulate this ball of energy around for a few moments . . . and allow its circulation to move you into even deeper states of relaxation and comfort . . .

Each time you inhale and exhale, you may be surprised to find yourself twice as relaxed as you were a moment before . . . Twice as comfortable . . . Twice as peaceful . . . For with each breath, every cell of your body becomes at ease . . . as all the tension, tightness, pain, or discomfort drains down your spine, down your legs, and into the ground . . . Continue to circulate this ball of energy around for a few moments . . .

As you allow your body to enjoy this nice state of deep, peaceful relaxation, I'd like you to think of a favorite place . . . It can be a real place or an imaginary place . . . It makes no difference . . . Think of a place that's outdoors . . . that's beautiful . . . peaceful . . . serene and secure . . . A magical, special place . . .

With your eyes closed, you may not see anything, but experience what it would feel like to be at this imaginary place . . . Sense it as fully as you can . . . Notice the time of day . . . Can you see a bright yellow sun blazing in the sky? . . . Can you feel its golden warmth beating down on your body? . . . How good it feels . . . Is the sky a brilliant, dazzling blue with white puffy clouds gently floating by? . . . Smell the air . . . fresh and alive.

As you sense the beauty all around you, listen to the sounds of nature, as the animals and insects lazily go about their day's work . . . Feel a gentle breeze softly waft against your face . . . and take a big, deep breath of the clean, fresh air around you . . . As you exhale . . . let your rib cage collapse in total, utter relaxation . . . How good it feels to be here at one with the natural world . . . Enjoy it . . .

Look around and fully sense this place . . . and see if you can find a favorite spot . . . a place where you can sit down for a few moments to sense fully the peaceful beauty all around you . . . Go over to the spot and sit down . . . Feel the earth firm and warm beneath you . . . Stretch out . . . relax . . . and enjoy it . . .

In this beautiful place in your mind's eye, you can more fully sense the interconnections of everything around you . . . And within you . . . As you rest and relax, you can sense the incredible regenerative forces at work . . . restoring . . . nourishing . . . energizing . . . healing . . . Take a few moments to enjoy your favorite place . . . It's special to you . . .

(Long pause)

As you relax and enjoy how wonderful it feels to be here, tell yourself that you can return anytime you wish . . . simply by taking a few moments to relax yourself and letting your imagination carry you here . . . Each time you come to visit, you will find it even more beautiful, more serene, and more peaceful as new horizons are opened for you to experience. It's so easy . . . so accessible . . . so available to you . . .

Before leaving, tell yourself that when you end this exercise, you will feel not only rested, relaxed, and comfortable, but also energized with such a powerful sense of well-being that you will be able to respond easily to any demands that may arise in the times ahead . . .

To end this experience for now, open your eyes and take the signal breath. Exhale . . . Inhale deeply through your nose . . . Blow out through your mouth . . . And be well . . .

© 1977 by David E. Bresler, Ph.D.

How did this exercise work for you? What did you see? Are you looking forward to returning to the spot you have found?

Take a few minutes to make a record of this experience by answering the questions below.

Exercise Thirty-four: Meeting an Inner Adviser

Now that you've found your favorite place, it's time to locate your adviser. There's no better place to seek out your adviser than in the calm, peaceful, personal place that you've just discovered. Not only do you feel

SAMPLE

EXERCISE THIRTY-THREE: Finding a Personal Place

DATE: <u>June 20</u>

TIME: <u>11 a.m.</u>

---

1. Where was your favorite place?

A park.

---

2. Describe what your favorite place looked like.

There are many tall trees, and a brook running through the park. The grass is green and lush. Flowers are everywhere. Children are playing.

---

3. During what season of the year did you visit it?

Spring.

---

4. What time of day was it?

Mid-afternoon.

---

5. What sounds could you hear?

The sounds of the brook splashing as it goes downstream. There is the laughter of children, and wind blowing through the trees.

---

6. What aromas could you smell?

The fresh smell of splashing water and the aroma of flowers.

---

7. What other experiences related to your favorite place did you enjoy?

The exhilaration of being outdoors and feeling part of nature.

**EXERCISE THIRTY-THREE: Finding a
Personal Place**

DATE: _____

TIME: _____

1. Where was your favorite place?

2. Describe what your favorite place looked like.

3. During what season of the year did you visit it?

4. What time of day was it?

5. What sounds could you hear?

6. What aromas could you smell?

7. What other experiences related to your favorite place did you enjoy?

comfortable in this imaginary place, but it's also a pleasant atmosphere in which to meet and communicate with your adviser for the first time.

Once again I suggest that you first make or purchase a tape recording of the following text, and find your adviser as the tape is being replayed. Be sure that the text is read slowly and deliberately. Don't rush through it. Take your time and give yourself as long an opportunity as possible to meet and become acquainted with your adviser.

Now let's begin.

Meeting an Inner Adviser

This tape contains a guided imagery exercise which will help you to make contact with an inner adviser who resides in your mind's eye . . .

Before beginning, take a moment to get comfortable and relax . . . Sit upright in a comfortable chair, with your feet flat on the floor, and close your eyes . . .

Take a few slow, deep, abdominal breaths . . . Inhale . . . Exhale . . . Inhale . . . Exhale . . . Focus your attention on your breathing for a few minutes . . . And recognize how easily slow, deep breathing alone can induce a nice state of deep, gentle relaxation . . .

Let your body breathe itself . . . according to its own natural rhythm . . . slowly . . . easily . . . and deeply . . .

Now take a signal breath . . . a special message that tells the body you are ready to enter a state of deep relaxation . . . Exhale . . . Breathe in deeply through your nose . . . and blow out through your mouth . . .

Remember your breathing . . . slowly and deeply . . . As you concentrate your attention on your breathing, imagine a ball of pure energy or white light that starts at your lower abdomen and as you inhale, it rises up the front of your body to your forehead . . . and as you exhale, it moves down your spine, down your legs, and into the ground . . .

Again . . . imagine this ball of pure energy or white light rise up the front of your body to your forehead as you inhale . . . and as you exhale, it goes down your spine, down your legs, and into the ground . . . Circulate this ball of energy around for a few moments . . . and allow its circulation to move you into even deeper states of relaxation and comfort . . .

Each time you inhale and exhale, you may be surprised to find yourself twice as relaxed as you were a moment before . . . Twice as comfortable . . . Twice as peaceful . . . For with each breath, every cell of your body becomes at ease . . . as all the tension, tightness, pain, or discomfort drains down your spine, down your legs and into the ground . . . Continue to circulate this ball of energy around for a few moments . . .

As you allow yourself to enjoy this nice state of deep, peaceful relaxation, return in your mind's eye to your personal place . . . Let your imagination become reacquainted with every detail of this beautiful spot . . . Sense the peaceful beauty all around you . . . Stretch out . . . Relax . . . And enjoy it.

(Long Pause)

As you relax in your favorite spot, put a smile on your face . . . and slowly look around . . . Somewhere, nearby, some living creature is waiting for you . . . smiling and waiting for you to establish eye contact . . . This creature may immediately approach you or it may wait a few moments to be sure that you mean it no harm . . . Be sure to look up in the trees or behind bushes, since your adviser may be a bit timid . . . But even if you see nothing, sense his or her presence and introduce yourself . . . Tell your adviser your name, and that you mean no harm, for you've come with only the friendliest intentions. Find out your adviser's name . . . The first name that comes to your mind . . . Right now . . .

Sprinkle some food out before you . . . and ask your adviser if he or she is willing to come over and talk with you for a few moments . . . Don't be alarmed if your adviser becomes quite excited and starts jumping up and down at this point . . . Often, advisers have been waiting a long time to make this kind of contact . . . Until now, your adviser has only been able to talk to you sporadically through your intuition . . . Tell your adviser you're sorry you haven't listened more in the past, but that you'll try to do better in the future . . .

If you feel silly talking in this way, tell your adviser that you feel silly . . . that it's hard for you to take this seriously . . . But if you sincerely want your adviser's help, make that very, very clear . . . Tell your adviser that you understand that like in any friendship, it takes time for feelings of mutual trust and respect to develop . . .

Although your adviser knows everything about you—since your adviser is just a reflection of your inner life—tell your adviser that you won't push for any simple answers to important questions that you may be dealing with . . . Rather, you'd like to establish a continuing dialogue . . . so that anytime you need help with a problem, your adviser can tell you things of great importance . . . things that you may already know, but you may have underestimated their significance . . .

If there's a problem that's been bothering you for a while, ask your adviser if he or she is willing to give you some help with it . . . Yes or no? . . . Your adviser's response is the first answer that pops into your mind . . . Pose your questions as you exhale . . . And the first response that comes into your mind as you inhale is your adviser's reply . . . An inspiration . . . Ask your questions now . . . (pause).

What did your adviser reply? . . . Ask any other questions that are on your mind . . . (pause). Continue your dialogue for a few moments . . . asking your questions as you exhale . . . and listening to the response that pops into your mind as you inhale . . . (pause).

Remember, your adviser knows everything about you, but sometimes— for a very good reason—he or she will be unwilling to tell you something . . . This is usually to protect you from information you may not be ready to deal with . . . When this occurs, ask your adviser what you need to do in order to make this information available to yourself . . . Your adviser will usually show you the way . . . (pause).

If there is something that you'd like your adviser to be thinking about between now and the next time you meet, tell this to your adviser now . . . (pause) . . . If there is anything your adviser would like *you* to think about

SAMPLE

EXERCISE THIRTY-FOUR: Meeting an Inner Adviser

DATE: June 20

TIME: 11 a.m.

---

1. Briefly describe "your favorite place"

a park with large trees, with a
brook running through it.

---

2. What was the first thing to approach you? Was this your adviser?

A chipmunk. Yes, it was my adviser.

---

3. Describe your adviser's physical appearance.

He was small and very animated.
Physically, he was very attractive.

---

4. Describe your adviser's personality.

Very outgoing, talkative, smiles a lot,
very likeable.

EXERCISE THIRTY-FOUR: Meeting an Inner Adviser

DATE: _____

TIME: _____

1. Briefly describe "your favorite place"

2. What was the first thing to approach you? Was this your adviser?

3. Describe your adviser's physical appearance.

4. Describe your adviser's personality.

SAMPLE

EXERCISE THIRTY-FOUR—*Continued*

---

5. Indicate your adviser's name, species, and sex (if known); if you met more than one adviser, include information for all.

Billy; chipmunk; male.

---

6. Did your adviser(s) tell you something that you already know is important in your life?

Yes. He knows how important it is for me to get rid of my pain so I can enjoy the park and other pleasant places.

---

7. Did your adviser(s) tell you something that you hadn't known or thought about before?

He said I should talk more to my spouse about my pain, because he can offer special insights into my discomfort.

---

8. Do you think you will continue to communicate with your adviser?

Yes, definitely.

---

9. Other notes of interest

I was surprised by how good this exercise made me feel.

EXERCISE THIRTY-FOUR—*Continued*

5. Indicate your adviser's name, species, and sex (if known); if you met more than one adviser, include information for all.

6. Did your adviser(s) tell you something that you already know is important in your life?

7. Did your adviser(s) tell you something that you hadn't known or thought about before?

8. Do you think you will continue to communicate with your adviser?

9. Other notes of interest

between now and the next time you meet, find out what that is now . . . (pause) . . .

Set up a time to meet again . . . a time that's convenient for you and a time that's convenient for your adviser . . . Be specific as to exact time and place . . . Tell your adviser that although these meetings are important to you, part of you is lazy or even reluctant to follow through . . .

One way your adviser can help motivate you to continue to meet periodically is by giving you a clear demonstration of the benefits you can gain . . . a demonstration so powerful that you will be moved to work even harder in getting to know yourself . . . If you are in pain, for example, ask your adviser if he or she will be willing to take away that pain completely . . . right now, just for a few moments, as a demonstration of power . . . If so, tell your adviser to do it . . . now . . . (long pause) . . .

Notice any difference? . . . If you're willing to do your share of the work, by relaxing yourself and meeting periodically to set things straight, there's no limit to your adviser's power . . . Ask for any reasonable demonstration that will be undeniably convincing to you of this power . . .

You might be, for example, somewhat forgetful . . . And although you want to continue these meetings with your adviser, you might forget the exact time and place that you agreed to meet . . . If so, ask your adviser to help you by coming into your consciousness just a few moments before it's time to meet, to remind you of the meeting.

Before leaving, tell your adviser you're open to having many different kinds of advisers . . . And that you will leave this totally up to your adviser's discretion . . . If your adviser wants to bring other advisers along the next time you meet, fine . . . Is there anything your adviser would like you to bring along with you the next time you meet? . . . If so, find out what that is . . . (pause).

See if your adviser will allow you to establish physical contact . . . This is very important . . . Just about every animal on the face of the earth loves to have its face stroked and its back scratched . . . See if your adviser will allow you to make this contact now . . . (pause) . . . While making this contact, find out if there's anything else that your adviser would like to tell you . . . If so, what is it? . . . (pause) . . .

Is there anything that you would like to tell your adviser before you leave? . . . If so, do it now . . . (pause) . . .

In a moment, you will take the signal breath to return from this meeting . . . But before you do, tell yourself that each time you make contact with your adviser the communication will flow more and more smoothly . . . more and more easily . . . more and more comfortably . . . Tell yourself that when this experience is over, you will feel not only relaxed, rested, and comfortable, but also energized with such a powerful sense of well-being that you will be able to respond easily to any demands that may arise . . .

To end this exercise for now, take the same signal breath that you used to begin it . . . Exhale . . . Breathe in deeply through your nose . . . Blow out through your mouth . . . And be well.

How did this exercise proceed? Were you pleased with the results? Did you find an adviser that you really like?

As I will emphasize later, it is very important for you to keep a record of your meetings with your adviser for future referral. To start you in this process, complete the following chart.

How Can Your Adviser Help?

Now that you have an adviser—whether it's a cat, a squirrel, a deer, or a dolphin—what should you do when you meet in the upcoming weeks and months? What should you talk about?

Very simply, you should discuss *anything* that's on your mind—or anything that your adviser might like to talk about. There are no limits, except that the dialogue should be kept totally honest on both sides. Your adviser can provide you with an endless number of insights—not only about your pain, but about other aspects of your life as well.

In working with hundreds of pain patients using this guided imagery technique, I find that the adviser can be helpful in at least four distinct ways.

1. *The adviser can provide advice on how to reduce stress and pain.* When you're in need of pain relief or stress reduction, ask your adviser for suggestions. Let your adviser play the role of an "imaginary doctor," as Mike Samuels, M.D., and Hal Bennett recommend in *The Well Body Book*. Talk your pain problem over with this make-believe doctor or adviser. He or she knows you better than anyone, and thus may be able to provide you with insights that no one else can.

Sometimes your adviser's thoughts may surprise you. But listen to them carefully; they are coming from within the deepest parts of you. Sylvia, an ulcer victim with terrible stomach pains, described a meeting with Shorty, her adviser, and the surprising revelation she received: "Shorty's sweet and darling, and the last time I talked with him he said I needed to keep my pain for a while longer so I'll continue working on myself. He said if I didn't have pain, I'd quit the relaxation exercise and become too anxious again. When I've learned to relax myself more consistently, he says the pain will go away."

2. *The adviser can provide support and protection.* Your adviser can supply encouragement for decisions on a course of action that you've decided upon, with an enthusiasm that friends or family members are either unable or unwilling to offer. Your adviser can also shield you from danger by warning you—in advance—when you are about to do something that is not in your best interest.

3. *The adviser has the power to give total and complete pain relief.* One way your adviser can demonstrate his potency is to provide total pain relief for a few moments. Of course, once you recognize that the adviser's

powers are, in essence, your own powers, then you can begin to understand the enormous control that you do have over your pain.

4. *The adviser can help you discover the message behind your pain.* Because pain is a message that something is wrong, it is essential for you to identify that message if you wish to overcome your discomfort completely. Often, the message has been repressed and is not available to the conscious mind. But your adviser can help you to uncover it in a gentle, loving, nonthreatening way. Your adviser can not only tell you why your body hurts, but also why your life hurts.

Improving Communication

A few people go through the guided imagery exercise time and time again and are still not able to find an adviser. If you're one of them, don't lose hope. Your adviser *is* there and will come to you when you least expect it. You're probably looking too hard.

Go back to your favorite place and in a state of relaxation, just begin enjoying the environment of that beautiful spot—the sights, the smells, the tastes, the sounds, the tactile sensations. If you wait patiently, something will ultimately attract your attention—a rabbit, a deer, a chipmunk, a dog, or some other living creature. It will happen. I have not yet worked with even one person who wasn't eventually able to find an adviser.

Some people feel that, at least in the beginning, they literally have to see their adviser in order to communicate in a meaningful way. For them, I often turn one of their thumbnails into their first adviser—using a felt pen to draw a mouth, a nose, and two eyes. Once they become accustomed to relating to this make-believe character, they then usually find it easier to move on to an imaginary adviser that exists only in their mind's eye.

Even if your adviser was located quickly and easily, you still may occasionally have communication problems. And actually, that's really not surprising. When you have a dialogue with your adviser, it's just a reflection of what's going on inside of you. If your adviser acts timid or frightened, perhaps you are feeling insecure. If your adviser won't talk to you, maybe it's a reflection of your unwillingness to open up about what's really going on inside.

Keep in mind that advisers always work on behalf of your best long-term interest. If an adviser won't cooperate with you, it may be a test of your sincerity. Try to determine the reason for this unwillingness to work together.

Let's assume, for instance, that you ask your adviser, "Why do I hurt?" and the reply is, "Hmm, I don't know." Well, your adviser—by his or her very nature—*does* know everything about you. A proper kind of follow-up question might be, "Are you reluctant to tell me something about my pain—yes or no? If so, what must I do in order for you to open up to me?" Your adviser will then probably respond very clearly. Typical responses include, "You have to learn to relax," or "You have to stop being so negative," or "You must stop being so aggressive."

If this strategy fails, let your adviser know that this inner dialogue is very important to you, and unless the two of you can work closely together, you're going to have to find another adviser. Sometimes advisers are stubborn, but if you're firm with them and show them that you are sincere, your adviser will eventually begin to open a dialogue.

Advisers test people in other ways as well. Irving Oyle tells the case history of a psychiatrist who suffered from severe migraine headaches. Though highly skeptical of guided imagery, he found an adviser—a mermaid named Ethel—who insisted that in order for them to talk he would have to swim out to her in the imaginary ocean where she lived. He refused at first, but at Dr. Oyle's urging, finally agreed. Once he had swum several hundred yards offshore, Ethel asked him to dive with her into the depths of the water so that their dialogue could begin. The psychiatrist began feeling even more silly. "How corny!" he exclaimed. "Sinking down into the sea of the subconscious. This whole thing is ridiculous!" Ethel responded curtly, "So sue me! Not only do I know about your headaches, but you deserve worse! You're even more ridiculous than I am."

Later, after they had become friends, the psychiatrist asked Ethel why she had been so hostile initially. Ethel replied, "You were hostile, too, and it was the only way I could get your attention."

Some patients have difficulty communicating because they simply don't like the physical forms their advisers take. Mary's first adviser was a snake, and frankly she was terrified of snakes. Although the snake was friendly, congenial, and interested in helping, Mary had trouble getting close to the snake because of her phobia.

Still, Mary tried her hardest, and eventually she and the snake became good friends. Not long thereafter, the snake introduced her to a second adviser—a wise old owl. The owl told her, "The reason for the snake was to see if you were sincere. You were being tested. Your sincerity is now clear, and I am here to help you in place of the snake."

Sincerity is difficult for some people, because they feel silly talking to an imaginary creature. If that's your problem, admit to yourself that, yes, the situation is silly. But even if you sometimes find it difficult to be *serious,* you can still be *sincere.* Don't play a game—establish a relationship. If you are talking, say, to a mouse, it may be silly on one level, but try to talk to the mouse as if the meeting is real and has personal meaning to you. For, if you do, it almost certainly will.

Some patients tell me that through their adviser they can program themselves while they're asleep. If you'd like to try this, talk with your adviser before you retire for the night, and say, "I'd like you to work with this particular problem tonight and have some recommendations for me tomorrow morning when I wake." See how effectively this works for you.

Finally, never be concerned if, in your particular case, your adviser appears to be totally uncooperative. This is an easy matter to resolve. If a sincere attempt to develop a close relationship with your adviser fails, warn your adviser that you have the power to dematerialize him or her. All you need to do is to stop thinking about your adviser, go back to your favorite place, and find a new one. When this is given as a sincere warning, and not just an idle threat, most advisers quickly become more cooperative.

Maintaining a Good Relationship

Once you've started meeting with your adviser, it's important to keep your relationship as genial as possible. Treat your adviser the same way you would any valued, trusted friend. If you make an appointment at a given time, keep it. If something unexpected happens—that is, you get caught in traffic and are unable to keep your seven o'clock appointment— be sure to contact your adviser as soon thereafter as possible and report what happened. Be honest in your explanation; remember, your adviser knows everything about you, and your sincerity counts.

A good way to lose your adviser is by neglecting to explain why you failed to keep an appointment. Just think of parallel situations in interpersonal relationships. What do you think would happen if you invited a very close friend to meet you for cocktails at 5:00 P.M., and you never showed up—nor did you call to explain or apologize? Months passed, and there was no communication between the two of you. Finally, a year later, you called him up, and said, "Hi, let's meet for cocktails at five P.M. tomorrow." What would happen? Your friend would probably be offended and indignant.

In the same way, a good relationship with an adviser must be nurtured. Make an effort to develop mutual trust and respect. People who take good care of their advisers receive the same kind of loving attention in return. And they never need to doubt the advice their advisers offer. Your adviser, like any good friend, would never deliberately mislead you.

I also encourage you to keep your relationship with your adviser on a fifty-fifty basis. If you ask for something from your adviser, be sure also to give something in return. What should you give? Ask your adviser. The most common request is, "Stop! Rest! Take it easy. Give me a chance to help heal you!" If that's the message you're receiving from your adviser, try to make a deal like, "If I rest and relax myself for a few minutes each day, will you talk to me and help me out?" Advisers almost always agree to this.

Also, make a continuing effort to maintain physical contact with your adviser. As with your friends and family, adding physical contact to a relationship places it on an entirely different level. Stroke your adviser's face if you can, and ask your adviser to do the same to you. It will help to promote a closer, more intimate relationship.

Another bit of advice—keep a careful record of your continuing dialogues with your adviser. Just jot down a few sentences about what transpired during each meeting. Sometimes your adviser will pour out large amounts of material all at once, and you may not appreciate or understand all of it until you have a chance to work it through. By the time you get around to that, you may have forgotten much of what happened.

For instance, your adviser might say, "Love yourself," or "Don't be so self-critical." You might dismiss those thoughts and only later realize that they are central to your attempts to restructure your life in a more positive way. So be sure to write these experiences down and to reevaluate them several days or weeks later.

Exercise Thirty-five: Chronicling Your Adviser Meetings

As with dreams, the significance of your adviser's recommendations may not become apparent until much later. However, unless you keep a record of them, they may be quickly forgotten and their meaning lost forever.

After each session with your adviser, write a few notes that describe the essence of it. What questions did you pose? What answers did your adviser give? What suggestions, warnings, or precautions were discussed?

The Creative Team

After you've developed a strong relationship with your adviser, I recommend that you find other advisers as well. Invite your adviser to bring a mate or other acquaintances along the next time you meet. The more help you get, the better.

Some people use multiadvisers to help resolve a particular conflict they may be experiencing. Their two advisers can debate the issue, taking opposing viewpoints, while the individual is able to evaluate their respective positions objectively.

Terry, a UCLA pain patient, was suffering from chronic endometritis

SAMPLE

**EXERCISE THIRTY-FIVE: Chronicling Your
Adviser Meetings**

DATE: _____

TIME: _____

During my meeting with my adviser
I asked
Why won't my pain leave?
My adviser responded
"Because you really want it to stay so your family will give you sympathy and attention."
Other suggestions given
"Try to go back to work so you can receive attention and praise in a more positive way."
Warnings and precautions
"Don't expect instant pain relief with a behavior change. But it will come gradually with time if you're committed to the new behavior."
Other notes
I think that Billy (the chipmunk) is right!

EXERCISE THIRTY-FIVE: Chronicling Your Adviser Meetings

DATE: _____

TIME: _____

During my meeting with my adviser

I asked

My adviser responded

Other suggestions given

Warnings and precautions

Other notes

(inflammation of the inner lining of the uterus). She asked her first adviser, a dog named Max, to recruit two other advisers to discuss her indiscriminate sexual activities, which she thought might be contributing to her problem.

One of the new advisers was a rabbit named Rachel, who told Terry, "You only live once, and life is very short. Why not make it as sweet as you can? Have as many different sexual experiences as possible, and don't worry about attachments. Just live loose and free!"

The other adviser was a deer named Bambi, who argued, "You have to respect yourself before others will respect you. Rather than having a lot of meaningless experiences, save yourself for the right person. It's quality not quantity that's important."

Terry felt that she received some very helpful insights from this debate. In a subsequent meeting with all three of her advisers, she decided she wanted to be more like the deer than the rabbit, and that while she still might occasionally allow herself to be sexually free (like the rabbit), it would never again be a permanent life-style.

I believe that, ideally, each individual should have three advisers—a male, a female, and a child—as a way of achieving symbolic balance. For each of us has masculine, feminine, and childlike qualities within us.

Our masculine side is verbal, aggressive, rational, and logical. Our feminine side is more receptive, creative, intuitive, and nourishing. And the childlike part of us is impulsive, trusting, open, naive, and irresponsible.

The child adviser, in many ways, can be the most interesting. This inner child is the part of us that watched the sky on summer nights, romped in the sunshine, and loved being held and touched. Its advice is always incredibly real and honest.

Some people create an image of themselves as their child adviser. They study childhood photographs to recall more clearly how they once looked. When you wish to know your real desires in the midst of confusion, ask your inner child. The answer will sometimes surprise you.

As you work more extensively with your advisers, you may find that conflicts arise between, say, your male and female advisers. If so, there may be a solution to this problem. Irving Oyle simply marries them! He performs a symbolic marriage of the two advisers and has them create a child to represent the neutral element. Very often, with the child's help, the conflict is cordially resolved soon thereafter.

There is one other technique you can try, in which all your advisers can participate. It was taught to me by Martin Rossman, M.D., a family physician in Mill Valley, California. At your personal place, join together with all of your advisers to symbolically plant a seed that will eventually produce the solution to your problems. Once the seed is planted, you should nourish it with your pain, your agony, your joy, and your ecstasy. Watch the seed grow and see what develops. As one patient told me, "I went through such agony last night. But this morning I went to my personal place and found that my tree had grown four inches. Suddenly, I felt wonderful, for the tree reminded me of my own growth through this experience."

Is Your Adviser Real?

As your experiences with your advisers continue, always keep in mind that they represent dialogues between different parts of your nervous system. Although you may feel, "I'm just talking to myself. How can that help me?" it's the unique content and symbolism of the dialogue that is important. Why did only certain responses pop into your head? Why did your adviser assume the name Roger? Why was he a frog? Why did he tell you to love yourself more? All of these have relevance and meaning to your life.

A surprising number of people have told me and other investigators that their advisers have actually materialized in their lives. Consider the case of Peter, whose adviser was a robin named Mandy. One day, while working at his desk near an open window of his house, a robin flew into the window. It perched on Peter's desk and stared at him for several minutes. In Peter's mind, the bird was saying, "Hi, I'm Mandy." Coincidence? Probably. But I can tell you of at least two dozen similar stories.

One of the most unusual adviser stories was told to me by a relatively unimaginative patient named Dorothy, whose adviser was a leprechaun named Faith. One day she told her adviser, "I just made you up in my head. How do I know that you're important and have anything to offer me?" The adviser replied, "This is something you're going to have to learn on your own, but perhaps I can help you toward this understanding in the following way."

Faith then instructed Dorothy to hold out her hand, and when she did, he gave her a ball. As she held it, the ball began to spin. As its velocity increased, it also started changing from one color to another. Faster and faster the colors changed. Then the ball began to shrink, then expand, shrink, expand. Suddenly the ball exploded and was replaced by a lightning bolt that extended from her hand "up into the cosmos." As she stood there, Faith told her, "This is your connection with infinity." Needless to say, Dorothy had never experienced anything like this before.

What doors of perception can your advisers open for you? Only you can find out. As with other techniques in this book, the adviser approach is not for everyone, but for those it helps, the results can be ecstatically inspiring.

Ultimately, guided imagery boils down to making friends with your nervous system. Many people in pain have found it to be incredibly rewarding. Why not see if it can work for you?

12 *Pain, Pleasure, and Love*

Go placidly amid the noise and haste, and remember what peace there may be in silence. As far as possible without surrender be on good terms with all persons. Speak your truth quietly and clearly; and listen to others, even the dull and ignorant; they too have their story. Avoid loud and aggressive persons, they are vexations to the spirit. If you compare yourself with others, you may become vain and bitter; for always there will be greater and lesser persons than yourself. Enjoy your achievements as well as your plans. Keep interested in your own career, however humble; it is a real possession in the changing fortunes of time. Exercise caution in your business affairs; for the world is full of trickery. But let this not blind you to what virtue there is; many persons strive for high ideals; and everywhere life is full of heroism. Be yourself. Especially, do not feign affection. Neither be cynical about love; for in the face of all aridity and disenchantment it is perennial as the grass. Take kindly the counsel of the years, gracefully surrendering the things of youth. Nurture strength of spirit to shield you in sudden misfortune. But do not distress yourself with imaginings. Many fears are born of fatigue and loneliness. Beyond a wholesome discipline, be gentle with yourself. You are a child of the universe, no less than the trees and the stars; you have a right to be here. And whether or not it is clear to you, no doubt the universe is unfolding as it should. Therefore be at peace with God, whatever you conceive Him to be, and whatever your labors and aspirations, in the noisy confusion of life keep peace with your soul. With all its sham, drudgery and broken dreams, it is still a beautiful world. Be careful. Strive to be happy.

—Desiderata

Found in Old Saint Paul's Church,
Baltimore, Maryland; dated 1692

More than a century ago, British physician Peter Mere Latham proclaimed, "It would be a great thing to understand pain in all its meanings."

Unfortunately, pain remains a major mystery both to doctors and laymen. This book has presented a different perspective of pain, which, it is hoped, has given you a better appreciation of its complexity.

For instance, can you now clearly understand the difference between a painful sensation and the pain experience? Do you understand the importance of pain in conveying the message that "something is wrong"? Have you started examining your own beliefs and expectations, changing the ones that are unrealistic? Can you now see the power of the mind in the healing process?

In guiding you toward answering pain's message, most of my recommendations have been directed at changing your life, rather than at symptomatic suppression of pain. If you've pursued a sincere self-exploration of your life, and made the changes you felt were necessary, I hope your pain has been eased in the process.

For example, I hope you have begun to divest yourself of the negative ritualistic behaviors that have imprisoned you. For until you recognize and give up the gains you may be receiving from your pain, your body will not be able to maximize its ability to cure you.

Also, try hard to continue your efforts to nourish yourself as fully and positively as possible. Not only should your meals be healthy, but you can also enhance your well-being by filling your life with the activities you enjoy—raising your serum fun levels through cooking, traveling, reading, or attending sporting events. Review Exercise Twenty-three for other suggestions. If you saturate your life with pleasure and happiness, you'll be taking an important step toward crowding pain out.

Also, don't underestimate the nourishment provided by "four hugs a day." A successful businessman, tormented by six years of agonizing pain in his right shoulder blade, recently told me, "These hugs have been tremendous. I used to give my wife a peck in the morning before leaving for work, and another one at night when I got home. It was a routine thing instead of a loving thing. But now we hug each other with feeling and affection. And what a difference. It just makes me feel so good."

It is also important for you to stay on top of the depression that you may still feel periodically. Too often, when chronic pain patients lapse into a state of depression, they close the doors on the sources of positive energy in their lives. Don't let that happen to you. Whenever you find yourself lost in depression, mobilize to resist it. You should react by saying, "There are feelings of depression welling up within me. Although I am aware of them, I will not identify with them. I will simply let them pass through me, as if I'm invisible. In addition, I will counterbalance them by doing something that's fun, or practicing the relaxation exercise, or . . ."

In the upcoming weeks, I hope you'll also continue to use the power of your imagination, relying on your adviser for guidance and counsel. As you learned in Chapters 10 and 11, the imagination can be the key that unlocks the body's amazing healing powers, even for people who have abandoned all hope.

Be sure to review periodically all the exercises in this book. By doing so, you may find yourself arriving at new insights, or reaffirming old ones. For example, when you return to Exercise Two on page 37, determine how many of your goals you have already reached and which ones you should now be channeling your energy toward. In Exercise Fifteen on page 229, have you resolved many of your bad habits? Have you developed any new ones? In Exercise Sixteen on page 244, has your Life Change Score changed significantly in recent weeks or months, and if so, are you more susceptible to illness or less? Continue to use the information from all the exercises in planning your pain-alleviation strategy.

If you have diligently practiced the techniques I have recommended in this book, your discomfort may now have eased or even been eliminated. Even if the intensity of your pain is the same, I hope your pain experience is better in some way. For example, perhaps now you can dissociate the pain sensation from the pain experience. Even if the injury or stimulus is still present, you may find yourself thinking, It still hurts, but it doesn't bother me, or I still feel it, but it doesn't hurt.

The Transformational Process

Adlai Stevenson, the political statesman, once philosophized, "There are no gains without pains." I hope this book has convinced you that your pain, however unpleasant, has had some positive effects on your life. Your discomfort may have forced you to make some healthy changes and transformations that you would not have otherwise made. Perhaps you're dealing better with stress now than you did before. Maybe you're nourishing yourself more positively. Possibly you're relating better to family and friends.

Chronic pain was the motivating force behind these changes—the energy that prompted you to embark upon the transformational process. Were it not for the desperate urgency of your discomfort, you may never have been stimulated toward making these important life transitions. After all, as you'll recall from Chapter 2, growth is a difficult process that requires you to surrender the security and comfort of old situations and habits.

More often than not, the most important change for the pain patient to make is to abandon negative attitudes like "Why did this happen to me?"

or "I know I'll never get better." To me, people with beliefs like these are victims of "cancer of the attitude," a malignant, metastatic, and infectious disease that can quickly spread to others around them. However, if these victims can change their attitudes, there is still hope. Remember: *Your pain doesn't make your life unbearable; rather, your life makes your pain unbearable.*

Also, keep in mind that change is a fluid, moving process. Even though you may not yet be in the place where you ultimately want to be, you should feel encouraged if you're making progress. Even the smallest degree of improvement is a step in the right direction—a step in the transformation from a life of pain to one that is more positive and fulfilling. Happiness is a journey, not a destination. If you're moving, you're growing. Only if you're stuck in your pain, doing nothing and going nowhere, do you need to worry.

The entire transformational process is well summarized by Erich Fromm, who said:

> Man is always torn between the wish to regress to the womb and the wish to be fully born. Every act of birth requires the courage to let go of something, to let go of the breast, to let go of the lap, to let go of the hand, to let go eventually of all certainties, and to rely only upon one thing: one's own power to be aware and to respond; that is, one's own creativity. To be creative means to consider the whole process of life as a process of birth, and not to take any stage of life as a final stage. Most people die before they are fully born. Creativeness means to be born before one dies.

The Power of Love

> All you need is love.
>
> —The Beatles

André had suffered from severe headaches for nearly six years. He described his life as "purposeless," and the more he wallowed in pain, the less interested he was in living.

But at a Christmas Eve party, André met a woman with whom he soon fell in love. As their emotional attachment grew, André's headaches began to subside until they eventually disappeared altogether. André believes that his headaches were cured by the power of love.

There are many definitions of love. Paul Brenner, M.D., says, "Love is the acceptance of all things." I would expand that definition to say, "Love is the acceptance of all things, including your power to change all things."

In my opinion, love may be essential to the healing process. Unfortunately, many people with chronic pain have forgotten (or have never learned) how to love. For example, many have learned to hate and mistrust their bodies, for throughout their illness they have perceived their bodies as an enemy that has turned on them. This, of course, is hardly the case. If, instead, these patients would only learn to trust and care for their bodies—to love and nourish them with relaxation, good food, and positive energy—they might suddenly find themselves moving down the road to health.

Think for a moment about the best possible analgesic for a child. I know of nothing that promotes self-healing faster or more effectively than a mother's kiss and the love that accompanies it. If you apply the same principle to your own illness, you can see why it's so important to love your body, your emotions, and your mind—in short, to love all of you.

If you have a dog, you know how loyal and loving it can be. No matter what kind of mood you're in, your dog is always there, no questions asked. As Bill Lyon, sportswriter for the Knight-Ridder newspapers wrote: "Dogs never ask why. They know. They know when you want sympathy, they know when you want joy. Dogs never say, 'I'm too busy right now', or 'Give me a call next week', or 'I'll get back to you later'. . . Maybe that's what dogs are for—to remind us of all the things we tend to forget about getting along with each other."

In much the same way, you must learn to love and be loyal to yourself. Give yourself sympathy, give yourself joy. Never be too busy to love yourself, no questions asked. And once you've learned self-love and self-acceptance, then it's easy to cultivate the love of others and, ultimately, the love of life. In short, love is often the best medicine of all.

Reaching Your Goal

If you've been helped by the program presented in this book, I'm sure you're very pleased. But don't stop now.

Many of my patients at UCLA have reported to me that they have helped their friends to achieve better health by teaching them some of the techniques they've learned. Perhaps you've heard the old county hospital motto, "See one, do one, teach one." That's the attitude I'd like you to have. Share this book and the ideas in it with people whom you think might benefit from it.

In self-improvement programs like Weight Watchers, the participants who enjoy the most success are those who remain as staff members—that is, those who teach the technique to others. So to achieve the greatest benefits from this program, one of the best things you can do is to teach others what you yourself have learned.

However, if you still have more progress to make yourself, don't be discouraged. Few good things in life come quickly. Like almost everything else of value, pain relief requires a lot of hard work—an incredible amount of hard work. The techniques presented in this book have to be practiced again and again and again. Pain control in the modern world is often an acquired talent that demands a sustained effort. Ask yourself if you really want to change, and if you do, continue devoting at least thirty minutes a day to this program until you obtain the results you desire.

I've seen hundreds of patients come to the UCLA Pain Control Unit with weakened bodies and weary minds. When they've left, many have said good-bye with smiles that had been absent from their faces for years.

Like them, you have the potential for making dramatic changes in your life. Most of the tools you need are already within you. John H. Knowles, president of the Rockefeller Foundation, recently predicted, "The next major advance in the health of the American people will result only from what the individual is willing to do for himself."

How much responsibility are you ready to assume for your own well-being? If you're sincerely committed to a future free of chronic pain, that dream can become a reality.

Perhaps you recall the opening paragraphs of this book, in which Linda, an advertising executive, vividly described the terribly painful situation in which she found herself. Time and again, she tried to overcome it, and failed. But with great determination and a willingness to work, Linda eventually transformed her life in a positive way. Here is how she subsequently described the remnants of her discomfort:

> I see it through the windows of my mind. The courtyard waits for me. My ballet slippers whisper to the beautiful old bricks; my eyes seek and find the tree. Has it ever been quite so graceful, quite so peaceful, its leaves so green? Why is it there never is quite so perfect a moment as now? The branches sweep almost to the ground, then lift again in the breeze like Grandmama's parasol. It too was lace, like the leaves; but these are handwrought by God. As I let myself drift down onto the chaise I think again, "Whose hands, whose love, could have made such a chair. It bends up a little, just here, to hold my knees; there's a little lift to hold my toes, a curved and cushioned spot to hold my head." And it's so much a part of me my eyes would close except I must first see what flowers are left. The pink azalea is still in bloom, the begonias never end, the baskets I thought so big are about to overflow with fern. The moss is moist on the hill that curves round the tree and at its top the bougainvillea spills, gold and coral blossoms borne like baby kisses on the wind. Breathe in, Linda, breathe in. She is there, behind me, her lovely face framed in its white coif, her eyes serene. How cool, those slender fingers on my forehead, how sure their touch. That jagged rock beneath my brow—where is it now? My eyelids close . . . I could not wait for this. There is that tiny finger pressure against my nose, under my eyebrows, just back of my ears. Breathe in. Breathe in. Let it go. The fire back of my eye is dying of its own accord; there was just enough ice on those fingertips to put it out. The day was so bright, so ghastly bright, and

now the light is filtered shade through the leaves, through the tree, through the hands that hold my face. Oh, yes, there, there, under the cheekbone. Breathe out, shoulders down, let it go. The color is all around me. The flowers, the moss, the trailing fern, the air. The sky is not above, but in me. I am floating, floating. Aware. In just a tiny wisp of time, this peace shall end and I'll be gay, and young again. The pain? Oh, yes, the pain. It's there. Somewhere.

Appendix

Professionally recorded cassette tapes of the relaxation and guided imagery exercises described in this book can be ordered from the Center for Integral Medicine if you do not wish to record your own. These include:

CIM No.	Title
DB 101	Conditioned Relaxation
DB 102	Mind-Controlled Analgesia
DB 103	Glove Anesthesia
DB 104	Finding a Personal Place
DB 105	Meeting an Inner Adviser

For information concerning these tapes and any other resources available from the Center, write to:

Center for Integral Medicine
P.O. Box 967
Pacific Palisades, California 90272

Reference Notes and Sources

(For complete publishing information, consult the Bibliography.)

Chapter 1 The Control of Pain

For patients with chronic pain, particularly recommended are general books by Melzack (1973), Freese (1974), and Shealy (1976), which describe the nature of pain and the various approaches to treat it.

The statistics concerning the incidence of migraine headaches in most Western countries were reported in Paulley and Haskell (1975). The information on arthritis was obtained from the Arthritis Foundation (1976). The Krebiozen story was reported by Shapiro (1963). The research by the Simontons is documented in their book (1978).

Information on endorphins can be found in Goldstein (1976) and Guillemin (1977). The relationship of endorphins and acupuncture was described in Pomeranz and Chiu (1976), Pomeranz (1977), and Pomeranz, Cheng and Law (1977). Also see Kosterlitz and Hughes (1976) and Restak (1977) for a further discussion of endorphins.

For an exploration of the journal technique, see the book by Progoff (1975). The book by Smith (1978) focuses on the journal process as it relates to dreams. Letter-writing to one's pain is a commonly used technique. For an illustration of its use by a nurse, see Cady (1976). Specific dialogues with a painful or troublesome bodily area have been studied by Belknap, Blau and Grossman (1975).

Chapter 2 What Is Pain?

Further analysis of the language of pain can be found in Melzack and Torgerson (1971). A description of the research on soldiers wounded in battle and their need for analgesic medication can be found in Beecher (1946) and Beecher (1959). A detailed review of the abilities of Vernon Craig is presented by Steiger (1976).

For a discussion of social and cultural factors in the pain experience, see Zborowski (1952, 1969), Sternbach (1968), Sternbach (1974), Gonda (1962), and Wolff and Langley (1968).

A personal approach to the integration of Eastern philosophy and modern theoretical physics and their relationship to modern medicine is provided by Oyle in three books (1973, 1974, 1976). Koestler (1972) discusses the relationship between parapsychology and modern theoretical physics, quantum mechanics and relativity theory. Related information is also presented by Davies (1977) and Toben (1975). Capra (1975) describes the relationship between Taoism and physics. A general discussion of Taoist thought is presented in Fung (1968), Lao

Tzu (1955), Christie (1968), and Rawson and Legeza (1973). A further explanation of Heisenberg's work can be found in his book (1958). A general review of the powers of the mind appears in Smith (1975). See also Dychtwald (1977), Brown (1974), Lilly (1972, 1973, 1975), Samuels and Samuels (1975), Pelletier (1977), and Oyle (1973, 1975, 1976).

An elaboration of Illich's philosophy is contained in his book (1976). Congenital insensitivity to pain is discussed in Critchley (1956) and Ervin and Sternbach (1960).

Chapter 3 Why Do You Hurt?

Many contemporary books on nutrition, including Arnow (1972), discuss the risks of food additives. More specific investigations of additives can be found in Longgood (1969) and Winter (1972). Also see Verrett (1974) and Jacobson (1972). A worthwhile magazine article on the subject is by Jenkins (1977).

The research of Feingold is addressed in his book (1974). He also published an article (1968) on the relationship between food additives and symptoms of allergies. The *FDA Consumer* periodically reviews governmental actions concerning food additives, including an article on the GRAS list by Hopkins (1978) and an article on food and drug interactions by Lehmann (1978).

A study on environmental allergies is reviewed in "Environmental Allergies" (1976). MacLeod (1969) discusses the National Tuberculosis Association and U.S. Public Health Service conclusions on the quality of the air. The study involving coronary patients was discussed by Levin (1974).

The definitive review of research into sensory deprivation is by Solomon, et al. (1961). Also see Vernon (1963). Studies of German psychiatrists concerning music and medicine is reviewed by Ryan (1976).

The dangers of airplane noise are discussed by Navarra (1969). Juby (1977) describes the health hazards of noise.

Cheek's research has been published in various medical journals. His most important papers are listed in the reference section. Also see reports by Scott (1972), Cherkin and Harroun (1971), and Trustman, et al. (1977).

Hill (1975) addresses the issue of ultra-high voltage lines in Indiana. Information on Project Sanguine and Seafarer can be found in Larkin and Sutherland (1977), Carter (1977), and Southern (1975).

Research by Becker is reviewed in his articles (1963a, 1963b, 1969). See also a report by Bentall (1976) presenting a physiological theory of how electromagnetism may promote healing. For more general works, consult books by Davis and Rawls (1974, 1975), Burr (1972), and Presman (1970). A discussion of magnetic fields generated by the human body is presented in Cohen (1975).

Although George Starr White's book, *Cosmo-Electric Culture,* is no longer in print, an excerpt from the book can be found in Gallert (1966). Electromagnetic influences on health are discussed by Kaufer (1978) and Brodeur (1977), who emphasize microwave radiation contamination. Also see Ott (1973) and Herndon and Freeman (1976).

Luce (1973), Raloff (1975), and Scheving (1976) provide useful information on biological clocks and their effects upon health. Numerous studies about seasonal birth have been conducted. Parker and Neilsen (1976), Cowgill (1966), and Hare

(1975) are of particular interest. Tasso and Miller (1976) and Lieber and Sherin (1972) researched the effects of the full moon on human behavior.

Many papers have been published addressing the effects of circadian rhythms on pain sensitivity, including Procacci, et al. (1974), Folkard, Glynn and Lloyd (1976), and Glynn, Lloyd and Folkard (1976).

"Life energy" is discussed in several books. Particularly recommended are Moss (1975), Krippner (1975), and Mann (1973). The life work of Wilhelm Reich is described by Raknes (1970) and Boadella (1973).

Research on Kirlian photography is discussed by Ostrander and Schroeder (1970, 1974), Krippner and Rubin (1974), Krippner (1975), and Moss (1975). Highly recommended is the journal, *Psychoenergetic Systems,* which publishes papers about consciousness, matter and energy interactions, and includes reports about acupuncture, bioelectric fields, Kirlian photography, unorthodox healing, paraphysics and other related fields. It is published by Gordon & Breach Science Publishers, 42 William IV St., London, England WC2.

For studies on "learned helplessness," consult Hiroto (1974), Seligman (1975), and Seligman and Beagley (1975).

Leboyer (1974) presents a beautifully moving discussion of the birth process. See also Miles (in press). Cheek (1975) describes the correlation between trauma at birth and the development of illness. Other discussions of changing attitudes toward the birth process are by Trotter (1975) and the October 1977 issue of *New Age,* published by New Age Communications, 32 Station St., Brookline Village, MA 02146.

Secondary gains are described by Sternbach (1974) and Shealy (1976). The statistics cited by Brena are included in Drew (1976).

A discussion of the interrelationship between genetic predispositions and psychosomatic disease, from an evolutionary point of view, appears in Simeons (1962). Maslow (1966, 1968, 1971) is highly recommended.

Chapter 4 What Can Traditional Medicine Do?

For a detailed examination of governmental expenditures for health care, consult *The Budget of the U.S. Government* (1978).

Weed (1971) discusses the "problem-oriented" approach to diagnosis. To understand medical diagnostic techniques further and how your body works, see Samuels and Bennett (1973). The functioning of the body is also discussed by Stonehouse (1974) and Frank and Frank (1972).

A widely respected work on auricular diagnosis is Nogier (1972). Also see Huang (1974), Nehemkis and Smith (1975), and Oleson, Kroening and Bresler (1978). Further information can be obtained from the German Academy for Auricular Medicine U.S.A., 3904 Bronson Blvd., Kalamazoo, MI 49008.

The validity of hair analysis is substantiated in Rees and Campbell (1974), Brown (1974), Chattopadhyay and Jervis (1974), Gordus (1973), and Hammer, et al. (1971).

The statistics on aspirin consumption are cited by Koenig (1973). Statistics of sleeping pill consumption are from a study by the National Institute on Drug Abuse, reported in "Study Links Sleeping Pills to 5000 Deaths a Year" (1977). The costs of drug promotion are discussed by Rucker (1972). Over-the-counter drug advertising is described by Silverman and Lee (1974). The role of "detail men" is addressed by Stetler (1973) and Silverman and Lee (1974). The number of prescriptions written each year is documented by Silverman and Lee (1974).

The definitive references on drugs—their uses and possible side effects—are Goodman and Gilman (1970) and *Physician's Desk Reference* (1978). (Your doctor receives a new edition of *Physician's Desk Reference* each year; ask him if you can have an old edition.) Other general sources of information on drugs include Breecher (1972), Goode (1972), Zinberg & Robertson (1972), Burack (1975), and DiCyan and Hessman (1972).

Information on poisoning deaths of children with aspirin can be found in Mann (1970). According to Menguy (1970), one out of every seven patients who enter hospital emergency rooms with massive stomach bleeding can attribute this malady to excessive aspirin consumption. Studies on the interaction of aspirin with other drugs is presented by Van Arman (1970). Articles on the consumption and death rate of Valium include Altman (1974), Cant (1976), "Psychiatrist Finds Big Rise in Deaths Linked to Valium" (1976), and "U.S. Ready to Propose Controls on Use of Valium and Librium" (1975). Barbiturate sales and death rates are documented in "Study Links Sleeping Pills to 5000 Deaths a Year" (1977). The effectiveness of sleeping pills is addressed in Kales, et al. (1974) and Kales, et al. (1977). The impact of sleeping pills upon REM sleep is discussed by Kales, et al. (1974).

There are many studies on adverse reactions to drugs, including Hurwitz and Wade (1969), Schimmel (1964), and Shapiro, Slone, Lewis and Jick (1971). The patient consuming twenty-four different drugs is documented by Halpern (1974). Melmon (1971) discusses drug problems in hospitals.

Norman Cousins' complete story of his successful battle against ankylosing spondylitis has been widely reprinted. It appeared originally in the *New England Journal of Medicine* (1976).

Ruedy's hospital studies are numerous, including Ogilvie and Ruedy (1967). Comparisons of the recovery of heart patients can be found in Cochrane (1974) and Mather (1971).

The lucid description of pain associated with dental drilling was provided (with thanks) by George Bernard, D.D.S. The information on nerve blocks was generously provided by Norman Levin, M.D. and Verne Brechner, M.D.

A review of surgical statistics and procedures appears in Rothenberg (1976) and Williams (1971). The mortality rate related to unilateral cordotomy is documented by Foer (1971). The risks of surgery are addressed by Evans (1968) and Gribbin (1972). The American College of Surgeons survey is cited by Gribbin (1972).

Beecher (1961) describes his surgical study with angina patients. A general review of the risks and costs of coronary bypass surgery is presented by Berlowe (1977).

In addition to Frank (1975), a more thorough discussion of the power of faith is available in Frank (1961). Gribbin (1972) documents the frequency of surgery. The report of the Congressional investigation on unnecessary surgery is presented in U.S. House of Representatives Subcommittee on Oversight Investigations (1974). Unnecessary surgery is also discussed by Williams (1971) and Gribbin (1972). Cabot addresses the subject of surgeons in Smith (1938).

Shealy (1976) discusses many of the risks and ramifications of surgery. See also Graham & Cooley (1970) and Williams (1971).

The Stanford study on electrical stimulation is described in "Stimulating the Brain to Prevent Pain" (1975). Shealy (1976) addresses his own research into DCS and TNS.

Sternbach (1974) and Merskey (1967) substantiate the link between pain, anxiety and depression. For a discussion of the role of the psychiatrist in treating the pain patient, see Kahn (1970) and Pilowsky (1976).

Shealy (1976) and Sternbach (1974) are sources for discussions of gains. Szasz (1975) addresses the plight of the pain patient. For a discussion of pain games, consult Shealy (1976), Sternbach (1974), and Berne (1964).

Chapter 5 *What About Unconventional Therapies?*

For a discussion of the benefits of heat, see DeLateur (1974). Cold therapy is described in Courage and Huebsch (1971), Faint (1971), DeLateur (1974), Mennell (1975), and Murphy (1960). Therapeutic pressure and massage is addressed by Beard and Wood (1964), Downing (1970), and Serizawa (1972).

The extent of chiropractic treatment in the United States is documented by Holden (1974). Opposition to chiropractic therapy from the AMA appears in Smith (1970). Sutherland (1975) cites the Cyriax study. The University of Utah study and the statements by Kane appeared in "Chiropractors Found More Understanding" (1974). For a general review of chiropractic therapies, consult Dintenfass (1970).

Orgone therapy is discussed by Reich (1949, 1961, 1970, 1973). Particularly recommended is Mann (1973). See also Boadella (1973), Cattier (1973), and Raknes (1970). Lowen (1966, 1969, 1971, 1972, 1973, 1975a, 1975b) describes Bioenergetics in depth. Nelson (1976) addresses the relationship between headaches and orgone therapy. For information on rolfing, see Rolf (1977) and Johnson (1977).

An explanation of yoga appears in Mishra (1973, 1974), Hittleman (1964, 1969), and Brena (1973). The Alexander and the Feldenkrais techniques are approached in Alexander (1971), Barlow (1973), and Feldenkrais (1949, 1972). Further information on movement can be found in Davis (1972).

Therapeutic touch is described by Montagu (1972) and Thie and Marks (1973). The research reports by Krieger (1975, 1976, in press) are highly recommended.

For a general overview of acupuncture, refer to Bresler, Kroening and Volen (1978a), Volen, Kroening, and Bresler (1978b), Palos (1972), Worsley (1973), Duke (1972), Huard and Wong (1968), McGarey (1974), Manaka and Urquhart (1972), Wallnoffer and von Rottanscher (1965), and Warren (1976).

The comments by Reston (1971) are from *The New York Times*. Diagnosis through acupuncture is reviewed in Kushi (1978), Toguchi (1974), Porkert (1974), and Veith (1949). Tongue diagnosis is discussed by Lu (1977). Information on auricular diagnosis appears in Nogier (1972), Huang (1974), Nehemkis and Smith (1975), and Oleson, Kroening and Bresler (1978). See Wu (1973) for information on Chinese pulse diagnosis.

Recommended acupuncture textbooks include Kao (1973), Matsumoto (1974), Wu (1962), Toguchi (1974), and especially the version written by the Academy of Traditional Chinese Medicine (1975). An English language translation of sections from the *Nei Ching* is authored by Veith (1949).

Research reprints on acupuncture and Chinese medicine appear in the *American*

Journal of Chinese Medicine (P.O. Box 555, Garden City, NY 11530), the *American Journal of Acupuncture* (1400 Lost Acre Dr., Felton, CA 95018), and *Acupuncture and Electrotherapeutics Research* (Pergamon Press, Ltd., Headington Hill Hall, Oxford, England OX30BW). The author's research on acupuncture can be found in Bresler (1973a, 1973b, 1974, 1975, 1977a, 1977b), Bresler, Cohen, Kroening, et al. (1975), Bresler and Kroening (1976a, 1976b), Bresler, Kroening and Volen (1978a, 1978b), Kroening, Volen and Bresler (1978), and Tashkin, et al. (1977).

The relationship between endorphins and acupuncture is addressed by Pomeranz and Chiu (1976), Pomeranz (1977), and Pomeranz, Cheng and Law (1977).

Information about the National Association for Veterinary Acupuncture can be obtained from the organization's headquarters (1905 Sunnycrest Drive, Fullerton, CA 92635). An informative article on acupressure is "Acupuncture: Myth or Miracle?" (1972). See Rosen (1971) for his experiences with acupuncture. For information on acupressure, consult Hart (1977), Cerney (1974), deLangre (1972), Serizawa (1976), Houston (1974), Namikoshi (1969), and Lawson-Wood (1963). Particularly recommended is Chan (1976).

An overview of hypnosis can be found in Morris (1974), Bowers (1976), Dengrove (1976), Powers (1961), and Miller (in press). Textbooks on the subject include Scott (1974) and Cheek and LeCron (1968). Particularly recommended is an outstanding clinical text by Kroger (1963). Early Mesmerism studies are documented by Ludwig (1964), Tomlinson & Perret (1975), and Wester (1976). The dangers of hypnosis are discussed by West and Deckert (1965), Nesbitt (1964), and Conn (1972).

For innovative application of guided imagery techniques, see Seligson (1977), Assagioli (1971), Samuels and Bennett (1973, 1974), Samuels and Samuels (1975), Shorr (1977), Jung (1964), Sommer (1978), McKim (1972), Singer (1975), Simonton and Matthews-Simonton (1978), and Oyle (1973, 1975, 1976). Research reports on imagery are published in the *Journal of Mental Imagery* (% Brandon House, P.O. Box 240, Bronx, NY 10471).

The concept of positive addiction is discussed by Glasser (1975).

General information on stress is included in Selye (1956, 1974), Pelletier (1977), Friedman and Rosenmann (1976), Spielberger and Sarason (1975), Simeons (1961), and Gunderson and Rahe (1974). For research articles, consult *The Journal of Human Stress* (82 Cochituate Road, Framingham, MA 01701).

Relaxation and meditation are discussed in White and Fadiman (1976), LeShan (1975), Benson (1976), Trungpa (1969), Walker (1975), Jacobson (1938, 1976), Shealy (1977), and Bloomfield, Cain, Jaffe and Kory (1975). Impressive studies on Transcendental Meditation were conducted by Wallace and Benson (1972).

For general references on autogenic training, see Pelletier (1977), Luthe (1969), Schultz and Luthe (1969), Lindemann (1973), and Rosa (1976). The use of autogenic training in pain therapy is described by Mitch, et al. (1976) and Sargent, et al. (1975).

An overview of research into biofeedback training is presented by Brown (1975), Pelletier (1975, and in press), Wickramasekera (1976), Barber (1972), and Karlins and Andrews (1973). Specific studies related to biofeedback and pain include Kentsmith, et al. (1976), Gessel (1975), Carlsson, Gale and Ohman

(1975), Medina, Diamond and Franklin (1976), Turin and Johnson (1976), Adler and Adler (1976), Budzynski and Stoyva (1969), Montgomery and Ehrisman (1976). Also see Werbach (1974) and Oliver (1976). Research reports on biofeedback can be found in the journal, *Biofeedback and Self-Regulation* (Plenum Publishing Co., 227 W. 17th St., New York, NY 10011).

General information on nutrition is presented in Arnow (1972), Davis (1954), Lappe (1971), and Rodale (in press). A discussion of the relative merits of breakfast cereals appears in "The Breakfast of What?" (1970). Food additives are discussed by Longgood (1969), Winter (1972), Verrett (1974), Jacobson (1972), Jenkins (1977), and Feingold (1968, 1974).

For information on various types of counseling, consult Jaffe (1979), Ferber, et al. (1972), Minuchin (1974), Kovel (1976), and Haley (1966).

The definitive works on faith healing and the placebo effect are Beecher (1955, 1959), Frank (1961), and more recently, Cousins (1977), Frank (1975), and Byerly (1976). Also see Shealy (1975) and Lasagna, et al. (1954). The article by Frank (1975) contains his commencement address. For a discussion of placebos and endorphins, consult *Science News* (1978).

Holistic medicine is addressed in Pelletier (1977) and Bloomfield and Kory (1978). Also see the *Holistic Health Review* (published by the Holistic Health Organizing Committee, P.O. Box 166, Berkeley, CA 94701), and the *New Health Catalyst* (published by Healthnet, P.O. Box 367, Mountain View, CA 94042). Also, consult the special Holistic Medicine issue of *New Realities* (2:1).

A discussion of bloodletting appears in "Blood-Letting and Purging" (1975).

Information concerning the developing field of integral medicine is available from the Center for Integral Medicine (P.O. Box 967, Pacific Palisades, CA 90272).

Chapter 6 What Can You Do to Help?

Pioneering work on the use of hypnosis as a surgical anesthetic has been conducted by Kroger (1960, 1963). Also see Doberneck (1959), Gentry (1960), Khalil (1976), Kroger and DeLee (1957), Mahren (1960), Marmer (1959), Mason (1955), and Werbel (1960).

Early studies exploring the physiological actions of morphine are described by Restak (1977). The relationship between morphine, periaqueductal gray matter (PAGM) stimulation, and pain was studied by Liebeskind (1976) and his colleagues and is summarized by Marx (1977).

Opiate (morphine) receptors were identified by Snyder (1977) and reported by Restak (1977). Endorphins were first reported by Goldstein (1976).

Pomeranz's research concerning endorphins and acupuncture can be found in Pomeranz and Chiu (1976), Pomeranz (1977), and Pomeranz, Cheng and Law (1977). The relationship of endorphins to the placebo effect has been reported in "Pain: Placebo Effect Linked to Endorphins" (1978).

For a fascinating explanation of the world inside the mind, see Lilly (1972, 1973, 1975). Discussions of locus of control appear in Hiroto (1974), Phares (1973, 1975), and Calhoun, Cheney and Dawes (1974). Highly recommended is a delightful book of insights by Brenner (1978).

The process of "nonidentification" with thoughts, emotions and sensations is discussed thoroughly in the writings of Gurdjieff (1950, 1963) and Ouspensky (1949, 1971a, 1971b, 1974). These readings are suggested for those interested in pursuing an extraordinary approach to understanding the nature of human consciousness.

For a unique approach to achieving self-awareness, see Ram Dass (1971, 1974, 1977).

Chapter 7 The Pause That Refreshes

The description of man as part of his universe is in Thomas (1974). Studies linking cancer to stress include Greene (1966). See also Greene and Miller (1958). See LeShan (1959, 1961, 1966) for reports of his cancer-related research.

Kissen (1967) describes his study with lung cancer patients. See also Kissen (1966). Pendergrass (1959) articulates his philosophy regarding psychological stress and cancer. A highly recommended book that covers these subjects is Simonton, et al. (1978).

Discussions of the link between stress and the diseases of civilization are included in Pelletier (1977), and Friedman and Rosenmann (1974). Dunbar (1974) presents his own findings on stress and disease.

Studies related to the "Schedule of Recent Experience" are included in Holmes and Masuda (1973) and Holmes and Rahe (1967a, 1967b). The Navy shipyard study is described in Rahe (1973). Cobb's research is addressed in Fier (1975).

General information on stress can be found in Selye (1956, 1974), Pelletier (1977), Spielberger and Sarason (1975), Simeons (1961), and Gunderson and Rahe (1974).

Studies citing the positive effects of relaxation on migraine and chronic tension headaches include Hay and Madders (1971) and Warner and Lance (1975).

The purpose, benefits and physiological processes of sleep are discussed by Trubo (1978) and Dement (1972). Dalmane was studied by Kales, et al. (1974) and Kales, et al. (1977).

General information on relaxation and meditation can be found in White and Fadiman (1976), Benson (1976), Jacobson (1938, 1976), Shealy (1977), and Bloomfield, Cain, Jaffe and Kory (1975). See Pavlov (1927) for a detailed explanation of his classic studies. The subject of yoga is addressed in Mishra (1973, 1974), Hittleman (1964, 1969), and Brena (1973).

Chapter 8 You Are What You Eat

Longgood (1969) and Arnow (1972) discuss additives extensively. Also see Mayer (1977) and Jenkins and Jenkins (1977). Arnow (1972) presents various statistics on additive consumption.

The GRAS list is discussed by Hopkins (1978). Feingold (1974) is also quoted in Jenkins and Jenkins (1977). Yudkin (1972) presents an array of information concerning sugar consumption.

For a detailed discussion of vitamins, consult Page and Abrams (1972), Rodale (1968), Null and Null (1972), and Arnow (1972). A thorough examination of minerals is presented in Rodale (1972), Page and Abrams (1972), Null and Null (1972), and Arnow (1972). See also the special minerals issue of Bestways (May 1978).

Vitamin C is explored in depth by Lewin (1976). Highly recommended is Pauling (1971). For a discussion of vitamin C as a treatment for cancer, see Pauling (1977) and Cameron and Pauling (1976).

An excellent overview of tryptophan is Feltman (1976), which cites many of the most significant studies of this amino acid. See also Jensen (1975), Blakeslee (1978), Hartmann (1967), and Clark (1978).

Chapter 9 It Never Hurts When You Laugh

Laughter is discussed in Cross and Cross (1977). Depression and its ramifications are discussed by Lowen (1972), Beck (1967), and Kushner (1978).

Highly recommended are the works of Maslow (1966, 1968, 1970, 1971). For guidance toward heightened sexual satisfaction, refer to Masters and Johnson (1966, 1970), Comfort (1972), and Kaplan (1975). For ideas on raising your serum fun level, see Yee (1974).

The subject of touching and human contact is addressed by Colton (1977), Montagu (1972), Thie and Marks (1973), and Kreiger (1975, 1976, in press). Massage techniques are discussed by Downing (1970), Serizawa (1972), and Beard and Wood (1964).

For an excellent book on innovative approaches to child rearing, see Bricklin (1975).

Chapter 10 Expanding Your Mind's Eye Through Guided Imagery

There are many excellent sources for information about imagery. Among the best are Oyle (1973, 1975, 1976), Simonton, et al. (1978), Schorr (1977), McKim (1972), Samuels and Bennett (1973, 1974), Samuels and Samuels (1975), Singer (1975), Richardson (1969), and Kroger and Fezler (1976). The technique of implosion is described by Astrup (1975).

Herrick (1956) computed the number of possible connections in the brain. The left and right hemispheres of the brain are discussed by Corballis and Beale (1976), Goleman (1977), Sage (1976), Buck (1976), Trotter (1976), and "The Right Brain: Surviving Retardation" (1977).

Many of the ideas in this chapter concerning the subjects of attention and consciousness were drawn from the writings of Gurdjieff (1950, 1963) and Ouspensky (1949, 1971a, 1971b, 1974).

Additional information on "organ language" appears in Cheek (1975). A well-documented history of imagery is presented by Samuels and Samuels (1975).

For a veritable catalog of guided imagery exercises, also see Kroger and Fezler (1976).

Chapter 11 Your Inner Adviser

For other applications of the inner adviser techniques, see Samuels and Bennett (1973, 1974) and Oyle (1973, 1975, 1976).

An interesting example of the use of guided imagery with insomniac children is described in Porter (1975).

Chapter 12 Pain, Pleasure, and Love

The statement on the transformational process is from Fromm (1956). Some honest and sensitive reflections upon the love experience appear in Paul and Paul (1975).

The quote from Lyon appears in Greenburg (1977). Knowles was quoted in Cooper (1977).

Bibliography

Academy of Traditional Chinese Medicine. 1975. *An Outline of Chinese Acupuncture.* Peking: Foreign Languages Press.

"Acupuncture: Myth or Miracle?" 1972. *Newsweek* 79:48-52.

Adler, C.S., and Adler, S.M. 1976. "Biofeedback Psychotherapy for the Treatment of Headaches: A 5-Year Follow-up." *Headache* 16:189-91.

Alexander, F.M. 1971. *The Resurrection of the Body.* New York: Dell Publishing Co., Inc.

Altman, L.K. 1974. "Valium, the Most Prescribed Drug." *The New York Times,* 19 May 1974, p. 1.

Anderson, M., and Savary, L. 1973. *Passages: A Guide for Pilgrims of the Mind.* New York: Harper & Row, Pub., Inc.

Arnow, L.E. 1972. *Food Power.* Chicago: Nelson-Hall Publishers.

Arthritis Foundation 1976. *Arthritis, the Basic Facts.* Atlanta: The Arthritis Foundation.

Assagioli, R. 1971. *Psychosynthesis.* New York: The Viking Press.

Astrup, C. 1975. "Psychological Mechanisms of Flooding (Implosion) Therapy." *Psychotherapy and Psychosomatics* 25:63-68.

Ballantine, H.T. 1972. "Will the Delivery of Health Care Be Improved by the Use of Chiropractic Services?" *New England Journal of Medicine* 286:237-242.

Barber, T.X., et al., eds. 1972. *Biofeedback and Self-Control.* Chicago: Aldine Publishing Co.

Barclay, W.R. 1976. "Unnecessary Surgery." *Journal of the American Medical Association* 236:387-88.

Barlow, W. 1973. *The Alexander Technique.* New York: Alfred A. Knopf, Inc.

Beard, G., and Wood, E. 1964. *Massage: Principles and Techniques.* Philadelphia: W.B. Saunders Co.

Beau, G. 1972. *Chinese Medicine.* New York: Avon Books.

Beck, A.T. 1967. *Depression: Clinical, Experimental, and Theoretical Aspects.* New York: Harper & Row, Pub., Inc.

Becker, R. 1963a. "The Biological Effects of Magnetic Fields: A Survey." *Medical Electronics and Biological Engineering* 1:293.

——— 1963b. "Relationship of Geomagnetic Environments to Human Biology." *New York State Journal of Medicine* 63:2215.

———1969. "The Effect of Magnetic Fields upon the Central Nervous System." In *Biological Effects of Magnetic Fields*, vol. 2, ed. M.F. Barnothy. New York: Plenum Publishing Corp.

Beecher, H.K. 1946. "Pain in Men Wounded in Battle." *Annals of Surgery* 123:96.

————1955. "The Powerful Placebo." *Journal of the American Medical Association* 159:1602-06.

————1959. *Measurement of Subjective Responses*. New York: Oxford University Press.

————1961. "Surgery as a Placebo." *Journal of the American Medical Association* 176:1102.

Belknap, M.M.; Blau, R.A.; and Grossman, R.N. 1975. *Case Studies and Methods in Humanistic Medical Care*. San Francisco: The Institute for the Study of Humanistic Medicine.

Benson, H. 1975. *The Relaxation Response*. New York: William Morrow & Co., Inc.

Bentall, R. 1976. "Healing by Electromagnetism—Fact or Fiction." *New Scientist*, 22 April 1976, 166-67.

Berlowe, R. 1977. "Coronary Bypass Surgery Will Not Prolong Life." *Caveat Emptor*, 7 February 1977, p. 3.

Berne, E. 1964. *Games People Play*. New York: Grove Press, Inc.

Bieler, H.G. 1965. *Food Is Your Best Medicine*. New York: Random House, Inc.

Blakeslee, A. 1978. "Studies Find Some Foods Affect Brain." *Los Angeles Times*, 9 April 1978, p. 2.

"Blood-Letting and Purging." 1975. *South African Medical Journal* 49: 1945-46.

Bloomfield, H.H.; Cain, M.P.; Jaffe, D.T.; and Kory, R.B. 1975. *TM: Discovering Inner Energy and Overcoming Stress*. New York: Delacorte Press.

Bloomfield, H.H., and Kory, R.B. 1978. *Health and Happiness: A New Approach to Complete Lifetime Wellness*. New York: Simon & Schuster.

Boadella, D. 1973. *Wilhelm Reich: The Evolution of his Work*. Chicago: Henry Regnery Co.

Bowers, K.S. 1976. *Hypnosis for the Seriously Curious*. Monterey, California: Brooks/Cole Publishing Co.

"The Breakfast of What?" 1970. *Newsweek*, 3 August 1970, p. 57-58.

Breecher, E.M. 1972. *Licit and Illicit Drugs*. Mount Vernon, New York: Consumers Union.

Brena, S.F. 1973. *Yoga and Medicine*. Baltimore, Maryland: Pelican Publishing Co., Inc.

Brenner, P. 1978. *Health Is a Question of Balance*. New York: Vantage Press, Inc.

Bresler, D.E. 1973a. "A Comparison of the Effects of Systemic and Local Anesthetic Drugs, Hypnosis and Acupuncture." In *Proceedings of the NIH Acupuncture Conference*, DHEW Publication no. 74-165.

————. 1973b. "Acupuncture in Oral Surgery." In *Proceedings of the NIH Acupuncture Conference*, DHEW Publication no. 74-165.

————. 1974. "Acupuncture and Hypnosis: A Comment." *Psychoenergetic Systems* 1:20.

————. 1975. "Scientific Approaches to the Study of Acupuncture Therapy." In *The Energies of Consciousness*, eds. S. Krippner and D. Rubin. New York: Gordon & Breach.

————. 1977a. "Acupuncture & American Physicians: A Comment." *Psychoenergetic Systems* 2:275.

————. 1977b. "Acupuncture, Taoist Thought and Healing." *Journal of Holistic Health* 2:66-69.

————. 1978. "Self-Control of Pain: The Use of Relaxation Training and Guided Imagery in a Self-Help Pain Control Program." *Pain Abstracts* 1:36.

Bresler, D.E.; Cohen, J.S.; Kroening, R.J.; et al. 1975. "The Potential of Acupuncture for the Behavioral Sciences." *American Psychologist* 3:411-14.

Bresler, D.E., and Kroening, R.J. 1976a. "Acupuncture: A Multidetermined Phenomenon." *Psychoenergetic Systems* 1:137-39.

————. 1976b. "Three Essential Factors in Effective Acupuncture Therapy." *American Journal of Chinese Medicine* 4:81-86.

Bresler, D.E.; Kroening, R.J.; and Volen, M.P. 1978a. *Acupuncture: Can It Help?* Pacific Palisades, California: Center for Integral Medicine.

————. 1978b. "Acupuncture in America." In *Healing Source Contact Directory*, ed. L. Kaslof. New York: Doubleday & Co., Inc.

Bresler, D.E., and Wisne, P.L. 1973. *Acupuncture: A Selected Bibliography*. Los Angeles: National Acupuncture Association.

Bricklin, A. *Mother Love*. Philadelphia: Running Press.

Brodeur, P. 1977. *The Zapping of America*. New York: W.W. Norton & Co., Inc.

Brooks, C. 1974. *Sensory Awareness: The Rediscovery of Experiencing*. New York: The Viking Press.

Brown, A.C. 1974. *The First Human Hair Symposium*. New York: Medcom Press.

Brown, B. 1974. *New Mind, New Body—Biofeedback: New Directions for the Mind*. New York: Harper & Row, Pub. Inc.

Buck, C. 1976. "Knowing the Left from the Right." *Human Behavior*, June 1978, pp. 29-35.

The Budget of the U.S. Government, Fiscal Year 1979. 1978. Washington, D.C.: United States Government Printing Office.

Budzynski, T.H., and Stoyva, J.M. 1969. "An Instrument for Producing Deep Muscle Relaxation by Means of Analog Information Feedback." *Journal of Applied Behavioral Analysis* 2:231-37.

Burr, H.S. 1972. *The Fields of Life*. New York: Ballantine Books, Inc.

Burton, C. 1972. "Neurosurgical Treatment of Intractable Pain." *Pennsylvania Medicine* 75:53.

Byerly, H. 1976. "Explaining and Exploiting Placebo Effects." *Perspectives in Biology and Medicine* 2:423-36.

Cady, J.W. 1976. "Dear Pain." *American Journal of Nursing* 76:960-61.

Calhoun, L.G.; Cheney, T.; and Dawes, A.S. 1974. "Locus of Control, Self-Reported Depression, and Perceived Causes of Depression." *Journal of Consulting and Clinical Psychology* 42:736.

Cameron, E., and Pauling, L. 1976. "Supplemental Ascorbate in the Supportive Treatment of Cancer I. Prolongation of Survival Times in Terminal Human Cancer." *Proceedings of the National Academy of Sciences USA* 73:3685-89.

Cant, G. 1976. "Valiumania." *The New York Times*, 21 February 1976, pp. 34-44.

Capra, F. 1975. *The Tao of Physics*. Berkeley, California: Shambhala Publications, Inc.

Carlson, R.J. 1975. *The End of Medicine*. New York: Wiley-Interscience.

Carlsson, S.G.; Gale, E.N.; and Ohman, A. 1975. "Treatment of Temporomandibular Joint Syndrome with Biofeedback Training." *Journal of the American Dental Association* 91:602-05.

Carter, L.J. 1977. "Seafarer: Project Still Homeless as Milliken Says No to Navy." *Science* 197:964-68.

Cattier, M. 1973. *The Life and Work of Wilhelm Reich.* New York: Avon Books.

Cerney, J.V. 1974. *Acupuncture Without Needles.* West Nyack, New York: Parker Publishing Co.

Chan, P. 1974. *Electro-Acupuncture.* Alhambra, California: Chan's Books.

Chan, P. 1976. *Finger Acupressure.* Alhambra, California: Chan's Books.

Chattopadhyay, A., and Jervis, R. 1974. "Hair as an Indication of Multi-Element Exposure of Population Groups." *Trace Substances in Environmental Health— VIII.* Columbia, Missouri: University of Missouri.

Cheek, D.B. 1959. "Unconscious Perception of Meaningful Sounds During Surgical Anesthesia as Revealed under Hypnosis." *American Journal of Clinical Hypnosis* 1:101-13.

———. 1960. "What Does the Surgically Anesthetized Patient Hear?" *Rocky Mountain Medical Journal* 57:49-53.

———. 1961. "Unconscious Reactions and Surgical Risk." *Western Journal of Surgery, Obstetrics and Gynecology* 69:325-27.

———. 1962a. "The Anesthetized Patient Can Hear and Remember." *American Journal of Proctology* 13:287-90.

———. 1962b. "Areas of Research into Psychosomatic Aspects of Surgical Tragedies Now Open Through Use of Hypnosis and Ideomotor Questionings." *Western Journal of Surgery, Obstetrics and Gynecology* 70:137-42.

———. 1962c. "Importance of Recognizing that Surgical Patients Behave as Though Hypnotized." *American Journal of Clinical Hypnosis* 4:227-36.

———. 1964. "Surgical Memory and Reaction to Careless Conversation." *American Journal of Clinical Hypnosis* 6:237-40.

———. 1975. "Maladjustment Patterns Apparently Related to Imprinting at Birth." *American Journal of Clinical Hypnosis* 18:75-82.

Cheek, D.B., and LeCron, L.M. 1968. *Clinical Hypnotherapy.* New York: Grune & Stratton, Inc.

Cherkin, A., and Harroun, P. 1971. "Anesthesia and Memory Processes." *Anesthesiology* 34:469-74.

"Chiropractors Found More Understanding." 1974. *Los Angeles Times*, 31 July 1974, p. 8.

Christie, A. 1968. *Chinese Mythology.* London, New York, Sydney and Toronto: Hamlyn House.

Clark, M. 1978. "Obsessive–Compulsive Behavior Linked to Low Serotonin Levels." *Medical Tribune*, 21 June 1978; p. 19.

Cochrane, A.L. 1974. *Effectiveness and Efficiency: Random Reflections on Health Services.* London: Nuffield Provincial Hospital Trust.

Cohen, D. 1975. "Magnetic Fields of the Human Body." *Physics Today* 28:34-43.

Colton, H. 1977. "Touch: It's as Vital as Food." *Forum*, December 1977, pp. 30-34.

Cooper, K. 1977. *The Aerobics Way.* New York: M. Evans Co., Inc.

Corballis, M.C., and Beale, I.L. 1976. *The Psychology of Left and Right.* Hillsdale, New Jersey: Lawrence Erlbaum Associates.

Courage, G.R., and Huebsch, R.F. 1971. "Cold Therapy Revisited." *Journal of the American Dental Association* 83:1070-73.

Cousins, N. 1976. "Anatomy of an Illness." *New England Journal of Medicine* 295:1457-62.

Cowgill, U.M. 1966. "Season of Birth in Man." *Ecology* 47:614-23.

Crile, G. 1976. "A New Way to Identify 'Inappropriate' Surgery Offered." *American Medical News*, 16 February 1976, pp. 11-12.

Critchley, M. 1956. "Congenital Indifference to Pain." *Annals of Internal Medicine* 45:737.

Cross, F., and Cross, W. 1977. "Cheers! A Belly Laugh Can Help You Stay Well." *Science Digest*, November 1977, pp. 15-20.

Dalén, P. 1975. *Season of Birth*. Amsterdam: North Holland Publishing Co.

Davies, P.C.W. 1977. *Space and Time in the Modern Universe*. Cambridge: Cambridge University Press.

Davis, A. 1954. *Let's Eat Right to Keep Fit*. New York: Harcourt Brace Jovanovich, Inc.

———. 1965. *Let's Get Well*. New York: Harcourt Brace Jovanovich, Inc.

Davis, A.R. and Rawls, W.C. 1974. *Magnetism and Its Effects on the Living System*. Hicksville, New York: Exposition Press.

———. 1975. *The Magnetic Effect*. Hicksville, New York: Exposition Press.

Davis, M. 1972. *Understanding Body Movement*. New York: Arno Press, Inc.

DeGroot, A., and Bresler, D.E. 1974. "Acupuncture: A Pilot Trial in Horses." *Journal of the American Veterinary Association* 164:367.

DeLangre, J. 1972. *Do-In*. Magila, California: Happiness Press.

DeLateur, B. 1974. "The Role of Physical Medicine in Problems of Pain." *Advances in Neurology* 4:495-97.

Delza, S. 1972. *T'ai Chi Ch'uan: An Ancient Chinese Way of Exercise to Achieve Health and Tranquillity*. New York: Cornerstone Library, Inc.

Dement, W. C. 1972. *Some Must Watch While Some Must Sleep*. San Francisco: W.H. Freeman & Co., Pub.

Dengrove, E. 1976. *Hypnosis and Behavior Therapy*. Springfield, Illinois: Charles C. Thomas, Pub.

Dintenfass, J. 1970. *Chiropractic: A Modern Way to Health*. New York: Pyramid Books.

Doberneck, R.C., et al. 1959. "Hypnosis as an Adjunct to Surgical Therapy." *Surgery* 46:299-304.

Dorland's Illustrated Medical Dictionary 1974. Philadelphia, London and Toronto: W.B. Saunders Co.

Downing, G. 1970. *The Massage Book*. New York: Random House, Inc.

Drew, C. 1976. "At New Pain Clinics, Groups of Specialists Aid Chronic Sufferers." *Wall Street Journal*, 13 September 1976, p. 1.

Dubos, R. 1959. *Mirage of Health*. New York: Doubleday & Co., Inc.

———. 1968. *Man, Medicine and Environment*. New York: Mentor Books.

Duke, M. 1972. *Acupuncture*. Moonachie, New Jersey: Pyramid Publications.

Dunbar, F. 1947. *Emotions and Bodily Changes*. New York: Columbia University Press.

Dychtwald, K. 1977. *Body Mind*. New York: Pantheon Books, Inc.

"Environmental Allergies." 1976. *Science Digest*, October 1976, pp. 15-16.

Ervin, F.R., and Sternbach, R.A. 1960. "Hereditary Insensitivity to Pain." *Transactions of the American Neurological Association* 85:70.

Evans, H.E. 1968. "Tonsillectomy and Adenoidectomy: Review of Published Evidence for and Against T. & A." *Clinical Pediatrics* 7:71-75.

Everson, T.C., and Cole, W.H. 1966. *Spontaneous Repression of Cancer.* Philadelphia: W.B. Saunders Co.

Faint, J. 1971. "Cold Comfort—for Alleviation of Pain." *Nursing Mirror* 132:32-33.

Farbman, A.A. 1973. "Neck Sprain, Associated Factors." *Journal of the American Medical Association* 223:9.

Feingold, B.F. 1968. "Recognition of Food Additives as a Cause of Symptoms of Allergy." *Annals of Allergy* 26:309-13.

——. 1974. *Why Your Child Is Hyperactive.* New York: Random House, Inc.

Feldenkrais, M. 1949. *Body and Mature Behavior: A Study of Anxiety, Sex, Gravitation and Learning.* New York: International Universities Press.

——. 1972. *Awareness Through Movement: Health Exercises for Personal Growth.* New York: Harper & Row, Pub., Inc.

Feltman, J. 1976. "Tryptophan—A New Natural Weapon Against Depression and Sleeplessness." *Prevention* 28:55-60.

Ferber, A.; Mendelsohn, M.; and Napier, A., eds. 1972. *The Book of Family Therapy.* New York: Science House.

Ferguson, M. 1973. *The Brain Revolution.* New York: Bantam Books, Inc.

Fier, B. 1975. "Recession Is Causing Dire Illness." *Moneysworth*, 23 June 1975.

Foer, W. H. 1971. "Percutaneous Cervical Radiofrequency Cordotomy." *The Journal of the Medical Society of New Jersey* 68:737-41.

Folkard, S.; Glynn, C.J.; and Lloyd, J.W. 1976. "Diurnal Variation and Individual Differences in the Perception of Intractable Pain." *Journal of Psychosomatic Research* 20:289-301.

Frank, A., and Frank, S. 1972. *The People's Handbook of Medical Care.* New York: Random House, Inc.

Frank, J.D. 1961. *Persuasion and Healing.* Baltimore: Johns Hopkins Press.

——. 1975. "The Faith that Heals." *The Johns Hopkins Medical Journal* 137:127-31.

Freese, A. 1974. *Pain.* New York: G.P. Putnam's Sons.

Friedberg, J. 1976. *Shock Treatment Is Not Good for Your Brain.* San Francisco: Glide Publications.

Friedman, M., and Rosenman, R. H. 1974. *Type A Behavior and Your Heart.* New York: Alfred A. Knopf, Inc.

Friedson, E. 1970. *Profession of Medicine.* New York: Dodd, Mead & Co.

Fromm, E. 1956. *The Art of Loving.* New York: Bantam Books, Inc.

Fung, Yu-Lan. 1958. *A Short History of Chinese Philosophy.* New York: Macmillan, Inc.

Galaburda, A.M.; LeMay, M.; Kemper, T.L.; and Geschwind, N. 1978. "Right–Left Asymmetries in the Brain." *Science* 199:852-56.

Gallert, M.L. 1966. *New Light on Therapeutic Energies.* London: James Clarke & Co.

Gary-Cobb, G. 1974. *The Miracle of New Avatar Power.* West Nyack, New Jersey: Parker Publishing Co.

Gentry, R.W. 1960. *Hypnosis in Surgery.* Paper delivered at the Pan American Medical Association, 10 May 1960.

Gessel, A.H. 1975. "Electromyographic Biofeedback and Tricyclic Antidepressants in Myofascial Pain-Dysfunction Syndrome: Psychological Predicters of Outcome." *Journal of the American Dental Association* 91:1048-52.

Glasser, W. 1975. *Positive Addiction*. New York: Harper & Row, Pub., Inc.

Glynn, C.J.; Lloyd, J.W.; and Folkard, S. 1976. "The Diurnal Variation in Perception of Pain." *Proceedings of the Royal Society of Medicine* 69:369-72.

Goldstein, A. 1976. "Opioid Peptides (Endorphins) in Pituitary and Brain." *Science* 193:1081.

Goleman, D. 1977. "Split-Brain Psychology: Fad of the Year." *Psychology Today,* October 1977, pp. 89-90, 149-51.

Gonda, T.A. 1962. "The Relationship Between Complaints of Persistent Pain & Family Size." *Journal of Neurology, Neurosurgery and Psychiatry* 25: 277-81.

Goode, E. 1972. *Drugs in American Society*. New York: Alfred A. Knopf, Inc.

Gordon, J.; Jaffe, D.; and Bresler, D.E., eds. 1978. *Mind, Body & Health: Toward an Integral Medicine*. Bethesda, Maryland: National Institute of Mental Health in cooperation with the Center for Integral Medicine, Pacific Palisades, California.

Gordus, A. 1973. "Factors Affecting the Trace-Metal Content of Human Hair." *Journal of Radioanalytical Chemistry* 15:229-43.

Grad, B. 1967. "The Laying-on of Hands: Implications for Psychotherapy, Gentling, and the Placebo Effect." *Journal of the American Society of Psychical Research* 61:286-305.

Graham, J., and Cooley, D.G. 1970. *So You're Going to Have Surgery*. New York: Hawthorn Books, Inc.

Greenberg, J. 1977. "Take Two Milkbone and Call Me in the Morning." *Science News*, 8 October 1977, p. 237.

Greenburg, D., with Jacobs, M. 1966. *How to Make Yourself Miserable*. New York: Random House, Inc.

Greene, W.A. 1966. "The Psychosocial Setting of the Development of Leukemia and Lymphoma." *Psychophysiological Aspects of Cancer*. E.M. Weyer and H. Hutchins, eds. New York: New York Academy of Sciences, pp. 794-801.

Greene, W.A., and Miller, G. 1958. "Psychosocial Factors and Reticuloendothelial Disease. Observations on a Group of Children and Adolescents with Leukemia. An Interpretation of Disease Development in Terms of the Mother–Child Unit." *Psychosomatic Medicine* 20:124-44.

Gribbin, A. 1972. "Senseless Surgery." *National Observer*, 29 July 1972, p. 1.

Guillemin, R. 1977. "Endorphins, Brain Peptides that Act like Opiates." *New England Journal of Medicine* 296:226-28.

Gunderson, E., and Rahe, R. 1974. *Life Stress and Illness*. Springfield, Illinois: Charles C. Thomas, Pub.

Gurdjieff, G.I. 1950. *Beelzebub's Tales to His Grandson, Books 1, 2, 3*. New York: E.P. Dutton & Co., Inc.

―――. 1963. *Meetings with Remarkable Men*. New York: E.P. Dutton & Co., Inc.

Haley, J. 1966. *Strategies of Psychotherapy*. New York: Grune & Stratton, Inc.

Halpern, L.M. 1974. "Psychotropic Drugs and the Management of Chronic Pain." *Advances in Neurology*. New York: Raven Press.

Hammer, D., et al. 1971. "Hair Trace Metal Levels and Environmental Exposure." *American Journal of Epidemiology* 93:84.

Hare, E.H. 1975. "Season of Birth in Schizophrenia and Neurosis." *American Journal of Psychiatry* 132:1168-71.

Hare, E.H., and Price, J.S. 1969. "Mental Disorder and Season of Birth:

Comparison of Psychoses with Neurosis." *British Journal of Psychiatry* 115:533-40.

Hare, E.H.; Price, J.S.; and Slater, E. 1974. "Mental Disorder and Season of Birth: A National Sample Compared with the General Population." *British Journal of Psychiatry* 124:81-86.

Harris, S. 1964. *The Econimics of American Medicine.* New York: Macmillan, Inc.

Hart, L.A. 1977. *Anybody Can Do It: Acupressure.* New York, New York: Lynn Mark Library.

Hartmann, E.L. 1967. "The Effect of L-tryptophan on the Sleep and Dream Cycle in Man." *Psychonomic Sciences* 8:479-80.

Hay, K.M., and Madders, J. 1971. "Migraine Treated by Relaxation Therapy." *Journal of the Royal College of General Practitioners* 21:664.

Hebb, D.O. 1949. *The Organization of Behavior.* New York: Wiley.

———. 1955. "Drives and the C.N.S. (Conceptual Nervous System)." *Psychological Review* 62:243-54.

———. 1958. *A Textbook of Psychology.* Philadelphia: W.B. Saunders Co.

Heisenberg, W. 1958. *Physics and Philosophy.* New York: Harper Torchbooks.

Herndon, J.H., and Freeman, R.G. 1976. "Human Disease Associated with Exposure to Light." *Annual Review of Medicine* 27:77-87.

Herrick, C.J. 1956. *The Evolution of Human Nature.* Austin: University of Texas Press.

Hill, G. 1975. "Ultrahigh-Voltage Lines Studied as Possible Peril." *The New York Times*, 10 November 1975, pp. 1, 65.

Hiroto, D.S. 1974. "Locus of Control and Learned Helplessness." *Journal of Experimental Psychology* 102:187-93.

Hittleman, R.L. 1964. *Yoga for Physical Fitness.* Englewood Cliffs, New Jersey: Prentice-Hall, Inc.

———. 1969. *Introduction to Yoga.* New York: Bantam Books, Inc.

Holden, C. 1974. "Chiropractic: Healing or Hokum? HEW is Looking for Answers." *Science* 185: 922-25.

Holmes, T.H., and Masuda, M. 1973. "Life Change and Illness Susceptibility, Separation and Depression." *American Academy for the Advancement of Science*, pp. 161-86.

Holmes, T.H., and Rahe, R.H. 1967a. "Schedule of Recent Experience (SRE)." Department of Psychiatry, University of Washington School of Medicine.

———. 1967b. "The Social Readjustment Rating Scale." *Journal of Psychosomatic Research* 11:213-18.

Hopkins, H. 1978. "The GRAS List Revisited." *FDA Consumer*, May 1978, pp. 13-15.

Houston, F.M. 1974. *The Healing Benefits of Acupressure.* New Canaan, Connecticut: Keats Publishing Co.

Huang, H.L., trans. 1974. *Ear Acupuncture.* Emmaus, Pennsylvania: Rodale Press.

Huard, P., and Wong, M. 1968. *Chinese Medicine.* New York: McGraw-Hill, Inc.

Hurwitz, N., and Wade, O.L. 1969. "Intensive Hospital Monitoring of Adverse Reactions to Drugs." *British Medical Journal* 1:531.

Illich, I. 1976. *Medical Nemesis.* New York: Pantheon Books, Inc.

"It's Time to Take Chiropractors Seriously." 1975. *Medical Economics*, 28 April 1975, p. 24.

Jacobson, E. 1938. *Progressive Relaxation.* Chicago: University of Chicago Press.

―――. 1976. *You Must Relax.* New York: McGraw-Hill, Inc.

Jacobson, M. 1972. *Eater's Digest.* New York: Doubleday & Co., Inc.

Jaffe, D.T. 1979. *Healing from Within.* New York: Alfred A. Knopf, Inc.

―――. "Family Therapy and Physical Illness." *Mind, Body and Health: Toward an Integral Medicine,* eds. J. Gordon, D. Jaffe, and D. Bresler, Pacific Palisades, California: Center for Integral Medicine.

Jaffe, D.T., and Bresler, D.E. 1978. "Diagnostic & Therapeutic Applications of Guided Imagery." In *Mind, Body & Health: Toward an Integral Medicine,* eds. J. Gordon, D. Jaffe & D. Bresler. Bethesda, Maryland: National Institute of Mental Health in cooperation with the Center for Integral Medicine, Pacific Palisades, California.

Janov, A. 1970. *The Primal Scream.* New York: Dell Publishing Co., Inc.

―――. 1971. *The Anatomy of Mental Illness.* New York: G.P. Putnam's Sons.

Janov, A., and Holden, E.M. 1975. *Primal Man: The New Consciousness.* New York: Thomas Y. Crowell Co., Inc.

Jenkins, J., and Jenkins, J. 1977. "The Chemical Fast." *Environmental Action,* 19 November 1977, pp. 4-7.

Jensen, K. 1975. "Tryptophan/Imipramine in Depression." *The Lancet* 2:920.

Johnson, D. 1977. *The Protean Body.* New York: Harper and Row, Pub., Inc.

Juby, M. 1977. "Noise—A Serious Health Problem." *Life and Health,* September 1977, pp. 9-11.

Jung, C. 1964. *Man and His Symbols.* New York: Doubleday & Co., Inc.

―――. 1972. *The Portable Jung.* Edited by Joseph Campbell. Translated by R.F.C. Hull. New York: The Viking Press.

―――. 1973. *On the Nature of the Psyche.* Translated by R.F.C. Hull. Princeton, New Jersey: Princeton University Press.

―――. 1973. *Synchronicity: An Acausal Connecting Principle.* Translated by R.F.C. Hull. Princeton, New Jersey: Princeton University Press.

Kahn, J.P. 1970. "How a Psychiatrist Looks at Pain." *Medical Times* 98:127-33.

Kales, A.; Bixler, R.; Kales, J.; and Scharf, C. 1977. "Comparative Effectiveness of Nine Hypnotic Drugs: Sleep Laboratory Studies." *The Journal of Clinical Pharmacology* 17:207-13.

Kales, A.; Bixler, R.; Tan, B.; Scharf, C.; and Kales, J. 1974. "Chronic Hypnotic-Drug Use." *Journal of the American Medical Association* 227:5.

Kao, F., and Kao, J. 1973. *Acupuncture Therapeutics—An Introductory Text.* San Mateo, California: Cadre.

Karlins, M., and Andrews, L. 1973. *Biofeedback.* New York: Warner Books, Inc.

Kaufer, S. 1978. "The Air Pollution You Can't See." *New Times,* 6 March 1978, pp. 29-37, 60-64.

Keleman, S. 1975. *Your Body Speaks Its Mind: The Bioenergetic Way to Greater Emotional and Sexual Satisfaction.* New York: Simon & Schuster.

Kentsmith, D.; Strider, F.; Copenhaver, J.; and Jacques, D. 1976. "Effects of Biofeedback upon Suppression of Migraine Symptoms and Plasma Dopamine-B-Hydroxylase Activity." *Headache* 16:173-77.

Khalil, G.A. 1976. "Hypnosis in Surgery—Why and When." *Southern Medical Journal* 69:1466-68.

Kissen, D.M. 1966. "The Significance of Personality in Lung Cancer in Men." In

Psycho-physiological Aspects of Cancer, eds. E. M. Meyer and H. Hutchins. New York: New York Academy of Sciences, pp. 933-45.

———. 1967. "Psychosocial Factors, Personality and Lung Cancer in Men Aged 55-64." *British Journal of Medical Psychology* 40:29.

Kitman, M. 1975. *The Coward's Almanac*. New York: Ballantine Books, Inc.

Koenig, P. 1973. "The Placebo Effect in Patent Medicine." *Psychology Today*, April 1973, p. 60.

Koestler, A. 1972. *The Roots of Coincidence*. New York: Random House, Inc.

Kosterlitz, H.W., and Hughes, J. 1976. "Possible Physiological Significance of Enkephalin, an Endogenous Ligand of Opiate Receptors." In *Advances in Pain Research & Therapy, Vol. I*, eds. J. J. Bonica and D. Albe-Fessard. New York: Raven Press, pp. 641-45.

Kovel, J. 1976. *A Complete Guide to Therapy*. New York: Pantheon Books, Inc.

Krieger, D. 1975. "Therapeutic Touch: The Imprimatur of Nursing." *American Journal of Nursing* 75:784-87.

———. 1976. "Healing by the Laying-on-of-Hands as a Facilitator of Bioenergetic Change: The Response of In-Vivo Hemoglobin." *Psychoenergetic Systems* 1:121-29.

———. in press. "Therapeutic Touch: A Reality Base for Alternative Health Practices." In *Mind, Body and Health: Toward an Integral Medicine*, eds. J. Gordon, D. Jaffe, and D. Bresler. Pacific Palisades, California: Center for Integral Medicine.

Krippner, S. 1975. *Song of the Siren*. New York: Harper & Row, Pub., Inc.

Krippner, S., and Rubin, D., eds. 1974. *The Kirlian Aura*. New York: Anchor Press.

———. 1975. *The Energies of Consciousness*. New York: Gordon and Breach.

Kroening, R.; Volen, M.P.; and Bresler, D.E. 1978. "Acupuncture: Healing the Whole Person." In *New Dimensions of Holistic Healing*, eds. H.A. Otto and J.K. Knight. Chicago: Nelson-Hall Pub.

Kroger, W.S. 1960. "Hypoanesthesia in Surgery." *Western Journal of Surgery, Obstetrics and Gynecology* 68:25-30.

———. 1963. *Clinical and Experimental Hypnosis*. Philadelphia: J.B. Lippincott Co.

Kroger, W.S., and DeLee, S.T. 1957. "Use of Hypnoanesthesia for Caesarean Section and Hysterectomy." *Journal of the American Medical Association* 163:442.

Kroger, W.S., and Fezler, W.D. 1976. *Hypnosis and Behavior Modification: Imagery Conditioning*. Philadelphia: J.B. Lippincott Co.

Kushi, Michio 1978. *Oriental Diagnosis*. Revised ed. 1978 by Sunwheel Pub. London: Abeta Press.

Kushner, R. 1978. "Depression: How to Cure It." *Forum*, February 1978, pp. 41-47.

Laing, R.D. 1969. *The Politics of the Family*. New York: Random House, Inc.

Langre, J. 1974. *Second Book of Do-In*. Magalia, California: Happiness Press.

Lao Tzu 1955. *The Way of Life*. Translated by R.B. Blakney. New York: Mentor Books.

Lappe, F. 1971. *Diet for a Small Planet*. New York: Ballantine Books, Inc.

Larkin, R.P., and Sutherland, P.J. 1977. "Migrating Birds Respond to Project Seafarer's Electromagnetic Field." *Science* 195:777-79.

Lasagna, L.; Mosteller, F.; von Felsinger, J.M.; and Beecher, H.K. 1954. "A Study of the Placebo Response." *American Journal of Medicine* 16:770.

Lawson-Wood, D., and Lawson-Wood, J. 1963. *First Aid at Your Fingertips.* Wellingborough, England: Thorsons Publishers Ltd.

Leboyer, F. 1974. *Birth Without Violence.* New York: Alfred A. Knopf, Inc.

Lehmann, P. 1978. "Food and Drug Interactions," *FDA Consumer*, March 1978, pp. 20-23.

LeShan, L. 1959. "Psychological States as Factors in the Development of Malignant Disease: A Critical Review." *National Cancer Institute Journal* 22:1-18.

―――. 1961. "A Basic Psychological Orientation Apparently Associated with Malignant Disease." *The Psychiatric Quarterly* 36:314-30.

―――. 1966. "An Emotional Life-History Pattern Associated with Neoplastic Disease." *Annals of the New York Academy of Science* 125:780-93.

―――. 1973. *The Medium, the Mystic, and the Physicist.* New York: The Viking Press.

―――. 1975. *How to Meditate: A Guide to Self-Discovery.* New York: Bantam Books, Inc.

LeShan, L., and Worthington, R.E. 1956. "Some Recurrent Life History Patterns Observed in Patients with Malignant Disease." *Journal of Nervous and Mental Diseases* 124:460-65.

Levin, A. 1974. "City Diseases That Can Kill You." *New York*, 7 October 1974, pp. 39-43.

Lieber, A.L., and Sherin, C.R. 1972. "Homicides and the Lunar Influence on Human Emotional Disturbance." *American Journal of Psychiatry* 129:101-05.

Liebeskind, J. 1976. "Pain Modulation by Central Nervous System Stimulation." In *Advances in Pain Research and Therapy, Vol. 1*, eds. J.J. Bonica and D. Albe-Fessard. New York: Raven Press.

Lilly, J. 1972. *Programming and Metaprogramming in the Human Biocomputer.* New York: Julian Press.

―――. 1973. *The Center of the Cyclone: An Autobiography of Inner Space.* New York: Julian Press.

―――. 1975. *Simulations of God: The Science of Belief.* New York: Simon & Schuster.

Lindemann, H. 1973. *Relieve Tension the Autogenic Way.* New York: Peter H. Wyden, Inc.

Longgood, W. 1969. *The Poisons in Your Food.* New York: Pyramid Books.

Lowen, A. 1966. *Love and Orgasm.* London: Staples Press.

―――. 1971. *The Language of the Body.* New York: Collier Books.

―――. 1972. *The Betrayal of the Body.* New York: Collier Books.

―――. 1973. *Depression and the Body.* Baltimore: Penguin Books, Inc.

―――. 1975a. *Bioenergetics.* New York: Coward, McCann & Geoghegan, Inc.

―――. 1975b. *Pleasure—A Creative Approach to Life.* Baltimore: Penguin Books, Inc.

Lu, Henry C. 1977. *Tongue Diagnosis in Color.* Vancouver, B.C., Canada: The Academy of Oriental Heritage.

Luce, G. 1973. *Body Time.* New York: Bantam Books, Inc.

Ludwig, A.M. 1964. "An Historical Survey of the Early Roots of Mesmerism." *The International Journal of Clinical and Experimental Hypnosis* 12: 205-17.

Luthe, W., ed. 1969. *Autogenic Therapy*, vol. 1-6. New York: Grune & Stratton, Inc.

MacLeod, H. 1969. "Our Polluted Air." *New York Post*, 11 November 1969, p. 45.

Mahren, F.J. 1960. "Hypnosis and the Surgical Patient." *American Journal of Proctology* 11:459-65.

Manaka, Y., and Urquhart, I. 1972. *The Layman's Guide to Acupuncture*. New York: Weatherhill.

Mann, J.B. 1970. "Treating Salicylate Intoxication." *California Medicine* 113:16.

Mann, W.E. 1973. *Orgone, Reich & Eros*. New York: Simon & Schuster.

Marmer, M.J. 1959. "Hypnoanalgesia and Hypnoanesthesia for Cardiac Surgery." *Journal of the American Medical Association* 171:512-17.

Marx, J.L. 1977. "Analgesia: How the Body Inhibits Pain Perception." *Science* 195:471-73.

Maslow, A. 1966. *The Psychology of Science: A Reconnaissance*. New York: Harper & Row, Pub., Inc.

————. 1968. *Towards a Psychology of Being*. Cincinnati: Van Nostrand Reinhold Co.

————. 1970. *Religions, Values, and Peak Experiences*. New York: The Viking Press.

————. 1971. *The Farthest Reaches of Human Nature*. New York: The Viking Press.

Mason, A.A. 1955. "Surgery under Hypnosis." *Anaesthesia* 10:295.

Mather, H.G. 1971. "Acute Myocardial Infarction: Home and Hospital Treatment." *British Medical Journal* 3:334-38.

Matsumoto, T. 1974. *Acupuncture for Physicians*. Springfield, Illinois: Charles Thomas Publishers.

Mayer, Jean 1977. "Let's Subtract Additives." *Family Health*, December 1977, pp. 42-43.

McGarey, W. 1974. *Acupuncture and Body Energies*. Phoenix, Arizona: Gabriel Press.

McKim, R.H. 1972. *Experiences in Visual Thinking*. Monterey, California: Brooks/Cole Pub. Co.

Medina, J.L.; Diamond, S.; and Franklin, M.A. 1976. "Biofeedback Therapy for Migraine." *Headache* 16:115-18.

Melmon, K.L. 1971. "Preventable Drug Reactions—Causes and Cures." *New England Journal of Medicine* 284:1361.

Melzack, R. 1973. *The Puzzle of Pain*. New York: Basic Books, Inc.

Melzack, R., and Torgerson, W.S. 1971. "On the Language of Pain." *Anesthesiology* 34:50.

Menguy, R. 1970. Paper presented at meeting of American College of Surgeons. Chicago, 13 October 1970.

Mennell, J. M. 1975. "The Therapeutic Use of Cold." *Journal of the American Osteopathic Association* 74:1146-58.

Merskey, H., and Spear, F.G. 1967. *Pain: Psychological and Psychiatric Aspects*. London: Bailliere, Tindall & Cassell.

Miles, R. in press. "Rituals of Childbirth." In *Mind, Body & Health: Toward an Integral Medicine*, eds. J. Gordon, D. Jaffe, and D. Bresler. Pacific Palisades, California: Center for Integral Medicine.

Miller, E. in press. "A Personal Exploration of Selective Awareness." In *Mind, Body & Health: Toward an Integral Medicine*, eds. J. Gordon, D. Jaffe, and D. Bresler. Pacific Palisades, California: Center for Integral Medicine.

Minuchin, S. 1974. *Families and Family Therapy*. Cambridge: Harvard University Press.

Mishra, R. 1973. *Yoga Sutras: The Textbook of Yoga Psychology*. New York: Doubleday & Co., Inc.

————. 1974. *Fundamentals of Yoga*. New York: Doubleday & Co., Inc.

Mitch, P.S.; McGrady, A.; and Iannone, A. 1976. "Autogenic Feedback Training in Migraine. A Treatment Report." *Headache* 15:267-70.

Montagu, A. 1972. *Touching: The Human Significance of Human Skin*. New York: Harper & Row, Pub., Inc.

Montgomery, P.S., and Ehrisman, W. J. 1976. "Biofeedback-Alleviated Headaches: A Follow-up." *Headache* 16:64-65.

Morris, F. 1974. *Self-Hypnosis in Two Days*. Berkeley: Intergalactic Publishing Co.

Moss, T. 1974. *The Probability of the Impossible*. Los Angeles: J.P. Tarcher, Inc.

Murphy, A.J. 1960. "The Physiological Effects of Cold Application." *Physical Therapy Review* 40:112.

Namikoshi, T. 1969. *Shiatsu: Japanese Finger Pressure Therapy*. Elmsford, New York: Japan Publications Trading Co.

Navarra, J.G. 1969. *Jet Aircraft Noise*. New York: Doubleday & Co., Inc.

Nehemkis, A.M., and Smith, B.R. 1975. *Ear Acupuncture Therapy*. Long Beach, California: Alba Press.

Nelson, A. 1976. "Orgone (Reichian) Therapy in Tension Headache." *American Journal of Psychotherapy* 39:103-11.

Nogier, P.F.M. 1972. *Treatise of Auriculotherapy*. Moulins-lés-Metz, France: Maisonneuve.

Null, G., and Null, S. 1972. *The Complete Handbook of Nutrition*. New York: Robert Speller & Sons.

Ogilvie, R.I., and Ruedy, J. 1967. "Adverse Drug Reactions During Hospitalization." *Canadian Medical Association Journal* 97:1450.

Ohasi, W. 1976. *Shiatsu*. New York: E.P. Dutton & Co., Inc.

Oleson, T.D.; Kroening, R.J.; and Bresler, D.E. 1978. "Diagnostic Accuracy of Examining Electrical Activity at Ear Acupuncture Points for Assessing Areas of the Body with Musculoskeletal Pain." *Pain Abstracts* 1:185.

Oliver, C. 1976. "Patient, Heal Thyself." *Canadian Doctor* 42:49-52.

Ostrander, S., and Schroder, L. 1970. *Psychic Discoveries Behind the Iron Curtain*. Englewood Cliffs, New Jersey: Prentice-Hall, Inc.

————. 1974. *Handbook of PSI Discoveries*. New York: Berkeley Publishing Corp.

Ott, J.N. 1973. *Health and Light*. Old Greenwich, Connecticut: Devin-Adair Co.

Ouspensky, P.D. 1949. *In Search of the Miraculous*. New York: Harcourt Brace Jovanovich, Inc.

————. 1971a. *The Fourth Way*. New York: Vintage Books.

————. 1971b. *A New Model of the Universe*. New York: Vintage Books.

————. 1974. *The Psychology of Man's Possible Evolution*. New York: Vintage Books.

Oyle, I. 1973. *Magic, Mysticism and Modern Medicine*. Bolinas: Mesa Press.

————. 1975. *The Healing Mind*. Millbrae: Celestial Arts.

————. 1976. *Time, Space, and the Mind*. Millbrae: Celestial Arts.

Page, M.E., and Abrams, H.L. 1972. *Your Body Is Your Doctor!* New Canaan, Connecticut: Keats Publishing.

"Pain: Placebo Effect Linked to Endorphins." 1978. *Science News* 114:164.

Palos, S. 1972. *The Chinese Art of Healing*. New York: Bantam Books, Inc.

Parker, G., and Neilson, M. 1976. "Mental Disorder and Season of Birth—A Southern Hemisphere Study." *British Journal of Psychiatry* 129:355-36.

Paul, J., and Paul, M. 1975 *Free to Love*. Los Angeles: J.P. Tarcher, Inc.

Pauling, L. 1971. *Vitamin C and the Common Cold*. New York: Bantam Books, Inc.

————. 1977. "On Vitamin C and Cancer." *Executive Health*, January 1977, pp. 1-4.

Paulley, J.W., and Haskell, D.J. 1975. "Treatment of Migraine without Drugs." *Journal of Psychosomatic Research* 19:367-74.

Pavlov, I. 1927. *Conditioned Reflexes: An Investigation of the Physiological Activity of the Cerebral Cortex*. New York: Oxford University Press.

Pelletier, K. 1977. *Mind as Healer, Mind as Slayer*. New York: Delta.

————. in press. "The Preventive Approach to Psychosomatic Medicine." In *Mind, Body & Health: Toward an Integral Medicine*, eds. J. Gordon, D. Jaffe, and D. Bresler. Pacific Palisades, California: Center for Integral Medicine.

Pelletier, K., and Garfield, C. 1976. *Consciousness East and West*. New York: Harper and Row, Pub., Inc.

Pendergrass, E. 1959. Presidential Address to the American Cancer Society Meeting.

Phares, E.J. 1973. *Locus of Control: A Personality Determinant of Behavior*. Morristown, New Jersey: General Learning Press.

————. 1975. *Locus of Control in Personality*. Morristown, New Jersey: General Learning Press.

Pilowsky, I. 1976. "The Psychiatrist and the Pain Clinic." *American Journal of Psychiatry* 133:752-56.

Pomeranz, B. 1977. "Brain's Opiates at Work in Acupuncture?" *New Scientist*, 6 January 1977, pp. 12-13.

Pomeranz, B.; Cheng, R.; and Law, P. 1977. "Acupuncture Reduces Electrophysiological and Behavioral Responses to Noxious Stimuli: Pituitary Is Implicated." *Experimental Neurology* 54:172-78.

Pomeranz, B., and Chiu, D. 1976. "Naloxone Blockade of Acupuncture Analgesia: Endorphin Implicated." *Life Sciences* 19:1757-62.

Porkert, M. 1974. *The Theoretical Foundations of Chinese Medicine*. Cambridge, Massachusetts: MIT Press.

Porter, J. 1975. "Guided Fantasy as a Treatment for Childhood Insomnia." *Australian and New Zealand Journal of Psychiatry* 9:169-72.

Powers, M. 1961. *A Practical Guide to Self-Hypnosis*. Hollywood: Wilshire Book Co.

Presman, A.S. 1970. *Electromagnetic Fields and Life*. New York: Plenum Pub. Corp.

Procacci, P.; Corte, M.D.; Zoppi, M.; and Maresca, M. 1974. "Rhythmic Changes of the Cutaneous Pain Threshold in Man." *Chronobiologia* 1:77-96.

Progoff, I. 1975. *At a Journal Workshop.* New York: Dialogue House Library.

"Psychiatrist Finds Big Rise in Deaths Linked to Valium." 1976. *The New York Times*, 30 March 1976, p. 18.

Rahe, R.H. 1973. "Life-Change Measurement as a Predictor of Illness." *Proceedings of the Royal Society of Medicine* 61:1124-26.

Raknes, O. 1970. *Wilhelm Reich and Orgonomy.* Baltimore: Penguin Books, Inc.

Raloff, J. 1975. "Biological Clocks." *Science Digest*, November 1975, pp. 62-69.

Rawson, P., and Legeza, L. 1973. *Tao· The Eastern Philosophy of Time and Change.* New York: Bounty Books.

Rees, E.L., and Campbell, J. 1974. "Patterns of Trace Minerals in the Hair and Relationship to Clinical States." *The Journal of Orthomolecular Psychiatry* 4:1-8.

Reich, W. 1949. *Character Analysis.* New York: Farrar, Straus & Giroux, Inc.

———. 1961. *The Function of the Orgasm.* New York: Farrar, Straus & Giroux, Inc.

———. 1970. *The Discovery of the Orgone.* New York: Noonday Press.

———. 1973. *Selected Writings: An Introduction to Orgonomy.* New York: Farrar, Straus & Giroux, Inc.

Reiter, B. 1957. *You and Your Operation.* New York: Macmillan, Inc.

Restak, R. 1977. "The Brain Makes Its Own Narcotics." *Saturday Review*, 5 March 1977, pp. 6-11.

Reston, J. 1971. "Now, About My Operation in Peking." *The New York Times*, 26 July 1971, p. 1.

Richardson, A. 1969. *Mental Imagery.* New York: Springer Publishing Co., Inc.

"The Right Brain: Surviving Retardation." 1977. *Science Digest*, 8 October 1977, pp. 229-30.

Rodale, J.I. 1968. *The Complete Book of Vitamins.* Emmaus, Pennsylvania: Rodale Books.

———. 1972. *Complete Book of Minerals for Health.* Emmaus, Pennsylvania: Rodale Books.

Rodale, R. in press. "A Framework for Nutrition Theory, Practice and Research in Holistic Health." In *Mind, Body & Health: Toward an Integral Medicine*, eds. J. Gordon, D. Jaffe, and D. Bresler. Pacific Palisades, California: Center for Integral Medicine.

Rogers, C. 1961. *On Becoming a Person.* Boston: Houghton-Mifflin Co.

Rogers, D.L. 1977. "Bypass, Boeing and Billions." *Western Journal of Medicine* 126:410-11.

Rolf, I. 1977. *Structural Integration: The Recreation of the Balanced Human Body.* New York: The Viking Press.

Rosa, K. 1976. *You and A.T.: Autogenic Training.* New York: E.P. Dutton & Co., Inc.

Rose, L. 1971. *Faith Healing.* New York: Penguin Books.

Rosen, S. 1971. "I Have Seen the Past and It Works." *The New York Times*, 1 November 1971, p. 41.

Rothenberg, R. E. 1976. *Understanding Surgery.* New York: New American Library.

Rucker, T.D. 1972. "Economic Problems in Drug Distribution." *Inquiry* 9:43.

Ryan, P. 1976. "Musical Medicine." *New Scientist*, 1 July 1976, 39.

Sage, W. 1976. "The Split Brain Lab." *Human Behavior*, June 1978, pp. 25-28.

Samuels, M., and Bennett, H. 1973. *The Well Body Book*. Berkeley and New York: Random House and Berkeley: Bookworks.

———. 1974. *Spirit Guides*. New York: Random House and Berkeley: Bookworks.

Samuels, M., and Samuels, N. 1975. *Seeing with the Mind's Eye*. New York: Random House and Berkeley: Bookworks.

Sargent, J.D.; Taylor; J.B.; Coyne, L.; Thetford, P.E.; Watler, E.D.; and Segerson, J.A. 1975. "Autogenic Feedback in Migraine Headache." *Journal of Kansas Medical Society* 76:266-67.

Scheving, L.E. 1976. "The Dimension of Time in Biology and Medicine— Chronobiology." *Endeavor* 35:66-72.

Schimmel, E.M. 1964. "The Hazards of Hospitalization." *Annals of Internal Medicine* 60:100.

Schultz, J.H., and Luthe, W. 1969. *Autogenic Therapy, Vol. 1*. New York: Grune and Stratton, Inc.

Scott, D.L. 1972. "Awareness During General Anaesthesia." *Canadian Anaesthesia Society Journal* 19:173-83.

———. 1974. *Modern Hospital Hypnosis*. Chicago: Year Book Medical Publishers, Inc.

Seligman, M. 1975. *Helplessness*. San Francisco: W.H. Freeman Co.

Seligman, M.E.P., and Beagley, G. 1975. "Learned Helplessness in the Rat." *Journal of Comparative and Physiological Psychology* 88:534-41.

Seligson, M. 1977. "The Physician of the Future: Freddie the Frog." *New West*, 3 January 1977, pp. 46-49.

Selye, H. 1956. *The Stress of Life*. New York: McGraw-Hill, Inc.

———. 1974. *Stress Without Distress*. Philadelphia: J.B. Lippincott & Co.

Serizawa, K. 1972. *Massage: The Oriental Method*. Tokyo: Japan Publications.

———. 1976. *Tsubo: Vital Points for Oriental Therapy*. Tokyo: Japan Publications.

Shapiro, A.K. 1965. Psychological Aspects of Medication. In *The Psychological Basis of Medical Practice*, eds. H.I. Lief, V.F. Lief, and N.R. Lief. New York: Hoeber Medical Division of Harper and Row, Inc., pp. 167-68.

Shapiro, S.; Slone, D.; Lewis, G.P.; and Jick, H. 1971. "Fatal Drug Reactions Among Medical Inpatients." *Journal of the American Medical Association* 216:467.

Shealy, C.N. 1975. *Occult Medicine Can Save Your Life*. New York: The Dial Press.

———. 1976. *The Pain Game*. Millbrae: Celestial Arts.

———. 1977. *90 Days to Self-Health*. New York: The Dial Press.

Sheehy, G. 1976. *Passages*. New York: E.P. Dutton & Co., Inc.

Shorr, J.E. 1977. *Go See the Movie in Your Head*. New York: Popular Library.

Silverman, M., and Lee, P.R. 1974. *Pills, Profits & Politics*. Berkeley and Los Angeles: University of California Press.

Simeons, A.T.W. 1962. *Man's Presumptuous Brain*. New York: E.P. Dutton & Co., Inc.

Simonton, O.C.; Matthews-Simonton, S.; and Creighton, J. 1978. *Getting Well Again*. Los Angeles: J.P. Tarcher, Inc.

Singer, J.L. 1974. *Imagery and Daydream Methods in Psychotherapy and Behavior Modification*. New York: Academic Press.

————. 1975. *The Inner World of Daydreaming*. New York: Harper & Row, Pub., Inc.

Smith, A. 1975. *Powers of Mind*. New York: Random House, Inc.

Smith, B. 1938. "Diagnosing the Doctors." *Reader's Digest*, August 1938, pp. 1-5.

Smith, D.L. 1978. *The Diary for Dreamers*. Ontario: The Shoreline Press.

Smith, R.L. 1970. "Chiropractic: Issues and Answers." *Today's Health*, January 1970, pp. 64-69.

Snyder, S.H. 1977. "Opiate Receptors in the Brain." *New England Journal of Medicine* 296:266-71.

Solomon, P. et al., eds. 1961. *Sensory Deprivation*. Cambridge: Harvard University Press.

Sommer, R. 1978. *The Mind's Eye*. New York: Delta.

Southern, W.E. 1975. "Orientation of Gull Chicks Exposed to Project Sanguine's Electromagnetic Field." *Science* 189:143.

Spielberger, C.D., and Sarason, I.G., eds. 1975. *Stress and Anxiety, Vol. 1*. New York: John Wiley & Sons, Inc.

Steiger, B. 1976. *Life Without Pain*. Westport, Connecticut: Bost Enterprises.

Sternbach, R.A. 1968. *Pain: A Psychophysiological Analysis*. New York: Academic Press.

————. 1974. *Pain Patients: Traits and Treatment*. New York: Academic Press.

Stetler, C.J. 1973. *Patterns of Prescription Drug Use: The Role of Promotion*. Washington, D.C.: Pharmaceutical Manufacturers Association.

"Stimulating the Brain to Prevent Pain." 1975. *Science Digest* 108:327.

Stone, I. 1972. *The Healing Factor: Vitamin C Against Disease*. New York: Grosset and Dunlap, Inc.

Stonehouse, B. 1974. *The Way Your Body Works*. New York: Crown Publishers, Inc.

"Study Links Sleeping Pills to 5000 Deaths a Year." 1977. *Los Angeles Times*, 28 November 1977, p. 4.

Sutherland, D.C. 1975. "Scientists from Around World Attend NINDS Conference." *The Journal of the CCA*, June 1975, pp. 18-22.

Tashkin, D.P.; Bresler, D.E.; Kroening, R.J.; Kerschner, H.; Katz, R.L.; and Coulson, A. 1977. "Comparison of Real and Simulated Acupuncture and Isoproterenol in Methacholine-Induced Asthma." *Annals of Allergy* 39:379-87.

Tasso, J., and Miller, E. 1976. "The Effects of the Full Moon on Human Behavior." *The Journal of Psychology* 93:81-83.

Thie, J., and Marks, M. 1973. *Touch for Health*. Santa Monica, California: De Vorss.

Thomas, L. 1974. *Lives of a Cell*. New York: The Viking Press.

Toben, B. 1975. *Space, Time and Beyond*. New York: E.P. Dutton and Co., Inc.

Toguchi, M. 1974. *The Complete Guide to Acupuncture*. New York: Frederick Fell Pub., Inc.

Tomlinson, W.K., and Perret, J.J. 1975. "Mesmerism in New Orleans: 1845-1861." *The American Journal of Clinical Hypnosis* 18:1-5.

Trotter, R.J. 1975. "Changing the Face of Birth." *Science News* 108:106-08.

————. 1976. "The Other Hemisphere." *Science News* 109:218-20.

Trubo, R. 1978. *How to Get a Good Night's Sleep*. Boston: Little, Brown & Co.

Trungpa, C. 1969. *Meditation in Action*. Berkeley: Shambala.

Trustman, R.; Dubovsky, S.; and Titley, R. 1977. "Auditory Perception During General Anesthesia—Myth or Fact?" *International Journal of Clinical and Experimental Hypnosis* 25:88-105.

Turin, A., and Johnson, W.G. 1976. "Biofeedback Therapy for Migraine Headaches." *Archives of General Psychiatry* 33:517-19.

U.S. House of Representatives Subcommittee on Oversight Investigations. 1974. *Cost and Quality of Health Care: Unnecessary Surgery*. Washington, D.C.: United States Government Printing Office.

"U.S. Ready to Propose Controls on Use of Valium and Librium." 1975. *The New York Times*, 31 January 1975, p. 42.

Van Arman, C.G. 1970. Cited in "Possible Interaction Occurs with Aspirin and Two Drugs." *Journal of the American Medical Association* 214:39.

Veith, I. 1949. *The Yellow Emperor's Classic of Internal Medicine*. Berkeley, California: University of California Press.

Vernon, J. 1963. *Inside the Black Room*. New York: Clarkson N. Potter, Inc.

Verrett, J., and Carper, J. 1974. *Eating May Be Hazardous to Your Health*. New York: Simon & Schuster.

Vickery, D.M., and Fries, J.F. 1976. *Take Care of Yourself*. Reading, Massachusetts: Addison-Wesley Pub. Co., Inc.

Volen, M.P., and Bresler, D.E. 1976. *A Guide to Good Nutrition*. Beverly Hills, California: Center for Integral Medicine.

Volen, M.P.; Kroening, R.J.; and Bresler, D.E. 1978. "Acupuncture: Current Status & Clinical Indications for American Medicine." In *Mind, Body & Health: Toward an Integral Medicine*, eds. J. Gordon, D. Jaffe, and D.E. Bresler. Bethesda, Maryland: National Institute of Mental Health in cooperation with the Center for Integral Medicine, Pacific Palisades, California.

Walker, C.E. 1975. *Learn to Relax*. Englewood Cliffs, New Jersey: Prentice-Hall, Inc.

Wallace, R.K., and Benson, H. 1972. "The Physiology of Meditation." *Scientific American*, February 1972, pp. 84-90.

Wallnofer, H., and Von Rottauscher, A. 1965. *Chinese Folk Medicine and Acupuncture*. New York: New American Library.

Warner, G., and Lance, J.W. 1975. *Relaxation Therapy in Migraine and Chronic Tension Headache* 1:298-301.

Warren, F.Z. 1976. *Handbook of Medical Acupuncture*. New York: Van Nostrand Reinhold Co.

Weed, L.L. 1971. *Medical Records, Medical Education and Patient Care*. Cleveland, Ohio: Case Western Reserve University Press.

Weil, A. 1972. *The Natural Mind: A New Way of Looking at Drugs and the Higher Consciousness*. Boston: Houghton Mifflin Co.

Werbach, M.R. 1974. "Psychiatric Applications of Biofeedback." *Psychiatry Digest*, April 1974, pp. 23-27.

Werbel, E. W. 1960. "Experiences with Frequent Use of Hypnosis in a General Surgical Practice." *Western Journal of Surgery, Obstetrics & Gynecology* 68:190-91.

Wester, W.C. 1976. "The Phreno-Magnetic Society of Cincinnati—1842." *American Journal of Clinical Hypnosis* 18:277-81.

White, J., and Fadiman, J. 1976. *Relax*. New York: Dell Pub. Co., Inc.

Wickramasekera, I., ed. 1976. *Biofeedback, Behavior Therapy and Hypnosis: Potentiating the Verbal Control of Behavior for Clinicians*. Chicago: Nelson-Hall Publishers.

Williams, R.J. 1971. *Nutrition Against Disease*. New York: Pitman Publishing Corp.

Winter, R. 1972. *A Consumer's Dictionary of Food Additives*. New York: Crown Publishers, Inc.

Wolff, B.B., and Langley, S. 1968. "Cultural Factors and the Responses to Pain." *American Anthropologist* 70:494.

Worsley, J. 1973. *Is Acupuncture for You?* New York: Harper and Row, Pub., Inc.

Wu Shui Wan. 1973. *The Chinese Pulse Diagnosis*. Alhambra, California: Chan's Books.

Wu Wei-Ping 1962. *Chinese Acupuncture*. Willingborough, England: Thorsons Publishers Ltd.

Yee, M.S., ed. 1974. *The Great Escape*. New York: Bantam Books, Inc.

Yudkin, J. 1972. *Sweet and Dangerous*. New York: Peter H. Wyden, Inc.

Zborowski, M. 1952. "Cultural Components in Responses to Pain." *Journal of Social Issues*. 8:16.

———. 1969. *People in Pain*. San Francisco: Jossey-Bass.

Zinberg, N.E., and Robertson, J.A. 1972. *Drugs and the Public*. New York: Simon & Schuster.

Index